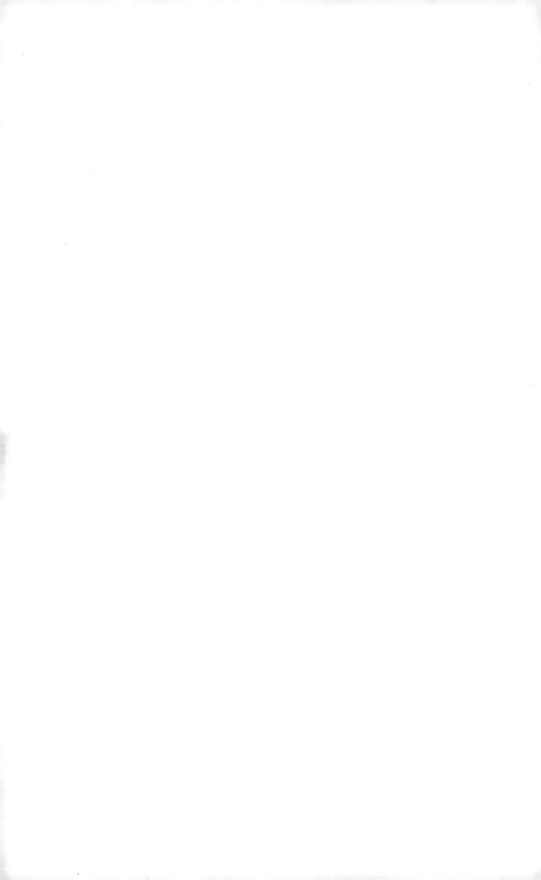

DEATH OF MEDICINE IN NAZI GERMANY

DERMATOLOGY AND
DERMATOPATHOLOGY
UNDER THE SWASTIKA

DEATH OF MEDICINE IN NAZI GERMANY

DERMATOLOGY AND DERMATOPATHOLOGY UNDER THE SWASTIKA

WOLFGANG WEYERS, M.D.
CENTER FOR DERMATOPATHOLOGY
FREIBURG, GERMANY

EDITED BY
A. BERNARD ACKERMAN, M.D.
INSTITUTE FOR DERMATOPATHOLOGY
JEFFERSON MEDICAL COLLEGE, PHILADELPHIA, PENNSYLVANIA

ARDOR SCRIBENDI, LTD. • PHILADELPHIA
MADISON BOOKS • LANHAM • NEW YORK • OXFORD

First Ardor Scribendi/Madison edition published in 1998.

Printed in the United States of America

9 8 7 6 5 4 3 2 1

The Lippincott-Raven edition of this book was previously catalogued by the Library of Congress as follows:

Death of medicine in Nazi Germany : dermatology and dermatopathology under the swastika / Wolfgang Weyers ; foreword by A. Bernard Ackerman.
    p.   cm.
    Includes bibliographical references and index
    1. Dermatology--Germany--History--20th century. 2. Medicine--
-Germany--History--20th century. 3. World War, 1939–1945
-Atrocities. 4. World War, 1939–1945—Medical care. 5. National
socialism. I. Weyers, Wolfgang.
RL46.D43   1998
616.5'00943'0904--dc21   97-52091
                                                    CIP

ISBN 1-56833-121-5 (cloth) and 1-56833-122-3 (paperback)

My father's father, Karl Weyers, was a member of the Social Democrats. When the Nazis assumed power, he was dismissed as director of an elementary school and from then on had to earn his living as a sales representative, a job for which he was entirely unsuited. After the war, the American military government wanted to appoint him mayor of the city of Homberg, but he asked only to return to his school. I remember him as a reserved, thoughtful man who liked to read, paint, and play with his dog. He loved music and could play on the piano any melody that came into his mind.

My mother's father, Jakob Weber, was a member of the Nazi party. He was a simple man who managed a pub in Cologne that was a favorite haunt of some Nazi groups, and I am sure he believed a lot of what he heard there. But what a lovable man he was! As a child, I was impressed by his mustache and his large hands that closed securely around mine. As an adult, when I visited him, he supplied me with sandwiches and biscuits so I would not be hungry on my return trip home.

Both of my grandfathers were, in their own way, wonderful persons. I knew them too little.

Virtue is thus concerned with both feelings and actions. But it is only those that are willing which are praised and blamed, whereas those that are unwilling are pardoned and sometimes even pitied. So it seems to be necessary for the student of ethics to define the difference between the willing and the unwilling.... Well then, it seems that actions are unwilling when they occur under compulsion or through ignorance.... But there is some dispute about whether to account as unwilling or willing those cases where something is done out of fear of something worse or for the sake of something fine.... So those actions are a mixture, though they seem to have more in common with the willing. For at the time when they are done they are chosen.... The agent acts willingly; for the origin of the movement of the parts of the body in such actions lies in him, and when the origin is in oneself it is in one's power to do it or not.

—ARISTOTLE
Nicomachean Ethics

Young Soldier: *I'm not going to listen. This is an injustice and injustice is something I will not endure.*

Mother Courage: *Oh really? Gives you a problem, does it? Injustice? How long can you put up with it for? Is an hour difficult? Or does it bug you for two? Because in the stocks, I tell you, there's this strange sort of moment when people suddenly think, oh perhaps I can put up with injustice after all.*

—BERTOLT BRECHT
Mother Courage and Her Children

CONTENTS

FOREWORD

COULD IT HAPPEN AGAIN? OF COURSE IT COULD—NOT ONLY TO JEWS, AND NOT ONLY AT THE HANDS OF GERMANS. In fact, it has happened, albeit on a smaller scale, many times since 1945: Witness the genocide of Bosnians, Rwandans, and Kurds, to mention but three memorable examples. And it will continue to happen until a profound change occurs in how nations throughout the world educate their children about the worth of individual human beings, irrespective of nationality, peoplehood, race, religion, or sex.

For that change to occur, the lessons of the excruciatingly painful effects of ultranationalism and racism on both the victims and the perpetrators must become ingrained in the minds of those who lead nations. The tale told by Wolfgang Weyers in these pages imparts some of those lessons. It should be required reading for all members of the human family who are determined to ensure that it does not happen again to any people or any group.

What makes Weyers' story so singular, riveting, alarming, instructive, and hopeful? For one, it is an unabridged, unflinching, and scrupulously factual account by a highly conscionable contemporary young German doctor of unconscionable behavior on the part of German doctors of one generation ago. For another, although a sense of outrage cries out from every line and even from between the lines of his narrative, Weyers engages the subject like the scientist he is, confining his study to the findings themselves (diagnosis), to the hows (pathogenesis), and to the whys (etiology), demonstrating critical yet dispassionate analysis throughout.

Weyers' book is a labor of the heart as well as of the mind. Unlike so many other chronicles of the years of madness between 1933 and 1945, when an ever escalating war was being waged against Jews in particular by the Nazis and their many European fascist collaborators, Weyers does not make the victims victims twice. He sympathizes, empathizes, and identifies with them, in stark contrast to the German physicians who are his subject and who, sixty years ago, regarded Jews in general, and Jewish medical colleagues in particular, as *Untermenschen.*

But Weyers goes further. He expresses, uninhibitedly, admiration and gratitude for the contributions of German and Austrian Jews to the enrichment of the culture of their native countries and to their profession of medicine. He uses the cooptation of medicine by the Nazis in 1933 to illustrate how what begins as seemingly small, relatively harmless events, such as enforced sterilizations in selected patients, can result in the perversion of a profession and of a society. He illustrates in full detail how the venality of all too many doctors and people of every vocation led to the corruption of behavior.

Caught between fear and greed, German physicians profited from the misfortunes of their Jewish colleagues and turned their backs on them. Weyers shows how individuals who seemed to be well educated and schooled in the Hippocratic oath could become accomplices to evil, both actively as committed Nazis who carried out with enthusiasm the diabolical dictates of the regime, and passively as indifferent onlookers who saw what was happening and did nothing to stop it. He directs attention forcibly to the importance of resisting wrongdoing of any kind as soon as it is identified as wrong.

Weyers' focus, at scanning magnification, is medicine in the Third Reich; at intermediate power, the fields of dermatology and dermatopathology; and at high magnification, the effects of the changes in medicine during the Nazi era on the individual lives of Jewish physicians and their Nazi counterparts and Jewish patients and their non-Jewish counterparts, and on the quality of patient care, teaching, and research in Germany during twelve years of Nazi rule.

But, at highest magnification, the implications of Weyers' work go far beyond that terrible time and place and extend to human beings everywhere and for all time. The lessons of Weyers' account cannot be misread. Had the physicians in Nazi Germany been true to their calling and to fundamental principles of moral conduct, the disaster that befell Jews and Gypsies, Poles and Russians, Belgians and French, Dutch and Czechs might have been averted. The many millions who died in the armies, navies, and air forces of the Allies and of the Axis powers might have been saved; the devastation visited on so many cities, among them London and Rotterdam, Dresden and Berlin, might have been prevented.

By their participation in the early 1930s in enforced sterilizations and "euthanasia"—the killing of defectives and the infirm—or by their acquiescence to it with barely a protest against those deplorable acts, the doctors of Germany gave the Nazis the go-ahead to the ever more brazen crimes of inhumanity that culminated in the mass murder of Jews. It is not by chance that in the annihilation camps established by the Nazis in Poland in the early 1940s for the expressed purpose of exterminating Jews, much of the equipment used for the killing, the personnel that did the killing, and the arguments that justified the killing came directly from the euthanasia program. For this reason, the doctors in Nazi Germany bear special responsibility for the calamity that befell humankind during little more than a decade, one from which the world has not recovered and never will.

Had the doctors of Germany resisted the euthanizing of the retarded, the deformed, and the feeble, as they should have as physicians, the Nazis—who were merely cowards and bullies in uniform—might have retreated, just as they might have done if Chamberlain and Daladier had had the spine to call their bluff on Czechoslovakia. But the doctors abandoned their trust and identified entirely with the aggressor. German doctors could have saved the world, including their own, but they did nothing.

What went awry with medical education in Germany that it produced physicians whose character was so flawed? The answer, in my view, is that physicians in Germany, like virtually all other elements in that society, were not really educated; they were indoctrinated. The word *education* comes from the Latin *educare*, which means to lead forth or draw out in the fashion of Socrates. Indoctrination, in contrast, denotes forcing ideas on others. Education seeks to encourage logical, critical, and incisive thinking, whereas indoctrination seeks to stifle it. Education may lead to the personal conviction that is indispensable to courage.

German doctors, like the rest of the members of that purportedly uniquely cultivated society, were indoctrinated with the principle of inordinate respect for authority, and for that reason were no more able to stand up to the Nazis than were the untutored and the unwashed. The doctors had no conviction and no guts. If physicians, inheritors of a noble tradition of a learned profession, could not utter a peep of protest against fundamental abuse of the rights of every human being, what could be expected from the rest of their society?

Weyers' work shows that the "German problem" is also a timeless human problem. Germany between 1933 and 1945 happened to be the cauldron, but no nation is exempt from being brought to a similar boil. The Germans are not disposed genetically to war and acts of brutality, or to accepting propaganda like that of Hitler, Goebbels, and Streicher. If the conditions are right, all peoples are susceptible to such behavior. Humaneness is not an inherent human quality; it is learned.

And what of young German dermatologists and dermatopathologists of today in a country in which neo-Nazism is on the rise, as it is throughout Western Europe? They are contributing to the advancement of their disciplines in university clinics and in laboratories, but all too many of them still stand by in silence as they witness, in a democratic society, what they perceive to be a system that tolerates violations of academic standards. During their training, and as junior faculty, they complain bitterly—though in private—about the arbitrary authority of those department chairs who put their names on articles and books they did not write a word of and who receive large incomes from patients they have not seen and from histopathologic sections they have not read.

Yet these young doctors do not utter or write a word of protest in public about a system that affects them profoundly. Not surprisingly, when they themselves become department heads, they perpetuate the system. And as department heads, they can be sure that no matter how patently wrong their statements are in scientific forums, no one will challenge them. These flaws are not confined to Germany, but wherever they exist, a society is at risk. Those who are unable to speak out on their own behalf will be impotent in the face of injustice to others.

As always, there are exceptions. In this work, Wolfgang Weyers has demonstrated that he is one of them.

The most rousing of the many lessons told in the pages that follow is simple to state but daunting to achieve. If genocide is not to happen again to any people anywhere, education must be designed and implemented in a way that encourages human beings to assert their individuality, to refute untruths, and to act against injustices. The lack of such a tradition led to the death of medicine in Nazi Germany and to the unnecessary deaths of more than fifty million individuals. Let the lessons of Weyers' story be an impetus to infuse new life into the education of people everywhere.

A. BERNARD ACKERMAN, M.D.
New York, New York

PREFACE

OW DO I BEHAVE AND HOW SHOULD I BEHAVE? WHEN IS IT RIGHT AND ESSENTIAL FOR ME TO UPHOLD MY personal convictions and inviolate standards, and when is it necessary to compromise for the greater good? At what point do compromises become concessions, and I become a wholly different person?

These questions—and how we choose to answer them—are at the moral and ethical foundation of every society, in every arena of life. They are posed in different ways, clearly articulated by the analytic mind or embedded in prayers, and demonstrated through action and the establishment of law. And they are important, especially for persons in responsible positions, such as politicians, lawyers, and physicians. Everyone who loves responsibility needs an ethical code to adjust their activities to that which is beneficial to society and to those human beings for whom they are responsible.

Unlike any other profession, medicine, for almost twenty-five hundred years, has been guided by an ethical code that attempts to answer some of these questions. According to the fundamental principles of the Hippocratic oath, which in many countries all physicians take, practitioners of medicine must carry out their duty with piety and purity, provide care that is never harmful to patients, refuse to administer deadly drugs, uphold the sanctity of patient confidentiality, and respect and support those who taught them medicine. Throughout history, the Hippocratic oath has been violated, but never more egregiously than under the Nazi dictatorship in Germany.

In National Socialist Germany, far from carrying out their duty with piety and purity, many physicians did not hesitate to inform the party about the undesirable activities of their patients. According to the Reich's Physicians' Ordinance of 1935, patient confidentiality could be disregarded if the "common sense of the people" demanded it, and by 1943, by virtue of Hitler's decision, the traditional privilege of confidentiality between patient and doctor was altogether abolished. Many reports attest that in their daily routines of changing dressings or performing minor surgical procedures, Nazi physicians made patients who were opposed to the party suffer. The administration of deadly drugs was commonplace, while the killing of mentally disabled patients became accepted procedure. The practice was casually extended to include patients who did not conform to the requirements of the state. Concentration camp internees were used for medical experiments and were often tortured to death in the process. Support and respect for mentors and teachers—many of whom were subjected to oppression and violence—were rare, and in acts motivated by opportunism, many physicians undermined their teachers in order to fill leading positions themselves.

How was it conceivable that physicians behaved in this way? How was it possible for them to neglect the ethical standards that had guided the practice of medicine until then? How could they so easily accept an ideology devoid of humanistic principles and common sense?

The questions have been asked often. The historical background has been examined, social circumstances considered, and the impact of political and economic decisions explored, yet the real answers lie within ourselves.

It is easy to condemn physicians who chose to conform to the rules of the Nazi dictatorship for their opportunistic and cowardly behavior; it may not be so easy to ask ourselves what we would do in the same situation. Of course, we do not torture patients, but do we perform our professional duties with piety and purity? Does the practice of medicine still obligate us to cure and give comfort, or is it a method to make money? Are patients treated like customers? Do we give up our independence when our ties with pharmaceutical companies become too strong? How important is an ethical component in medical education? How much attention is paid to education at all?

Given the current estrangement of medicine from its ethical roots, it is not hard to imagine that under similar circumstances, the average physician of today might behave even worse than the physicians in the Third Reich. Many years of relative stability have made us complacent, and perhaps we have accepted a decline in ethical standards too easily, without considering the consequences and the danger. In National Socialist Germany, there were some physicians who saw the danger early and were prepared. Through their actions, they demonstrated how essential the critical evaluation of one's own behavior is, and how an ethical code, professional and personal, must stand at the center of any life. By exploring the worst chapters in the history of medicine, we can prepare ourselves to meet future conflicts head-on.

When exploring a period in history, it may be more telling to concentrate on one aspect of it and describe it in its relationship to the general development than to try to discuss many different aspects at the same time. The Nazis considered the German people to be suffering from a decline in racial quality that was mainly caused by the poisoning effects of Jews, and they thought of themselves as physicians to the German people. Medicine, therefore, was of extreme importance to them, and the changes that afflicted medicine tell more about National Socialism than those in other fields of public life. Dermatology, in turn, was more obviously influenced by Jews than all the other medical specialties and, for that reason, attracted the Nazis' special interest. As a consequence, the changes in dermatology are excellently suited to serve as a model for the general development under the swastika, a development that turned an apparently cultivated nation into one that committed the most barbaric crimes in history and that demonstrates how low the threshold may be that prevents ordinary, educated people from becoming the accomplices of murderers. It is critical to remain exquisitely aware of the events of those years, and to realize the range of behavior that can exist under extraordinarily difficult circumstances.

WOLFGANG WEYERS, M.D.
Freiburg, Germany

ACKNOWLEDGMENTS

I WISH TO EXPRESS MY GRATITUDE TO SEVERAL MEN AND WOMEN I DO NOT EVEN KNOW, TO WIT, THOSE WHO HAVE studied the history of medicine in Nazi Germany before me. Their dismay was obvious, their inquiries thorough, their descriptions accurate; they provided a solid foundation for me to build on.

Studies have also been conducted on various aspects of the history of dermatology in Nazi Germany, especially by Albrecht Scholz and his co-workers at the University of Dresden. It was my objective to study that subject in depth and to discuss it in the broader context of medicine and society in its entirety, because the changes that affected dermatology and dermatopathology can only be fully appreciated in the context of the larger story. To this end, I received great help from some excellent books about the history of politics and the history of medicine in the Third Reich, including Kater's *Doctors Under Hitler*, Proctor's *Racial Hygiene*, Weindling's *Health, Race and German Politics Between National Unification and Nazism*, and Klee's *Auschwitz, die NS-Medizin und ihre Opfer*. I applaud those authors and thank them.

More specifically, for valuable information and courteous permission to use some of the pictures that have not been published previously, I thank Jost Benedum, Albrecht Günther, Ruth Jahn, Ursula Lang, and Wolfgang Meyhöfer (Giessen); Idamarie Eichert (Koblenz); Max Hundeiker (Hornheide); Paul Joachim Unna (Hamburg); Cathrin Schmidt (Gera); Albrecht Scholz (Dresden); Daisy Kopera and Peter Soyer (Graz); Karl Holubar and Heidrun Weiss (Vienna); Inga Silberberg-Sinakin (Vineland, New Jersey); and Rudolf Baer (New York).

I thank my parents, Paula and Siegfried; my wife, Imke; and my friend, Steffen Heussner, for their help in the preparation of this manuscript. I also thank my father-in-law, Werner Altekrüger, who searched for pictures and documents in Hamburg.

I thank my former chairman, Wolf-Bernhard Schill, for allowing me the opportunity to pursue my interest in the history of dermatology; my colleague, Frank-Michael Köhn, who was strolling around in the loft of our clinic one day and came across an old cupboard filled with numerous letters and documents from the Nazi period; and Elvira Erb, photographer of the skin clinic of the University of Giessen, who helped me prepare the pictures for the book.

I thank those who invested their efforts to bring this book to completion, editing the text, organizing the pictures, and making helpful suggestions. I am especially grateful to Elizabeth Willingham of Silverchair Science + Communications, who by extraordinary professionalism, combined punctiliousness with celerity in readying pages and revised pages for printing; Carol Field, who brought her splendid intellect, superb competence, and exquisite sensitivity to the task of converting a manuscript into a bound book that would comport with her exceptionally high standards; and Louise Fili and Mary Jane Callister, who shared those standards and oversaw every detail of the design of the book, including the cover and dust jacket.

Excerpts from the book appeared in the journal *Dermatopathology: Practical and Conceptual*, and I am grateful for permission to reprint them.

Last, I wish to express my deepest gratitude to A. Bernard Ackerman, who encouraged me to carry out this study and supported me from the beginning to the end. Without him, this book would not exist. Much has been said and written about Dr. Ackerman; the most important aspect is that *he cares*. He cares about the clarity of observation and the challenge of new ideas and about honesty, uprightness, and the welfare of his students and those who work for him. If education is about the teaching of responsibility—to self and others—then Dr. Ackerman is the perfect teacher and the perfect model.

When we ask ourselves how we would have behaved during the Nazi era, we would only have had to meet Dr. Ackerman's standards; in that way, we could not have done wrong.

DEATH OF MEDICINE IN NAZI GERMANY

DERMATOLOGY AND
DERMATOPATHOLOGY
UNDER THE SWASTIKA

INTRODUCTION

THE HISTORY OF DERMATOLOGY AND DERMATOPATHOLOGY IS CLOSELY CONNECTED TO THE POLITICAL HISTORY of Germany. The rise of the swastika in Germany in the early 1930s had a major impact not only on dermatology in Germany but on the development of dermatology worldwide.

At the beginning of the twentieth century, Germany was the leader of the international dermatology community, a status achieved mainly through the work of its Jewish practitioners. The most influential disciples of Ferdinand von Hebra in Vienna[1]—Heinrich Auspitz (fig. 1),[2] who described acantholysis and the Auspitz phenomenon in psoriasis; Moriz Kaposi (fig. 2),[3] who is best known for having identified Kaposi's sarcoma; Isidor Neumann (fig. 3),[4] who gave the first description of pemphigus vegetans; and Filip Josef Pick (fig. 4),[5] who was one of the founders of the German Dermatological Society—were Jewish. The leading dermatologists in the German Reich were Jewish as well: Heinrich Köbner (fig. 5),[6] remembered for his descriptions of the Köbner phenomenon and epidermolysis bullosa simplex; his successor in Breslau, Albert Neisser (fig. 6),[7] who discovered the causative microorganism of gonorrhea and was the first to succeed in staining the bacilli of leprosy; Edmund Lesser (fig. 7),[8] who founded the famous Berlin school of dermatology; and Paul Gerson Unna (fig. 8),[9] the Nestor of external pharmacotherapy and the genius of dermatopathology. Of fifty-one dermatologists born between 1850 and 1890, thirty-one were Jewish, and many of them had Jewish disciples who became famous in their own right.[10]

There are several reasons for the predominance of Jews in German dermatology. Traditionally, Jews have entered the profession of medicine in part because of the high honor bib-

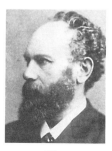

FIG 1
HEINRICH AUSPITZ
(1835–1886)

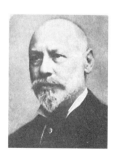

FIG 2
MORIZ KAPOSI
(1837–1902)

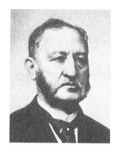

FIG 3
ISIDOR NEUMANN
(1832–1906)

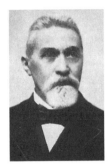

FIG 4
FILIP JOSEF PICK
(1834–1910)

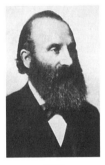

FIG 5
HEINRICH KÖBNER
(1838–1904)

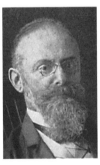

FIG 6
ALBERT NEISSER
(1855–1916)

lical texts bestowed on physicians. In addition, violent out-breaks of anti-Semitism throughout history have made it desirable for Jews to be highly skilled and highly mobile, conditions that are fulfilled by the medical profession.

In 1933, Jews constituted only 0.8 percent of the general population in Germany, yet they accounted for about 16 percent of all physicians. In large cities, the numbers were even higher; in Berlin, more than half of all physicians were Jewish.[11]

The number of Jews in dermatology was greater than in any other medical specialty. In 1934, one-fifth of all Jewish specialists were dermatologists, and one-fourth of all dermatologists in the German Reich were Jews.[12] The predominance of Jews in dermatology was a result of a widespread anti-Semitic attitude in Germany that hampered the careers of Jews in firmly established fields of science. Because dermatology was still a young, developing specialty, it offered career opportunities to Jews when few others existed.

Furthermore, the practice of dermatology was held in relatively low esteem among many physicians. They assiduously avoided the study of skin diseases because it meant constant exposure to "ugly" lesions, unesthetic and smelly forms of treatment, and a population of patients considered to be socially inferior.

At that time, the treatment of venereal diseases accounted for much of the practice of what then were known as dermatovenereologists. In public opinion, patients with venereal diseases were outcasts who should rightly suffer the consequences of their immoral lifestyle. Until 1900, the German government officially regarded venereal disease as a self-inflicted condition and therefore excluded it from coverage by health insurance. Because dermatologists were in contact with these "dirty" diseases and cared for these "immoral" patients, the opinion of the specialty was very low.

As a consequence, young Jewish physicians who had been turned down for residencies in internal medicine or surgery found opportunities open to them in dermatology. Some who became the most influential German practitioners of dermatology were forced into the specialty by the lack of opportunity elsewhere. Eugen Galewsky, known for the introduction of anthralin in the treatment of psoriasis, had originally applied for a position in a surgical department but was turned down repeatedly.[13]

Perhaps the single most important explanation for Jewish pre-eminence in German dermatology was the fact that by the first decade of the twentieth century, the predominance of Jews in the specialty was already a tradition. Young Jewish physicians who wanted to specialize often followed in the footsteps of their parents, relatives, or friends. The history of dermatology is replete with examples of well-known Jewish fathers and sons like Joseph and Werner Jadassohn, Samuel and Max Jessner, and Felix and Hermann Pinkus.[14] Furthermore, because many professors and even directors of dermatologic departments were Jewish, there was a greater willingness to accept Jewish assistants.

Finally, the public so closely identified Jews with the practice of dermatology that all dermatologists were regarded as Jews and were frequently referred to as *Felljuden*, a derogatory term that means "fur Jews."[15] For this

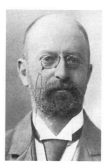

FIG 7
EDMUND LESSER
(1852–1918)

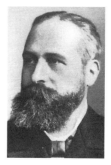

FIG 8
PAUL GERSON UNNA
(1850–1929)

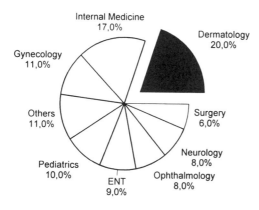

FIG 9 JEWISH MEDICAL SPECIALISTS IN GERMANY IN 1933.

very reason, many non-Jewish physicians chose not to specialize in dermatology (fig. 9).

The combination of these factors meant that the medical profession in general, with its many Jewish members, was more severely affected than most other fields by the rise of the Nazis. In no other medical specialty was this as true as in dermatology. Within a short period of time, most of the leading German dermatologists were fired and forced to emigrate. Of 2,078 dermatologists living in Germany in 1933, 566 were Jewish. The fate of about two-thirds of German Jewish dermatologists is known: 248 emigrated, most of them to the United States; fifteen survived within the confines of Nazi Germany; fifty-eight died in Germany, at least ten of them through suicide; and at least sixty-one dermatologists shared the fate of most other European Jews—death in a concentration camp.[16] Between 1933 and 1945, approximately six million Jews—two-thirds of European Jewry—were killed by the Nazis (fig. 10).

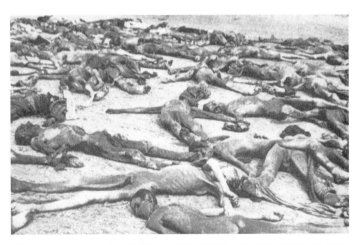

FIG 10 GERMAN CONCENTRATION CAMP AFTER ITS LIBERATION IN 1945.

THE HISTORY OF
ANTI-SEMITISM

ANTI-SEMITISM IS AN OLD PHENOMENON AND NOT ONE UNIQUE TO GERMANY. OUTBREAKS OF ANTI-SEMITISM have occurred for many centuries in many regions of the world. Resentment of minorities, not just Jews, is universal, evident in all social groups and cultures, and ever ready to escalate into hatred and persecution. Prejudice is one of the basic patterns of the human psyche and an ineradicable element of human society.

The struggle of life is a struggle for appreciation. If one's sense of being appreciated is threatened, the results are fear, envy, and aggression—fear of losing love or being set back in a professional career, envy of those who have been more successful, and aggression against them if they are weak. This universal pattern of fear, envy, and aggression influences the relationships of individuals, social groups, and nations. It presents itself as polemics in political campaigns, as aggressiveness against supporters of an opposing sports team, and as expressions of hostility against people of different color and culture, especially in times of economic recession. The results are most pronounced when the threat to sense of self and place can be attributed to an individual or a distinct group of people—usually a minority. For centuries, Jews were that targeted minority. They were considered different from non-Jews in many ways, were easily recognizable by certain physical attributes, and were extraordinarily successful. For these reasons, no other people in history have inspired more fear and envy or have been more often attacked than Jews.

The history of discrimination and persecution of Jews dates back to the second half of the first millennium B.C.E. As Greek ideas about the oneness of humanity spread, Jewish beliefs and practices were seen as increasingly antihumanitarian.

That Jews believed they were the chosen people, refused to respect other deities, tended to treat non-Jews and the foods that they ate as ritually unclean, forbade marriage to non-Jews, and observed dietary laws that prevented social intercourse with non-Jews contributed to this attitude. Judaism was called by its enemies "an inhospitable and anti-human form of living" and "inimical to humanity." Old stories about Jews—that they conducted secret human sacrifices in their temples, for example—originated during this period.[1]

With respect to religious beliefs, the Greeks and Romans were rather permissive; they had many different gods, and they tolerated the gods of other people. Tolerance decreased with the rise of Christianity. Originally, Christianity was a Jewish sect, and the polemics found in the gospels—such as Jesus' supposed rebuke of the Jews in the Gospel of John, "You are of your father the devil"—should be interpreted as arguments within Judaism. However, once Christianity became the state religion of the Roman Empire under Constantine the Great in the fourth century, the notion of the Jew as devil pervaded Roman Catholicism and determined Christianity's relationship with the Jews.

In contrast to other religions known to the Romans, Christianity claimed to be the only true faith. The conversion of dissenters was considered to be a Christian's moral obligation, not only because it spread Christianity but because it saved heterodox people from the fate of eternal hellfire. But many Jews did not convert. They could not accept the divinity of Jesus because they considered God to be unique and indivisible. Christianity and Judaism were therefore incompatible.

The tensions between Christianity and Judaism were aggravated by the fact that both religions shared the same foundation: the Old Testament of the Bible of Christians was the Hebrew scriptures of the Jews. Differences in the interpretation of those scriptures were a constant source of conflict, and the mere existence of a different view of the Bible challenged the authority of the Church of Rome. The refusal of Jews to convert, despite their familiarity with the Bible, was said to be proof of perfidy and falsehood, and prompted the Catholic Church to institute an increasing number of compulsory measures against Jews. The ostensible goal of these measures was to defend Christianity against the Jewish threat and to protect Christians from the ruinous consequences of contacts with Jews. The severity of those measures can be appreciated in the Canonical Laws: Jews were forbidden to marry Christians or to dine with them (Synod of Elvira, 306); Jews were not allowed to fill public offices (Synod of Clermont, 535); Christians were not allowed to consult Jewish physicians (Trullanian Synod, 692); Jews were restricted to circumscribed living areas (Synod of Breslau, 1267); and Jews could not acquire academic rank (Council of Basel, 1434). Many of these regulations were adopted later by the Nazis.[2]

Through its nearly complete control of spiritual life, the Roman Catholic Church was able to create a stereotype of Jews that was passed on, unquestioned, from generation to generation and that eventually became an integral part of European culture. Throughout Europe, Jews were perceived as creatures of the devil. Any misery or social conflict was blamed on the influence of Jews, even in places without a significant Jewish population. The fear of Jews acquired mystic, irrational dimensions; it was ubiquitous, sometimes subliminal, but omnipresent and always capable of becoming virulent in times of crisis, war, or religious incitement.[3]

The Crusades in the eleventh and twelfth centuries were associated with outbreaks of anti-Semitic violence. Massacres of Jews occurred in France and Germany. In the thirteenth century, Jews were expelled from England and in the fifteenth from Spain, where anti-Semitism, for the first time, had become racial rather than religious. Under the rule of the Spanish Inquisition, Jews were perceived as being so unfathomably duplicitous that even baptism did not prevent them from being persecuted. With the expulsions from England and Spain, many Jews moved to eastern Europe, particularly

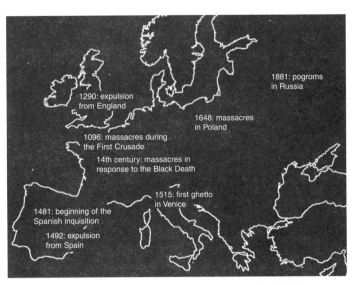

FIG 11 EVENTS IN THE HISTORY OF ANTI-SEMITISM.

to Poland. After major pogroms in 1648, a reverse trend of migration from the east to the west occurred, and many Jews settled in the German-speaking countries (fig. 11).[4]

In reaction to hostility and restriction, Jews adopted professions that not only made them economically viable but also allowed them mobility. They became physicians, tradesmen, moneylenders. Their worldwide connections enabled them to raise vast sums of money, which made them indispensable, especially in times of war, and Jews often prospered while the general population did not. This further strained the relationship between Jews and their neighbors. The typical Jew was thought by non-Jews to be ugly, obsequious, deceptive, avaricious, and completely possessed by thirst for money.

In 1543, Martin Luther (fig. 12) wrote in his treatise *About the Jews and Their Lies* that the Jews were "bloodhounds and murderers of the entire Christianity, fully intentionally, for more than 1,400 years, and they like to be that with their deeds, as they have often been burned because they were accused of poisoning water and wells, stealing and dissecting children, just to cool down their anger at the blood of the Christians. . . . They

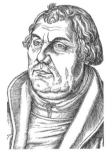

FIG 12

MARTIN LUTHER

(1483–1546)

detain us Christians in our own country, let us work in our wet sweat, get money and possessions, while they sit behind the stove, are lazy and pompous, bake pears, devour, booze, live sweetly and well from what we worked for, have captured us and our goods with their damned usury."[5]

Such prejudices, derived from ancient and medieval sources, became firmly anchored in the German mind. But the eighteenth century—the Enlightenment, with its ideas of religious tolerance—brought major changes. Common rights for citizens of all faiths were first established in the American Bill of Rights, the First Amendment guaranteeing the free practice of religion. The same rights were won in France and England. With the Napoleonic Wars in the first decade of the eighteenth century, the doctrines of the French Revolution were exported to Germany. Wherever the French occupied German lands, Jews became the beneficiaries of the Rights of Man, winning emancipation in most of southern and western Germany. The trend toward emancipation also reached Prussia, where Frederick William III (fig. 13), in despair after his country had been reduced to less than half its previous size, proclaimed in an edict in 1812 that Jews, after fighting and dying for their fatherland and sharing all the duties and hardships of their fellow citizens, should receive the privileges of full-fledged citizens.

After Napoleon's defeat and the Congress of Vienna in 1815, however, the rights that Jews had won were disavowed and rescinded. Throughout the nineteenth century, the only way for a Jew to have an ordinary professional career in German-speaking countries was through baptism. Many made use of it, among them great poets and musicians like Heinrich Heine and Gustav Mahler, as well as lawyers and physicians. Moriz Kaposi, the successor of Ferdinand von Hebra as chairman of dermatology in Vienna, not only changed his religious affiliation but also discarded his real name, Kohn, which is derived from *kohen*, the Hebrew term for priest.

Changing names was not uncommon among apostate Jews. At the beginning of the nineteenth century, in the process of

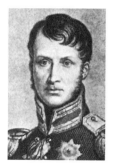

FIG 13
FREDERICK
WILLIAM III
(1770–1840)

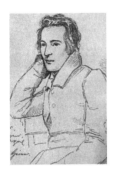

FIG 14
HEINRICH HEINE
(1797–1896)

Jewish assimilation, Jews had been obliged to choose permanent family names. Many Jews selected biblical names, such as Cohn, Levy, and Moses; others chose names that communicated their profession or provenance—e.g., Goldschmied or Dessauer—or they created new beautiful names, such as Rosenberg or Blumenthal. As a consequence, typical "Jewish names" eventually identified Jews and subjected them to discrimination. Jokes invoking Jewish names were common, the name Cohn being the most common target. Its bearers were attacked in little verses (many German words rhyme with Kohn). A *Kohn Lexicon* was even published for the purpose of making fun of the name by deliberate misspelling of words— "Kohn-Kurs" instead of "Konkurs," the latter being the German expression for bankruptcy. In 1910, a Berlin lawyer observed that "among large parts of the population, Christian as well as Jewish, 'Cohn' is a designation for those Jews who, to a high degree, have certain typically Jewish, unpleasant qualities. Thereby, the word has changed into an invective and slanderous term." Even the authorities, such as the president of the police of Berlin, conceded that the name Kohn was hardly tolerable for its bearer and opted for the possibility to have it changed himself.[6] As a consequence, no other name was changed more often than Kohn, and it is likely that among the reasons that prompted Moriz Kohn to have his family name changed to Kaposi was the negative connotation of the name Kohn.

The pressure on Jews in German-speaking countries to break with Judaism was so intense that by the middle of the nineteenth century, approximately two-thirds of those who had gained importance in social or cultural life had converted to Christianity. Heinrich Heine (fig. 14), one of the greatest German poets of that period, called baptism the "entrance ticket to European culture."[7]

Many of the Jews who had bought their "entrance ticket" professed anti-Semitic feelings themselves. Heine himself hated being Jewish, regarded Judaism as an antihuman force, and wrote of "three evil maladies, poverty, pain, and Jewishness."[8] Another example is the Jewish anatomist Jacob Henle (fig. 15), whose name is linked eponymically to more than a dozen structures of the human body, such as Henle's loop, a U-shaped turn in the medullary portion of a renal tubule, and Henle's layer in the inner sheath of a hair follicle. Henle, who had been baptized as a child, repeatedly made derogatory remarks about Jews, dissociated himself from his Jewish colleagues, and, in one letter to his father, even spoke of "filthy Jews."[9] Such anti-Semitic emotions soon became commonplace among apostate Jews. There was a peculiar kind of self-hatred among those who tried to become thoroughly assimilated but still could not escape their origin. In the process of assimilation, apostate Jews inevitably absorbed anti-Semitic feelings that were inherent in the mentality and culture of their country.

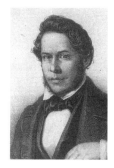

FIG 15
JACOB HENLE
(1809–1887)

Despite the obvious societal advantages gained through baptism, the majority of Jews refused to convert to Christianity. Consequently, they were forced to either tolerate major limitations on their careers or leave the country. Self-exile was chosen by David Gruby (fig. 16), a Hungarian Jew, who was offered a professorship at the University of Vienna under the condition that he embrace the Catholic religion. Gruby found this requirement unacceptable and emigrated to France. At the Foundling Hospital in Paris, Gruby gave courses in microscopy and was the first to describe trypanosomes and Microsporum.[10]

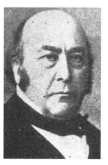

FIG 16
DAVID GRUBY
(1810–1898)

In contrast to David Gruby, the Jewish pathologist Robert Remak (fig. 17) stayed in Germany. Years before Rudolf Virchow, Remak recognized that cells could only be derived from other cells. He demonstrated that new cells form by cell division, developed the concept of specificity of the three germ layers of the embryo, proved the connection between nerve fibers and ganglion cells, and, working at the institute of Johann Lucas Schönlein,[11] discovered the causative organism of favus, now known as *Trichophyton*

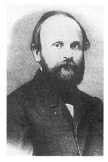

FIG 17
ROBERT REMAK
(1815–1885)

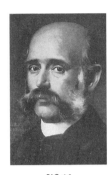

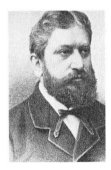

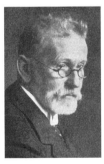

schoenleinii. As the first Jewish physician in Germany, Remak was appointed lecturer through an imperial decree in 1847. Despite his success, his determination to remain a Jew prevented him from acquiring an even higher academic rank. Throughout his lifetime, he struggled for recognition, which he has yet to be accorded even to this day. Instead he was vigorously attacked by his colleagues and was passed over as they were promoted.[12]

Likewise, the career of Carl Weigert (fig. 18) was hampered by his adherence to his faith. Weigert was one of the foremost pathologists of the nineteenth century. He is remembered especially for the introduction of various staining techniques into histology, the first successful attempt at staining bacteria in tissues, the first description of coagulation necrosis, and the first accurate description of infarction of the heart. Weigert was an assistant of Julius Cohnheim (fig. 19), Virchow's most distinguished pupil, who was famous for his studies on the mechanisms of inflammation and for his theory that neoplasms are derived from remnants of embryonic tissue that do not participate in the formation of surrounding normal tissues. Cohnheim, who was of Jewish descent, served as chairman of pathology at the University of Leipzig. When he died in 1884, Weigert hoped to succeed him and was superbly qualified for the position. Nevertheless, Weigert was not even considered as a candidate for the chair of pathology and never rose to the rank of full professor.[13] The discrimination against Jewish scientists also affected Weigert's cousin, Paul Ehrlich (fig. 20), the founder of histochemistry and chemotherapy and winner of the Nobel Prize for medicine in 1908, who was appointed full professor only in 1914, one year before his death.[14]

Nevertheless, Remak, Weigert, and Ehrlich had careers that would have been impossible for Jews merely half a century earlier. The process of emancipation of Jews in Germany was slow. Brief spells of liberalism and the expansion of rights were followed by long periods of conservatism and repression. Overall, however, in the late nineteenth century, the situation for Jews in Germany improved markedly; new possibilities opened up for ambitious Jewish men who previously would have become Talmudic scholars but now could enter German universities.

The Jews increasingly identified themselves with Germany and with Germans, and they recognized similarities between the German and Jewish mentalities. Many aspired to complete assimilation and contributed greatly to German culture. Jewish composers and conductors, such as Giacomo Meyerbeer, Felix Mendelssohn, and Gustav Mahler, carried on the long and venerable tradition of German music, and poets such as Heinrich Heine enriched German literature. Jews played a major role in the industrialization of Germany and were involved prominently in the liberal and socialist movements. Franz Boas founded the science of cultural anthropology; Ferdinand Julius Cohn, bacteriology; and Sigmund Freud, modern psychology. German Jews soon began to win Nobel prizes: two in physics, four in chemistry, and two in physiology and medicine, all for work done before the World War I.

The extraordinary success of Jews in all aspects of public life did not occur without a backlash. Because Jews were more visible than ever, they became subjects of increasing public interest and, in the process, the traditional anti-Semitism that had remained relatively dormant resurged. Fear and envy of Jews, especially among workers, farmers, and the poor middle class, were pervasive. Many blamed Jews for all the negative aspects of changing modern life and held them responsible for an increasing sense of insecurity that truly was an inevitable consequence of industrialization (figs. 21, 22).

Toward the end of the nineteenth century, a rise in anti-Semitism could be observed in many European countries, often aggravated by prominent representatives of social and cultural life. The German composer Richard Wagner sought to eliminate Jews entirely from the sphere of creative life: "I

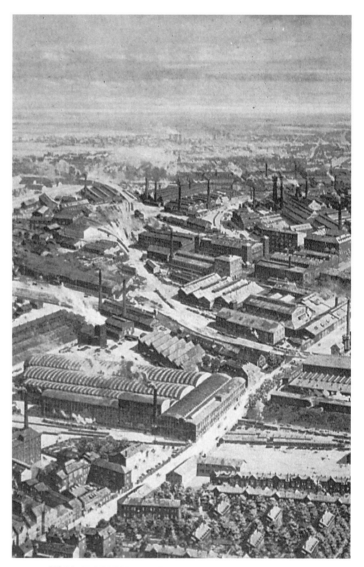

FIG 21 INDUSTRIAL AREA IN GERMANY AT THE END OF
THE NINETEENTH CENTURY.

hold the Jewish race to be the born enemy of pure humanity
and everything noble in it. I am perhaps the last German who
knows how to hold himself upright in the face of Judaism
which already rules everything."[15] Pierre-Joseph Proudhon,
the leading French socialist theoretician, wrote: "The Jew is
the enemy of the human race. One must send this race back

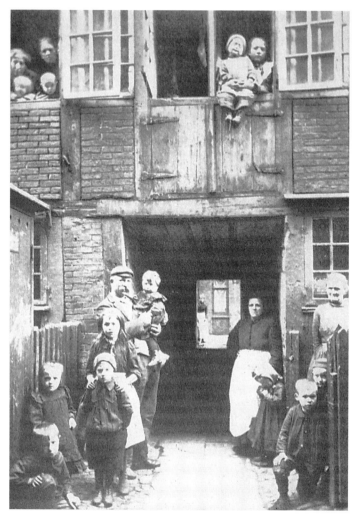

FIG 22 IMPOVERISHED FAMILIES IN GERMANY
AT THE END OF THE NINETEENTH CENTURY.

to Asia or exterminate it . . . by fire or fusion or by expulsion.
The Jew must disappear."[16]

These sentences illustrate a change in the character of anti-
Semitism. The religious anti-Semitism of previous centuries
did not deny Jews the right to live. Despite the unfathomable
hatred against them, Jews were accepted as fellow, if flawed,
human beings who could be redeemed by baptism. The objective of the Church was to induce Jews to convert and thereby

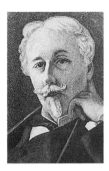

FIG 23
JOSEPH ARTHUR
DE GOBINEAU
(1816–1882)

confirm the superiority of Christianity. As old beliefs were challenged in the nineteenth century, anti-Semitism became adjusted to altered concepts of society and life. The religiously motivated hatred against Jews was complemented by political and social prejudices; Jews were said to be amoral subjects who conspired to undermine the country. Jews were no longer viewed as members of a religious group but as a nation and, eventually, as a distinct race that was biologically incompatible with other European peoples.[17]

From 1853 to 1855, the French aristocrat Joseph Arthur de Gobineau (fig. 23) published his *Essai sur l'inégalité des races humaines*, in which he defined the Aryan race[18] as the "most noble human family," superior to all other races. In Gobineau's view, the Aryan race was in decline and the European nations in a state of progressive degeneration. Fanaticism and superstition, luxury and immorality were only symptoms of this decline but not the underlying causes. Instead, Gobineau attributed the degeneration of a nation to the fact "that it no longer possesses the inherent quality which it had before, because it no longer possesses the same blood in its vessels, the value of which has been steadily diminished by continuous mixture."[19]

The inappropriate transfer of biological ideas to cultural and social issues was common in those years. Originally, the equation of biology and sociology was an attempt to maintain a unifying view of the world that had been challenged by the new concepts of biology, especially by Darwin's thesis of the evolution of species through selective propagation. The philosophy of monism, in which the material and the immaterial world, body and spirit, form an "indivisible universe, a realm of substance," found many followers, including Paul Gerson Unna, who published a journal devoted to that philosophy. The human spirit was no longer regarded as a gift of God but was thought to be a special form of energy, comparable to forces in the material world and subject to the same biological laws that determined the evolu-

tion of species. Ernst Haeckel (fig. 24), one of the main proponents of monism, applied the zoological concept of evolution by selection and counterselection to the history and
future of human societies in his effort to establish social
Darwinism.[20]

The equation of biological and sociological concepts was
fostered by the new findings of cell biology. After the discovery of cell division by Robert Remak in 1851, Rudolf Virchow (fig. 25) confirmed the theory that all cells grow from
pre-existing cells, and his ideas gave pathology an entirely
new basis and direction. In 1861, the Bonn anatomist Max
Schultze (fig. 26)[21] noted that the cell was more than a membrane around a structureless substance. He identified proto-
plasm as the basis of cellular organization. In the same year,
Virchow introduced the idea that an aggregate of cells
formed a cell state.[22] For Virchow, as one of the founders and
most prominent representatives of the German liberal party,
liberal principles were pre-eminent in biology and politics.
He compared the cell to an individual citizen and was
opposed to hierarchical concepts of control of either substances or regions.

In contrast, other biologists, such as Ernst Haeckel, contended that the more differentiated an organism was, the
more necessary control was. Just as higher organisms
required a more developed brain, more highly developed
societies needed control centrally by the state. This view
superseded liberal concepts of biology and of state and gave
legitimacy to authoritarian structures and strictures. The
development of bacteriology, which was accompanied by the
discovery of hordes of alien parasites invading the cell state
and being resisted by antibodies, reinforced the analogy of
body and state and the belief that central control was necessary to secure the health of individual citizens as a prerequisite for survival of a nation.[23]

The danger associated with those analogies was soon recognized by people like Virchow, who addressed it in these

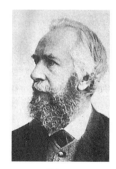

FIG 24
ERNST HAECKEL
(1834–1919)

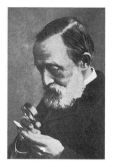

FIG 25
RUDOLF VIRCHOW
(1821–1902)

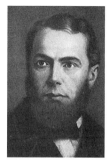

FIG 26
MAX SCHULTZE
(1825–1874)

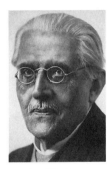

FIG 27
PAUL
SCHIEFFERDECKER
(1849–1951)

words: "Nothing is similar to life but life itself. One may call the state an organism because it is composed of living citizens; one may also call the organism a state, a society, a family, because it is composed of living members of the same origin. But that is the end of all comparison."[24] Virchow criticized especially the unhesitating acceptance of the new concept of the origin of humans and the far-reaching conclusions based on it. He stressed that this concept was still a theory rather than established scientific fact and expressed his concern that the theory "might come back to us in a frightening form. . . . It is very serious, and I hope that the theory of the origin of species will not bring us all the horrors that other theories . . . have created. After all, this theory, if applied consequently, has an extremely precarious side."[25]

The precarious side of Darwinism was expressed in the idea that different races had different value. At one time, that idea might have gone unnoticed, but in the late nineteenth century it fell on fertile soil and was fed by trends of nationalism, imperialism, and colonialism. As European nations tried to surpass one another in demonstrations of strength and power, the map of the world became their playing field. Foreign countries and foreign people were considered to be inferior.

This view of the world was so firmly rooted in the minds of Europeans that it was presented as an indubitable fact even in scientific publications. When the anatomist Paul Schiefferdecker (fig. 27)[26] presented the first description of apocrine glands, he found them to be more prevalent in animals than in humans, and in Negroes than in Caucasians. He interpreted his findings as evidence for a more advanced state of biological development of Caucasians, as compared to primitive peoples. Schiefferdecker also studied the distribution of elastic fibers of the skin in respect to races. He claimed that in the face of the Indo-Germanic race there was a special type of elastic fiber that was missing in inferior races. He referred to those fibers as *elastica mimica* and attributed their development genetically to the more expressive mimicry of more cultivated peoples. Of course, no such fibers exist.

Nevertheless, such bizarre speculations were incorporated, unquestioned, into the textbooks of the time. Their effect was to reinforce the fear of a decline of European nations through mixture of their peoples with those of inferior races. Internal problems of European countries were frequently attributed to the negative influence of alien elements.

This scapegoatism was especially prevalent in the multi-national Austro-Hungarian monarchy, which was afflicted by severe rifts among Germans, Czechs, Poles, Italians, Croatians, Romanians, and others. Each national group tried to hold its ground against the others, blamed the others for its trouble, and thought that it was denied rights that it deserved. In this tense nationalistic atmosphere, Jews remained outcasts. Because most of them spoke German or Yiddish, a German language written in Hebrew characters, they were generally reckoned among the German population. The Germans, however, perceived Jews as alien, with aspirations for domination over the German people and for destruction of "true" German culture.[27]

Such fears were boosted by the immigration of orthodox Jews from eastern Europe, especially to Vienna, whose Jewish population rose from 6,200 (2.2 percent) in 1860 to 72,600 (10.1 percent) in 1880. At the high schools and the University of Vienna, the percentage of Jews was much higher and exceeded by far that of other Austrian cities. In 1890, for instance, Jews accounted for 32.8 percent of students at the University of Vienna, as compared to 2.9 percent at Graz and only 0.2 percent at Innsbruck, where the climate was less cosmopolitan and more anti-Semitic. In 1861, the University of Vienna was the first in the Austro-Hungarian empire to appoint a Jew extraordinary professor—namely, the dermatologist Hermann Zeissl (fig. 28), who is still

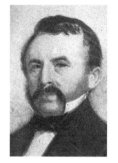

FIG 28

HERMANN ZEISSL

(1817–1884)

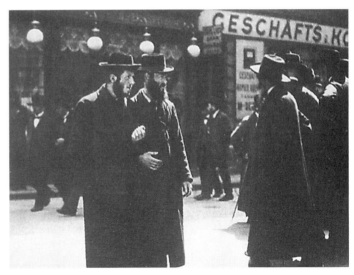

FIG 29 ORTHODOX JEWS IN VIENNA.

appreciated for his contributions to distinguishing syphilis from gonorrhea. The first Jews who were chairs of university departments were appointed in the 1890s. Academic careers for Jews, however, remained an exception. For most capable Jewish physicians of that time, attainment of a university career required a huge donation to the university, such as underwriting a scientific or clinical institute.[28] Such wealthy sponsors could be found among the most successful businessmen of the city, who owned palaces that exceeded in size and splendor those of the aristocrats and who had gained entrance into the highest circles of society. Whereas most influential Jews had become assimilated and could not be distinguished from other Germans, orthodox Jewish immigrants were eye-catching because of their black hats, caftans, and long sidecurls (fig. 29). The perception of orthodox Jews as being distinctly different from Germans was soon transferred to the entire Jewish community, including businessmen, students, and professors. The pre-eminence of Jews in public life was said to be a manifestation of domination of Germans by aliens (fig. 30).[29]

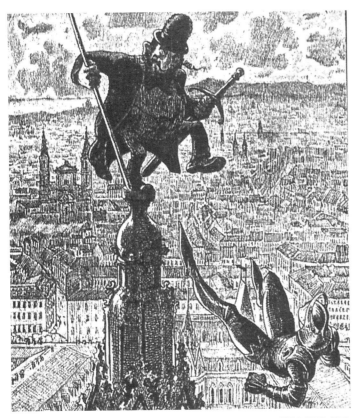

FIG 30 THE JEW ON THE CITY HALL OF VIENNA, REPLACING THE OLD
STATUE ON TOP OF THE BUILDING—A WARNING OF IMPENDING
JEWISH RULE OVER VIENNA.

Even moderate men who respected Jews and had Jewish
friends denied the possibility of complete assimilation by
Jews. Theodor Billroth (fig. 31), the famous pioneer of abdominal surgery and one of the earliest proponents of cellular
pathology, contended in 1876 that "a Jew cannot become a
German any more than a Persian, Frenchman, New Zealan-
der, or African; what one calls German Jews are Jews who
speak German only by chance, who have been educated in
Germany by chance, even if they write poetry and think in
the German language more beautifully and better than some
Germans of purest descent." According to Billroth, Jews were
devoid of true "German feelings" that were based on
"medieval romanticism." He wrote further that "despite all

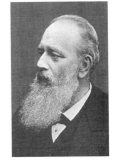

FIG 31
THEODOR
BILLROTH
(1829–1894)

21

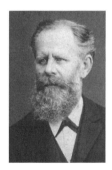

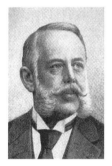

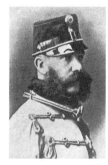

reflection and individual sympathy, I feel the abyss between pure German and pure Jewish blood as deep as a Teuton may have felt the abyss between himself and a Phoenician." With those remarks, Billroth inspired an outbreak of anti-Semitism at the University of Vienna. Its vigor surprised him and eventually induced him to join the League for Repulsion of Anti-Semitism.[30]

Other prominent Viennese physicians also tried to suppress the rising tide of anti-Semitism. The famous clinician and pathologist Hermann Nothnagel (fig. 32) was chairman of the League for Repulsion of Anti-Semitism. In one of his lectures in 1894, he criticized the anti-Jewish attitude of the student societies of Vienna; a violent response in the lecture hall resulted.[31] Hans von Hebra (fig. 33), the son of Ferdinand von Hebra and the successor of Heinrich Auspitz as head of the Skin Unit of Vienna General Polyclinic, wrote in 1892: "Engendered by hatred, born by stupidity, educated by wickedness, anti-Semitism represents a monstrosity of the human spirit."[32] Despite the efforts of Hans von Hebra and other like-minded men, however, the monstrosity of anti-Semitism could no longer be contained.

The word "anti-Semitism" was introduced in 1873 by Wilhelm Marr, an unsuccessful journalist who foretold the "victory of Jewry over Germandom." Within the next decade, the first anti-Semitic political parties were founded; their leaders had meteoric careers and became Hitler's models during his years in Vienna from 1907 to 1913. So prevalent was anti-Semitism in the Austro-Hungarian monarchy that Emperor Francis Joseph I (fig. 34) commented, "One does everything to protect the Jews, but who is not an anti-Semite?"[33]

In the German Reich, the situation was not very different. Anti-Semitism became fashionable and was accepted even in academic circles. Heinrich von Treitschke (fig. 35), National Liberal and professor of history at the University of Berlin, was a vocal advocate of anti-Semitism. In 1879 he coined the phrase "The Jews are our misfortune." It was a saying that persisted through succeeding generations of Germans and eventually became a favorite slogan of the Nazis.[34]

Prejudice against Jews was spread in anti-Semitic newspapers and pamphlets, but also in seemingly innocuous publications like children's books. In his story "Plisch and Plum," the famous cartoonist Wilhelm Busch (fig. 36) pictured a Jew by the name of Schmulchen Schievelbeiner. He described his countenance as crafty, his eyes as black, his soul as gray, and his entire appearance as ugly. The Jew is attacked by two little dogs, Plisch and Plum, loses the bottom of his pants, and frees himself in a clever but not very dignified manner. He then threatens the dog's owner by taking him to court and, finally, with a big smile, collects his smart money (see figs. 38, 39).[35] Stories such as this were present on the shelves of innumerable German playrooms —and still are. They shaped the picture of Jews in the German mind and contributed to the rise of more obvious forms of anti-Semitism.

In the 1870s and 1880s, anti-Semitism was boosted by several events, including the immigration of orthodox Jews fleeing pogroms in Russia. A lasting economic depression was evidence for anti-Semites that Jewish capitalists had engaged in financial manipulations to undermine the country. In the spring of 1881, a Petition by Anti-Semites with more than 200,000 signatures was presented to Germany's chancellor, Otto von Bismarck. It demanded "the emancipation of the German people from a form of alien domination which it cannot endure for any length of time." In Berlin, agitation at mass meetings about the petition led to street brawls, attacks on Jews, and smashing of windows of Jewish homes and shops.[36] Several prominent citizens, including well-known physicians like Paul Langerhans (fig. 37) and Rudolf Virchow stood up against this movement, signed counterpetitions, and deplored in public assemblies the fact that this kind of religious intolerance was still possible in Berlin. On January 12, 1881,

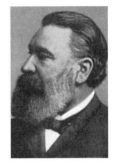

FIG 35
HEINRICH
VON TREITSCHKE
(1834–1896)

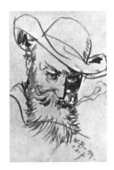

FIG 36
WILHELM BUSCH
(1832–1908)

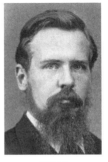

FIG 37
PAUL LANGERHANS
(1847–1888)

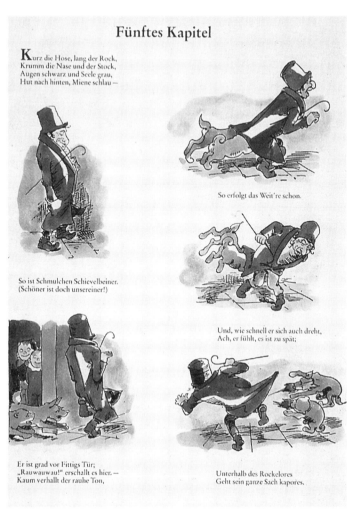

FIG 38 WILHELM BUSCH: "PLISCH UND PLUM."

Rudolf Virchow stated that "especially this big city, which houses the largest number of Jewish fellow citizens in Europe, is called upon to testify that the concurrence of Jewish elements in the life of the city as well as the state has taken place in a national sense, truly supportive of the state. The friendship to Jews is a special peculiarity of Berlin. I myself consider it an honor to have a large number of Jewish friends who surpass me in regard to intellect and sagacity so that I can learn from them. I really want to

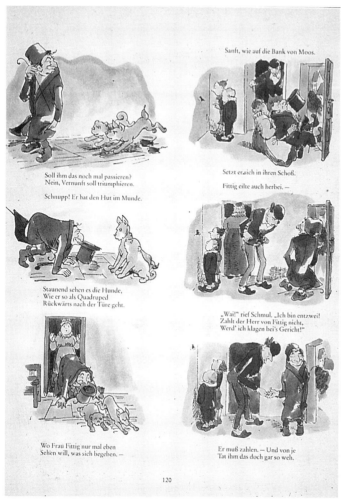

Sanft, wie auf die Bank von Moos.

Soll ihm das noch mal passieren?
Nein, Vernunft soll triumphieren.

Schnupp! Er hat den Hut im Munde.

Setzt er sich in ihren Schoß.

Fittig eilte auch herbei. —

Staunend sehen es die Hunde,
Wie er so als Quadruped
Rückwärts nach der Türe geht.

„Wai!" rief Schmul. „Ich bin entzwei!
Zahlt der Herr von Fittig nicht,
Werd' ich klagen bei's Gericht!"

Wo Frau Fittig nur mal eben
Sehen will, was sich begeben. —

Er muß zahlen. — Und von je
Tat ihm das doch gar so weh.

120

FIG 39 WILHELM BUSCH: "PLISCH UND PLUM."

know if there is a second city in the world where Jews have accomplished so much."[37]

Although Jews contributed immensely to the wealth and strength of the new German Reich, they were never awarded true emancipation. They suffered condescension from the authorities and obstruction to their careers. Nevertheless, they relished the opportunities that had opened to them and the climate in which intellectual achievement was measured justly and treated respectfully. Most educated Jews

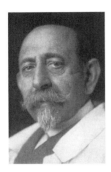

FIG 40
OTTO LUBARSCH
(1860–1933)

drew nourishment and delight from the writings of Kant and Hegel. They felt a strong link between the traditional Jewish spirit of rationality and the liberal spirit of modern Germany, which attempted to devise and apply rational solutions to all social problems. With its philosophical idealism, reverence for pure religion, and ethical humanism, Wilhelmine Germany, like no other nation in the world, seemed to be bound naturally to Judaism.

For this reason, most German Jews thought that at last they had found a haven. They considered Germany to be their home and fatherland, eagerly awaiting a future of even further emancipation and desiring a complete amalgamation of Jewry and Germandom. Many Jews even exceeded their non-Jewish compatriots in national pride. Otto Lubarsch (fig. 40), for instance, a successor of Rudolf Virchow as chairman of pathology at the University of Berlin, was a fervid admirer of the German spirit and of the great figures in German history. Although his family was Jewish, Lubarsch, since his early childhood, tried to suppress any specifically Jewish feature of himself or his lifestyle. As a medical student, he followed the ideal of the "strict, rough, and hardworking Prussian," was an active member of a dueling fraternity, and, because of his constant readiness for battle, acquired the nickname "Säbel-Lubarsch" ("saber Lubarsch"). He even had to serve a jail sentence for illegal dueling, which was considered an honor rather than a disgrace.[38] Throughout his lifetime, Lubarsch remained a monarchist and a loyal subject of the German kaiser, and in this regard he was not alone among Jews. Many Jews were "better Germans," and when it came to war, they demonstrated their patriotism with enthusiasm.

On August 1, 1914, the day the order for German mobilization was signed, the Central Association of German Citizens of Jewish Faith appealed to its members "to dedicate their strength to the fatherland above the measure of duty." The Jewish writer Ernst Toller recalled, "We live in an ecstasy of emotion. . . . The words Germany, fatherland, war have magic power; when we say them, they do not evaporate, they float in the air, spin around, inflame us."[39]

More than 10,000 Jews volunteered for the German army in World War I (fig. 41), thinking that this war would be the final chapter in the struggle for Jewish emancipation. They discovered just the opposite.

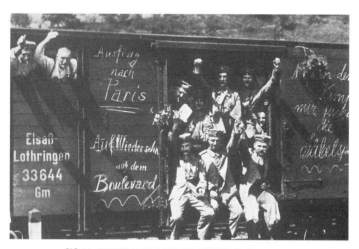

FIG 41 GERMAN TROOPS ON THEIR WAY TO THE FRONT AT THE BEGINNING OF WORLD WAR I.

THE ASSUMPTION
OF POWER

WORLD WAR I ENDED IN 1919 WITH GERMANY'S CAPITU-
LATION. AFTER THE GERMAN DEFEAT, THE VICTORIOUS
Allied powers forced Germany to sign the Treaty of Versailles,
which imposed severe penalties on Germany, including loss of
one-seventh of its territory and one-tenth of its population,
confiscation of industrial equipment, and enormous reparations. The harshness of these measures resulted in years of
economic and political chaos in Germany.

Politically, the degradation of Germany led to increased
nationalism. The Democrats who signed the Treaty of Versailles were defamed as traitors, and the legend of the "stab in
the back" accused Socialists and, most prominently, Jews of
being responsible for the defeat of the brave German soldier
by fostering antiwar agitation at home (see fig. 44).

Walther Rathenau (fig. 42), the Jewish foreign minister of
the Weimar Republic, had foreseen that development. As early
as in 1916, he had predicted, "The more Jews die in this war,
the more emphatically will their enemies prove that all of
them stayed behind the front to engage in war usury. The
hatred will double and treble."[1] Rathenau himself became a
victim of the hatred; he was killed by right-wing terrorists in
June 1922. Several putsches against the Weimar Republic, one
led by Adolf Hitler, were unsuccessful (see fig. 45).

The economic consequences of paying reparations resulted
in astronomical inflation. In October 1923, one dollar equaled
twenty-five billion reichsmarks. Wages had to be delivered in
sacks or baskets (see figs. 47, 48). It took two days for a skilled
worker to earn the billions of Reichsmark needed for a single
pound of butter, and those who had saved for a pension lost
everything within a few months. Karl Touton (fig. 43), who is
invoked to this day because of his original description of the

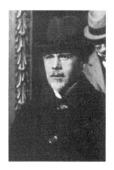

FIG 42
WALTHER
RATHENAU
(1867–1922)

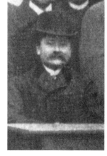

FIG 43
KARL TOUTON
(1858–1934)

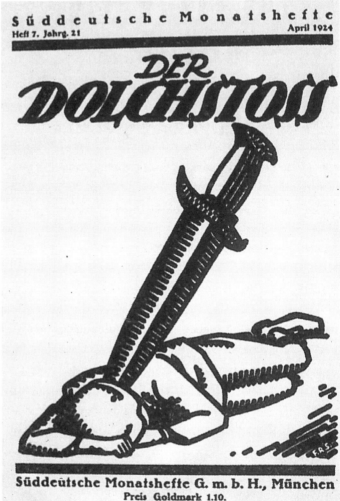

FIG 44 DOLCHSTOSS ("STAB IN THE BACK").

giant cell named after him, had a busy dermatologic practice in Wiesbaden. During this period, he lost his entire fortune and was left with almost nothing.[2]

Although inflation had disastrous consequences for the majority of Germans, it proved highly profitable for industrialists, who could pay off their debts faster and produce their goods cheaper than ever. The proportion of Jews among the industrialists was high, and anti-Jewish sentiment was easy to galvanize as a result (fig. 49).

Ostensibly rational arguments that explained, defended, and fostered the rising tide of anti-Semitism were mere pretenses. The true causes of anti-Semitism were irrational feelings that had been instilled in the minds of most Germans during early childhood and were constantly reinforced in later life—by jokes at the expense of Jews, by anti-Semitic phrases that had become part of colloquial language, and by anti-Semitic undertones in newspapers, magazines, movies, and political discussions. Some Germans were aware of those feelings and tried to suppress them, whereas others tried to integrate them into a seemingly rational view of the world. Still others made no attempt to conceal the irrationality of their convictions.

According to anti-Semitic doctrine, Jews were responsible equally for capitalistic exploitation and Communist agitation, and their involvement in both was seen as evidence of a "secret Jewish conspiracy for world domination." Jews were thought to call the shots in Western democracies as well as in Bolshevist Russia, where they were believed to be attempting to establish worldwide Bolshevism under Jewish leadership. These fables were shared in political meetings, pamphlets, and caricatures like that of the "eternal Jew" (fig. 50). Accord-

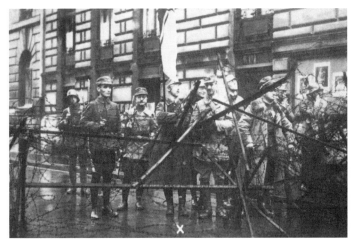

FIG 45 PUTSCH IN MUNICH IN 1923. IN THE CENTER
WITH THE FLAG IS HEINRICH HIMMLER.

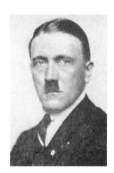

FIG 46
ADOLF HITLER
(1889–1945)

ing to Hitler (fig. 46), Jews had many techniques for achieving world mastery, including control of the press and trade unions, Marxism, and the democracies. As for democracy itself, Hitler held that "only the Jew can praise an institution which is as dirty and false as he himself."[3]

In the first years of the Weimar Republic, Hitler's National Socialist party—the Nationalsozialistische Deutsche Arbeiterpartei (NSDAP)—was nothing but an insignificant fringe group on the very far right of the political spectrum. The democratic parties and the press were amused rather than fearful of Hitler; in their view, his anti-Semitic convulsions were ridiculous, and they considered him a clown (fig. 53).

The situation began to change in late 1929 as the world suffered an economic crisis. Heavily obligated to foreign banks and denied further credit abroad, the German government instituted a program of economic retrenchment in a vain attempt to meet its reparation obligations. The result was rapidly rising unemployment and a call for a strong leader to guide Germany out of its desperate situation. To many, Hitler was their last hope (fig. 54). As if in synchrony with the increase in the unemployment rate, the percentage registered by the Nazi

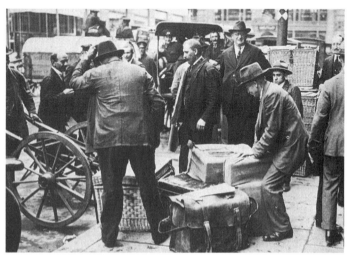

FIG 47 DELIVERY OF WAGES DURING
POSTWAR INFLATION IN GERMANY.

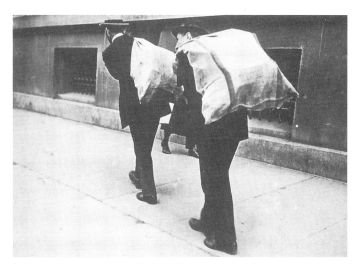

FIG 48 DELIVERY OF WAGES DURING
POSTWAR INFLATION IN GERMANY.

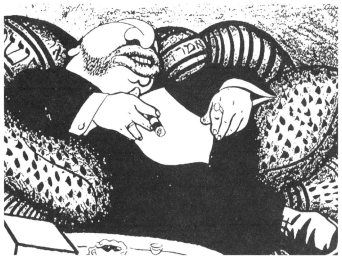

FIG 49 ANTI-SEMITIC PROPAGANDA IN THE
YEARS OF THE WEIMAR REPUBLIC.

party in the elections for the German parliament, the Reichstag, rose from 2.6 percent in 1928 and 18.3 percent in 1930 to
37.4 percent in 1932.[4]

The Nazis recruited their followers from all social groups.
They were supported by workers, by industrialists who donated

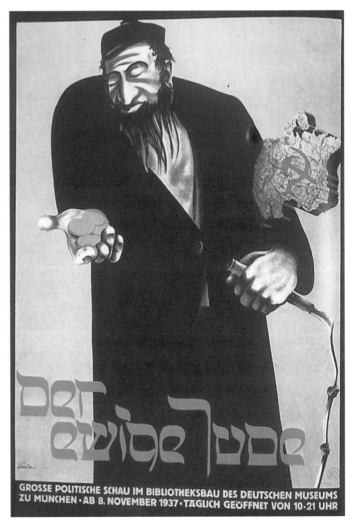

FIG 50 NAZI PROPAGANDA POSTER: "THE ETERNAL JEW."

vast sums of campaign money, and especially by the impoverished middle class, which included many physicians (fig. 55).

In 1926, nearly half of all doctors in Germany earned a
salary only slightly above that of the average industrial
worker, and the world economic crisis only made the situation
worse. Even in 1929, before the economic havoc, 48 percent of
German doctors earned less than what was considered to be
the minimum necessary for survival. By 1932, this number

had jumped to 72 percent, and it was reported that 10 percent of all German physicians were "starving" during the years of the Depression.[5] Furthermore, the future for physicians did not look bright, and that bleak circumstance was complicated by an excess of medical students that threatened to increase competition in the profession. An increasing number of young physicians remained unemployed, and official statisticians predicted that by 1936, 4,900 German medical school graduates would be unable to find work.[6] The Nazi party offered a solution to these medical students and unemployed doctors when it announced in 1930 that the "misery of the rising generation of German physicians . . . will immediately be solved when, in the future Third Reich, fellow Germans will be treated only by physicians of German descent."[7]

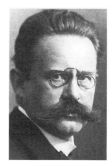

FIG 51
ALBERT JESIONEK
(1870–1935)

The medical profession in Germany was not the only one to call for the exclusion of Jews. In fact, Jews, on average, suffered less from the disastrous economy than did the population at large. The unemployment rate for them was relatively low because close to 46 percent of them—compared to 16 percent in the general population—were self-employed. Three percent of all self-employed people in Germany were Jewish. Furthermore, the high level of education of many Jews assured a certain job security. Although less than 1 percent of the German population was Jewish, Jews accounted for 2.6 percent of schoolteachers and for almost one-sixth of all lawyers and physicians.

In an environment of poverty and distress, the relative wealth of many Jews led to envy and discrimination on the part of non-Jews. At the University of Giessen, for instance, the non-Jewish chairman of dermatology, Albert Jesionek (fig. 51), was criticized for employing Stephan Rothman (fig. 52), a Hungarian Jew. Under extreme pressure, in 1926 Jesionek was forced to terminate the contract of Rothman, who still continued to work in Giessen for some time without pay. In 1928 Rothman returned to Hungary and in 1935 was appointed secretary general of the International Congress of Dermatology that was to

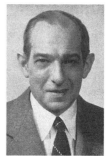

FIG 52
STEPHAN ROTHMAN
(1894–1963)

be convened in Budapest. Anticipating the coming of war, he emigrated to the United States in 1938, became chair of dermatology at the University of Chicago, and was one of the most esteemed dermatologists in the world. Among other contributions, Rothman was the first to demonstrate large quantities of the precursor to vitamin D, 7-dehydrocholesterol, in human

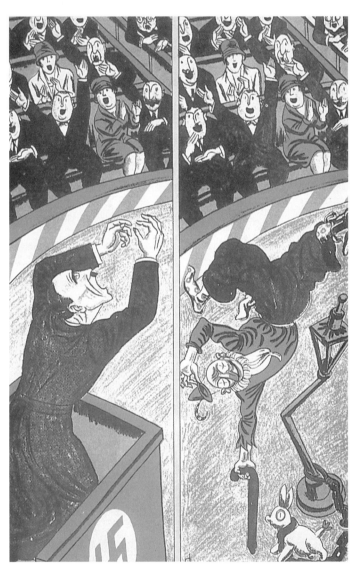

FIG 53 CARICATURE OF HITLER AS A CLOWN
IN THE NEWSPAPER *SIMPLICISSIMUS*.

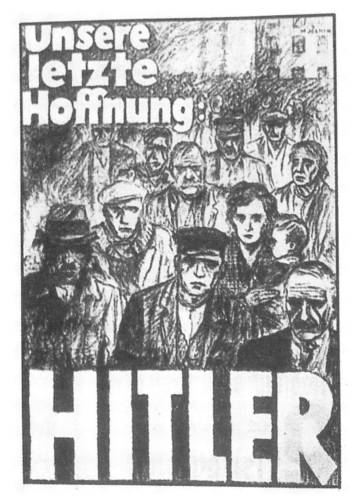

FIG 54 POSTER STATING "OUR LAST HOPE. HITLER."

epidermis. In numerous physiological and biochemical studies, he delineated the relationship between microflora and lipids of the skin, explored the relationship between squalenes and cholesterol in human sebum, and demonstrated the sun-protective effect of *para*-aminobenzoic acid, which continues to be the most widely used compound in sunblocks. Rothman's most important work was his classic textbook *Physiology and Biochemistry of the Skin*, which he poignantly dedicated "to the memory of my teacher, Albert Jesionek."[8]

The discrimination against Jewish physicians in the Weimar Republic also is illustrated by their failure to secure

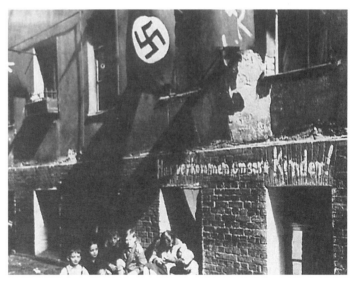

FIG 55 POLITICAL RADICALIZATION IN THE WEIMAR REPUBLIC. FLAGS OF COMMUNISTS AND NAZIS ARE SEEN SIDE BY SIDE. THE GRAFFITI READS: "HERE OUR CHILDREN GO TO THE DOGS!"

leading positions. In the mid-1920s, for example, Oscar Gans was a possible candidate for a chair in dermatology after having published the first volume of his textbook on dermatopathology, *Histologie der Hautkrankheiten.* He recalled the situation in these words:

> *My friends congratulated me and held that this work had secured for me a chairmanship. In consideration of my being Jewish, however, I was absolutely sure that this would not be the case. And I was right: several chairs of dermatology became vacant and were filled with younger colleagues. Then I received a call to the Mayo Clinic in Rochester for the winter term of 1926/27 and, henceforth, it was more difficult to ignore me. Nevertheless, none of the smaller German faculties ever put me on a list until Frankfurt became vacant after K. Herxheimer's retirement in 1929. When the list for Frankfurt appeared (1929) with the names (1) Bruno Bloch— Zürich, (2) O. Gans—Heidelberg and Rost—Freiburg*

(aequo loco), *there was an outburst of fury at the Congress of the German Dermatological Society in Königsberg in August 1929, especially by W. Scholtz . . . Spiethoff—Jena, Mulzer—Hamburg, who thought they had more right to that position.*[9]

The atmosphere at German medical schools became increasingly tense for Jews, not only for faculty but for students as well. In the mid-1920s, medical students refused to allow Jews into their organizations, and in Königsberg, Jews and foreign students were thrown out of classrooms. At the Technical University of Hannover, the students' assembly demanded, by a two-thirds majority, the exclusion of all students of Jewish descent. In Giessen, right-wing fraternities threatened to boycott certain pubs if Jewish students were served there, and in several instances, Jews were physically attacked by Nazi rowdies.

The rapid rise of virulent anti-Semitism proved to be a powerful tool for Hitler. His radical propaganda and call for a national uprising soon attracted increasing numbers of followers, turning the NSDAP into the strongest party in the German parliament (fig. 56). Yet, instead of closing ranks against Hitler, the Democratic parties tried to use him for their own aims, chummed up to him, and refrained from taking stern measures against illegal encroachments by storm troopers. Socialists and Communists neglected the danger of the Nazis and instead continued to fight one another. Some of them even opted for Hitler's participation in the government, arguing that once Hitler failed, their own time surely would come. Like Rudolf Breitscheid—spokesman for foreign affairs of the Social Democratic party, who died in a concentration camp in 1944—many lost their lives because of their own irresponsible, selfish, myopic tactics.[10]

In the elections for the Reichstag in November 1932, the NSDAP became the strongest party, but for the first time, it also suffered major losses. Liberal journals exulted that Hitler's time was over, and Joseph Goebbels, head of the Nazi

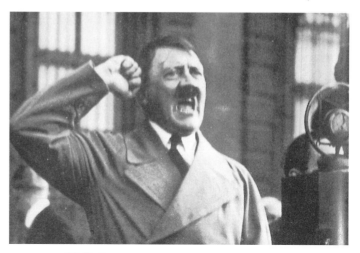

FIG 56 HITLER DELIVERING A SPEECH IN 1932.

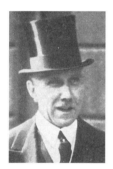

FIG 57
FRANZ VON PAPEN
(1879–1969)

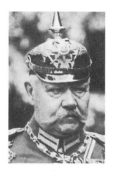

FIG 58
PAUL VON
HINDENBURG
(1847–1934)

propaganda machine, wrote in his diaries: "The year 1932 was a real run of bad luck. . . . The past was difficult, and the future is dark and sad, all hopes and prospects have vanished completely." Power-hungry leaders of several right-wing parties, however, turned the Nazis' defeat into a victory by offering themselves for positions in a government under Hitler's leadership, among them Franz von Papen (fig. 57), the intellectually lightweight, arrogant chancellor in the year 1932. On January 30, 1933, Adolf Hitler was appointed chancellor of the German Reich by the Reich's president Paul von Hindenburg (fig. 58), a former World War I general who was not a Democrat himself but was still loyal to the former monarchic system.[11]

At the time of his appointment, Hitler's base of power was small (figs. 59, 60). The new chancellor was head of a coalition cabinet that had only a minority of seats in the Reichstag. Nevertheless, he obtained absolute power within fifty-two days. By setting the Reichstag on fire and accusing the Communists of the crime, he compelled President von Hindenburg to sign a Decree for the Protection of the People and the State. This edict suspended the seven sections of the constitution that guaranteed individual and civil liberties.

The decree became effective on February 28. Within the next few days, leaders of the Communist and Socialist parties were arrested, leftist and liberal publications were halted, and Democratic party meetings were either broken up or banned (fig. 61). With all the resources of propaganda now available to them, the Nazis went into a new general election on March 5, 1933, yet they again failed to win a majority of votes. By this time, however, so many of their political opponents were already in prison that Hitler had the two-thirds majority in the Reichstag needed for passing the Law for Removing the Distress of People and Reich—the so-called Enabling Act. On March 23, 1933, Hitler at last acquired the legal basis for his dictatorship.

With incredible speed, the Nazis set out to reshape all organizations and institutions according to the edicts of their party. Within two weeks, the parliaments of all German states were dissolved and replaced by Reich's governors, who received their orders directly from the Reich's minister of the interior in Berlin. On May 1, the Nazis celebrated Labor Day with a mass demonstration in Berlin. For the event, leaders of

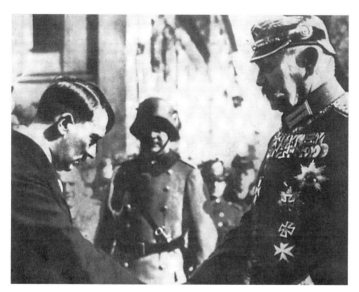

FIG 59 HITLER SHAKING HANDS WITH PAUL VON HINDENBURG.

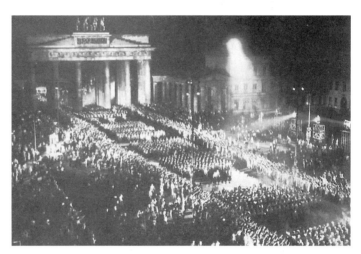

FIG 60 NAZI CELEBRATION IN BERLIN AFTER HITLER'S
APPOINTMENT AS CHANCELLOR OF THE GERMAN REICH.

the trade unions had been flown to Berlin from all over Germany and were exceedingly impressed by the friendliness of
the Nazis to the working class. One day later, the very same
labor leaders were arrested. Many were beaten and placed in
concentration camps. The trade unions were banned, their
headquarters occupied, and their funds confiscated. By July
14, all political parties except the NSDAP had been eliminated. Party members were installed in crucial positions in
every public office.[12]

In those few weeks, it became abundantly clear that democratic rules and civil rights would no longer be respected. It
was still possible, however, to save the nation from the tyranny
that followed. Most Germans were opposed to the Nazis, as
they had demonstrated in the last regular election in November 1932. President von Hindenburg could have dismissed
Hitler with the full support of the armed forces, but he was
elated to see Socialists and Communists in jail. He closed
ranks with Hitler, and called him his comrade. Socialists,
Communists, and trade unionists could have called for a general strike, as they had done before when the democratic constitution was at stake, but instead they appealed for calm and
caution, arguing that a general strike should only be a last

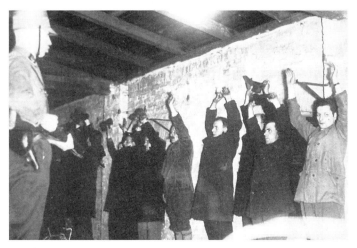

FIG 61 ARRESTED SOCIALIST AND COMMUNIST PARTY MEMBERS.

resort. Shortly thereafter, that option no longer existed. Professional groups such as administrative officers, judges,
lawyers, and physicians could have refused to cooperate with
the Nazis, but they preferred to do "business as usual." The
representatives of the German states who protested the violation of their constitutional rights could have ordered the
police to arrest Nazi governors, but they did not have the
courage to resist. Most Democrats adopted the spineless policy
of "wait and see." It was not long before they were to rue
their indifference, but by then it was too late.

THE REORGANIZATION OF MEDICINE

THE RAPID ESTABLISHMENT OF A TOTALITARIAN STATE NOT ONLY AFFECTED GOVERNMENT INSTITUTIONS, POLITICAL parties, and trade unions, it also transformed professional organizations, most notably those involving the practice of medicine. According to Martin Bormann (fig. 62), the secretary of Adolf Hitler, "the Führer holds the cleansing of the medical profession far more important than, for example, that of the bureaucracy, since in his opinion the duty of the physician is or should be one of racial leadership."[1]

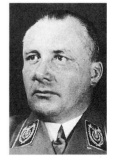

Gerhard Wagner (fig. 63), the future Reichsführer of physicians, was assigned by the Nazi party the task of gaining control of the medical sector. He set out to accomplish this by absorbing traditional physicians' organizations into the party's own physicians' league. In addition, he created two powerful new organizations, the German Panel Fund Physicians' Union (Kassenärztliche Vereinigung Deutschlands, or KVD), which included all physicians working in the area of public health insurance,[2] and the Reich's Chamber of Physicians, in which membership was compulsory for every practicing physician in Germany. The KVD and the Reich's Chamber of Physicians served legitimate purposes, including medical organization and medical education, mediation between sickness funds and insurance-panel doctors, and the establishment of social insurance schemes for physicians and their families. Disciplinary courts within each organization, however, soon seized political and professional control over German physicians—and in totalitarian fashion.

The Reich's Physicians' Ordinance of December 13, 1935, established that both the professional life and the private life of physicians were subject to the approbation of the Reich's Chamber of Physicians. Gerhard Wagner praised the chamber

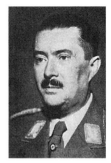

as an instrument that enabled the German medical community "to maintain discipline and order in the ranks by virtue of our own professional jurisdiction." "Discipline and order in the ranks" meant that physicians were obligated to practice their profession in the interest of the community of the people as it was defined in the National Socialist sense. Any deviation from National Socialist doctrines could result in penalties that ranged from fines to withdrawal of a license to practice medicine.[3]

That the new professional organizations tended to restrict the freedom and independence physicians had previously enjoyed was not grasped immediately by medical doctors. Gerhard Wagner, favoring persuasion over force, had little difficulty gaining the full cooperation of the old bourgeois physicians' unions, which welcomed the Nazis and the end of the Weimar Republic. On March 12, 1933, Karl Haedenkamp, executive director of the leading physicians' lobby—the so-called Hartmannbund—expressed his joy thus: "The time for a calm and continuous development has come at last. The overthrow of party politics has opened the way for genuine statesmanship. The opposition has no possibility of overturning the plans of the Reich's government. The parliamentary methods of the period following the First World War have suffered a decisive defeat, the horse trading of the political parties is at an end."[4]

On March 22, 1933, Alfons Stauder, the democratically elected president of the Hartmannbund and the Deutscher Ärztevereinsbund, met in "intimate talks" with Gerhard Wagner and then telegraphed Hitler that "the principal professional organizations in Germany gladly welcome the firm determination of the Government of National Renewal to build a true community of all ranks, professions, and classes, and they gladly place themselves at the service of this great patriotic task."[5] Two days later, the old medical organizations and the National Socialist Physicians' League were unified under Wagner's command.

The prime objective of the new medical organization was the "de-jewification of medicine." Only one week after Hitler's takeover, a pediatrician and founder of the National Socialist Physicians' League, Kurt Klare, wrote to a colleague that "Jews and philosemites ought to take note of the fact that Germans are masters of their own house once more and will control their own destiny."[6] Three weeks later, Leonardo Conti (fig. 64), the Prussian commissar of health and Wagner's successor as leader of German physicians, explicitly warned Jews not to be surprised if German physicians began ridding the profession of alien influence. Alfons Stauder, the highest representative of all German physicians in the last four years of the Weimar Republic, advised insurance companies "as soon as possible to replace Jewish doctors enrolled in their programs" and urged Jewish colleagues within the professional organizations to resign immediately from any office that they might hold by election or appointment.[7]

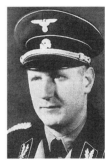

FIG 64
LEONARDO CONTI
(1901–1945)

On March 23, 1933, the day of the Enabling Act, the Nazi party newspaper, *Völkischer Beobachter*, published on its front page a proclamation by Gerhard Wagner, who addressed fellow physicians and stated:

> *There is hardly any profession more important for the greatness and the future of the nation than the medical; no other has been so strictly organized for decades. And yet, no other is so Jewified and so hopelessly involved in unsociable thinking. Jewish lecturers dominate the chairs of medicine, disgrace medical science, and have saturated generations of young physicians with a mechanistic attitude. Jewish "colleagues" installed themselves in the managing boards of professional organizations; they debased the medical conception of honor, and undermined race-specific ethics and morality. Jewish "colleagues" gained control over our professional policy; thanks to them, a*

bargaining mentality and unworthy commercial atti-tude has increasingly established itself in our ranks. And the end of this dreadful development is the eco-nomic bankruptcy, the loss of our esteem with the people, and the continuously decreasing influence in state and administration.... Honor and sense of duty demand from us to put an end to this untenable situa-tion. Therefore, we call upon all German physicians: Clean up the boards of our organizations, sweep away all who do not want to understand the signs of our time, make our profession German again in leader-ship and spirit.[8]

Wagner did not hesitate to put these ideas into action. On March 24, on the occasion of the unification of the physicians' organizations under his leadership, he ordered the "removal of Jews and Marxists from boards and committees."[9] Only three weeks later, Leonardo Conti criticized the German Der-matological Society for not having moved fast enough to exclude Jewish members. "Also in those scientific societies," Conti wrote, "it is an unbearable circumstance and cannot be accepted, that, because of a pathologic accumulation of Jewry in the centers of science, the leadership is in the hands of peo-ple of an alien race."[10] To correct this "unbearable" situation, Conti appointed Josef Schumacher, an unknown dermatolo-gist from Berlin, to reorganize the society.

Schumacher had been a student of Paul Gerson Unna and had published with him a short book about the physiology of the skin of humans and animals. Schumacher had then opened a private practice in Berlin but had not been engaged in any scientific or educational work. His sole qualification for the job of reorganizing the German Dermatological Soci-ety was his active membership in the Nazi party.

The second man in charge was Bodo Spiethoff, director of the skin clinic in Jena. Spiethoff, who had been a member of the Nazi party since 1931, was appointed chairman of the

German Society for the Fight Against Venereal Diseases. In May 1933, he informed the members of the society that the old board had been forced to resign. He phrased the news diplomatically and obtusely: "The board of the society, the boards of the subdivisions, and the members of the committees have placed their positions at disposal. In this, I may see the proof that every single one who has worked in a responsible position is convinced that the work of the German Society for the Fight Against Venereal Diseases has to be completely adapted to the new conditions."[11]

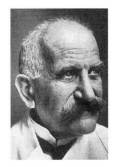

Among the former members of the managing board were Leopold Ritter von Zumbusch, Felix Pinkus, and—as chairman of the society—Joseph Jadassohn (fig. 65), at the time probably the most famous dermatologist in the world. As the successor of Albert Neisser, Jadassohn had turned the skin clinic of Breslau into one of the world's leading dermatological centers. He had given original descriptions of several conditions, such as nevus sebaceus and pachyonychia congenita; had introduced patch testing for the detection of the causes of contact dermatitis; and had just published his enormous *Handbuch der Haut- und Geschlechtskrankheiten*, the most comprehensive text on dermatology ever written. Despite his resignation in 1931, Jadassohn continued to work until 1934 at the skin clinic in Breslau with his successor and former associate Max Jessner. As a Jew, Jadassohn's tenure was difficult and problematic. His international fame did not prevent him and his family from being subjected to the countless measures of oppression that befell Jews in Germany. His son-in-law, the non-Jewish philologist Kurt Jäckel, was denied academic promotion because he was married to Jadassohn's daughter.[12] In 1934, Jadassohn moved to Switzerland, where he died two years later. His death was not noted in a single German medical journal.[13]

Jadassohn not only had been chair of the German Society for the Fight Against Venereal Diseases but also secretary and treasurer of the German Dermatological Society, and on

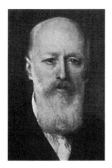

FIG 66
GUSTAV RIEHL, SR.
(1855–1943)

April 12, 1933, he was forced to give up that position as well. In an obituary published in Czechoslovakia in 1936, the former chairman of the Prague section of the German Dermatological Society, Viktor Bandler, deplored the fact that "Jadassohn, who was accepted as representative of the German Dermatological Society for decades, who carried the fame of German dermatology to all countries, across all oceans, who was loved and respected throughout the world, was deemed by the ruling gang of German dermatologists, through a disgraceful, mendacious judicial decision, not to be entitled and qualified to represent the German Dermatological Society."[14] Bandler was referring to a decision by the Superior Court of Breslau naming Josef Schumacher as the new legal representative of the German Dermatological Society. The arrogant tactics of the "ruling gang of German dermatologists" is illustrated further by the fact that the acting president of the German Dermatological Society, Gustav Riehl from Vienna, was not even informed of forthcoming changes. When Riehl (fig. 66)[15] finally learned of Jadassohn's resignation, he ordered Jadassohn not to deliver any documents of the society to Schumacher. A few months later, however, Riehl himself was persuaded to resign.

The German Dermatological Society, traditionally the central organization of dermatologists from all German-speaking countries, ceased to exist in its traditional form. The new representatives of German dermatology were no longer interested in collaborating with colleagues from the Netherlands, Switzerland, Czechoslovakia, or Austria. According to Bodo Spiethoff, these colleagues were "either Jewish or Christian Socialist, in other words, directed openly against our state."[16] The upcoming congress, scheduled for Vienna in the spring of 1933, was canceled, and instead the Seventeenth Congress of the German Dermatological Society was held in Berlin in October 1934. The meeting was opened by the new chairman of the society, Karl Zieler from Würzburg, who demanded that "it is the will of all of us that our society shall be firmly embedded into the requirements of the new National Socialist State, which is based on people and race. This has been accomplished yesterday in the general assembly: reorganization according to the leadership principle. Like the other scientific societies, the German Dermatological Society is now integrated into the Reich's Central Office for Health Leadership, and thereby closely connected to the Reich's Ministry of the Interior."

Zieler explained the exclusion of prominent representatives of the society by arguing that "it is only natural that reforms are associated with certain hardships" and that "new times demand new men." In closing his speech, he asked all congress participants to join him in a unified cheer: "The Leader of our German People, our Reich's Chancellor Adolf Hitler, Sieg Heil!"[17]

Exactly how reform of the German Dermatological Society was to happen was not a matter for debate. The new board of the society was not elected by the general assembly but was appointed by Schumacher, the legal representative of the society. It consisted of Karl Zieler (president), Bodo Spiethoff (vice president), Josef Schumacher (secretary), Erhard Riecke (vice secretary), Ernst Heinrich Brill (treasurer), and Paul Mulzer (vice treasurer). Except for Riecke, all were members of the Nazi party.

In addition to the new board, Schumacher also appointed an executive committee, among whose members were Friedrich Bering from Cologne, Georg Birnbaum from Dortmund, Walter Frieboes from Berlin, and Egon Keining from Hamburg. The duties of the executive committee were outlined clearly in a note by Schumacher that was published in the *Dermatologische Wochenschrift* a few months before the opening session of the congress: "In accordance with the statute, the executive committee, which is now invested with the capability to act, will convoke a general assembly of the society in which the new statutes must be accepted."[18]

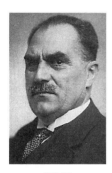

FIG 67
ERICH HOFFMANN
(1868–1959)

The only prominent German dermatologist to publicly protest these measures was Erich Hoffmann (fig. 67), chairman of the skin clinic in Bonn, renown for his discovery, together with Fritz Schaudinn, of the spirochete of syphilis in 1905. Hoffmann wrote numerous letters to the ministry in Berlin complaining about the inappropriate behavior of Schumacher. The letters were ignored, but Hoffmann himself was not. His criticism and irreverent ideas often professed in lectures to medical students—"I prefer a white vest to a brown shirt," for example—brought about his dismissal as director of the dermatological department of the University of Bonn. (In German parlance, a "white vest" is a symbol of a clear conscience; brown shirts were part of the Nazi uniform.) Although the dismissal of Hoffmann was known to be solely motivated by politics, it was explained in an official note in the *Zentralblatt für Haut- und Geschlechtskrankheiten* in an obtuse, misleading way:

> *Following a suggestion by the Prussian Minister for Sciences, Arts, and People's Education, Prof. E. Hoffmann has been called by the board of the foundation Georg-Speyer-House in Frankfurt to become an external member of this research institute in order to give him the opportunity to devote himself exclusively to his research in the field of cutaneous and venereal diseases, exempt from official duties. At the same time, Prof. Hoffmann, who has accepted this invitation with the understanding that he will maintain his residence and private medical office in Bonn, will be released from his official duties as full professor of the medical faculty of Bonn and director of the Department of Dermatology.*[19]

In addition to reorganization of the medical societies, the Nazis also moved to change the editorial boards of the most prestigious medical journals. This task was given to Kurt

Klare, who, for his efforts as chief censor of medical publications, was rewarded with the honorific title of "professor." Immediately after his appointment, Klare made it known that German medical journals should "henceforth be edited only by physicians of German descent."[20]

To achieve this aim, medical publishers were put under massive pressure. Ferdinand Springer, the head of Germany's largest scientific publishing house, was instructed bluntly by Leonardo Conti to dismiss one of his chief editors, the pharmacist Ernst Urban, "in default of which the publishing house would be occupied by an already available group of a hundred." Urban was neither Jewish nor involved politically, but at one point he had refused to publish Nazi political propaganda in a pharmaceutical journal and had continued to employ Jews. In addition, he had provoked the Nazis by printing a poem that, reading between the lines, was a rebuff to the Nazis.

Although Conti's order to dismiss Urban was technically illegal, compliance was enforced through a state-sanctioned threat, and Springer had no choice but to let Urban go after thirty-three years of service to the publishing house. Urban was soon replaced by a man from Conti's staff. The legal consequences that followed were to be borne by the publishing house alone, and in a lawsuit that ultimately granted Urban a severance pay of 45,000 reichmarks, Conti's directive was never mentioned.[21]

Between 1933 and 1936, many editors and authors of dermatological journals were informed that their efforts and contributions were no longer needed, and the results soon became clear. Until 1936, the leading German periodical, the *Archiv für Dermatologie und Syphilis*, was edited by Jadassohn, Frieboes, and von Zumbusch. The list of contributors included many Jews: Abraham Buschke, Wilhelm Siegmund Frei, Leopold Freund, Karl Herxheimer, and Felix Pinkus (fig. 68). In subsequent editions, these names were no longer mentioned. The only man who remained on the editorial

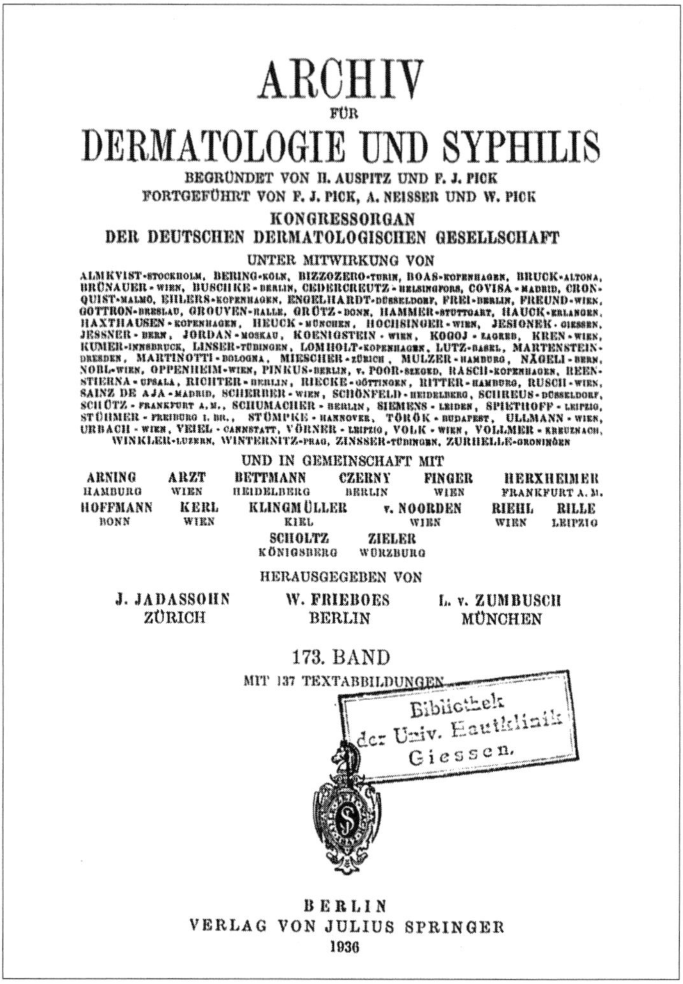

ARCHIV
FÜR
DERMATOLOGIE UND SYPHILIS
BEGRÜNDET VON H. AUSPITZ UND F. J. PICK
FORTGEFÜHRT VON F. J. PICK, A. NEISSER UND W. PICK
KONGRESSORGAN
DER DEUTSCHEN DERMATOLOGISCHEN GESELLSCHAFT
UNTER MITWIRKUNG VON

ALMKVIST-STOCKHOLM, BERING-KÖLN, BIZZOZERO-TURIN, BOAS-KOPENHAGEN, BRUCK-ALTONA, BRÜNAUER - WIEN, BUSCHKE - BERLIN, CEDERCREUTZ - HELSINGFORS, COVISA - MADRID, CRON-QUIST-MALMÖ, EHLERS-KOPENHAGEN, ENGELHARDT-DÜSSELDORF, FREI-BERLIN, FREUND-WIEN, GOTTRON-BRESLAU, GROUVEN-HALLE, GRÜTZ-BONN, HAMMER-STUTTGART, HAUCK-ERLANGEN, HAXTHAUSEN-KOPENHAGEN, HEUCK-MÜNCHEN, HOCHSINGER-WIEN, JESIONEK-GIESSEN, JESSNER - BERN, JORDAN-MOSKAU, KOENIGSTEIN - WIEN, KOGOJ - ZAGREB, KREN-WIEN, KUMER-INNSBRUCK, LINSER-TÜBINGEN, LOMHOLT-KOPENHAGEN, LUTZ-BASEL, MARTENSTEIN-DRESDEN, MARTINOTTI-BOLOGNA, MIESCHER-ZÜRICH, MULZER-HAMBURG, NÄGELI-BERN, NOBL-WIEN, OPPENHEIM-WIEN, PINKUS-BERLIN, v. POOR-SZEGED, RASCH-KOPENHAGEN, REEN-STIERNA-UPSALA, RICHTER-BERLIN, RIECKE-GÖTTINGEN, RITTER-HAMBURG, RUSCH-WIEN, SAINZ DE AJA-MADRID, SCHERBER-WIEN, SCHÖNFELD-HEIDELBERG, SCHREUS-DÜSSELDORF, SCHÜTZ - FRANKFURT A.M., SCHUMACHER - BERLIN, SIEMENS - LEIDEN, SPIETHOFF - LEIPZIG, STÜHMER - FREIBURG i. BR., STÜMPKE - HANNOVER, TÖRÖK - BUDAPEST, ULLMANN - WIEN, URBACH - WIEN, VEIEL - CANNSTATT, VÖRNER - LEIPZIG, VOLK - WIEN, VOLLMER - KREUZNACH, WINKLER-LUZERN, WINTERNITZ-PRAG, ZINSSER-TÜBINGEN, ZURHELLE-GRONINGEN

UND IN GEMEINSCHAFT MIT

ARNING	ARZT	BETTMANN	CZERNY	FINGER	HERXHEIMER
HAMBURG	WIEN	HEIDELBERG	BERLIN	WIEN	FRANKFURT A. M.
HOFFMANN	KERL	KLINGMÜLLER	v. NOORDEN	RIEHL	RILLE
BONN	WIEN	KIEL	WIEN	WIEN	LEIPZIG
		SCHOLTZ	ZIELER		
		KÖNIGSBERG	WÜRZBURG		

HERAUSGEGEBEN VON

| J. JADASSOHN | W. FRIEBOES | L. v. ZUMBUSCH |
| ZÜRICH | BERLIN | MÜNCHEN |

173. BAND
MIT 137 TEXTABBILDUNGEN

BERLIN
VERLAG VON JULIUS SPRINGER
1936

FIG 68 TITLE PAGE OF THE *ARCHIV FÜR DERMATOLOGIE UND SYPHILIS* BEFORE REMOVAL OF JEWISH EDITORS.

board was Frieboes, and among the new editors were Ernst Heinrich Brill and Karl Zieler, both prominent members of the Nazi party (fig. 69).

The changes in the editorial board resulted in a serious decline in the quality of the journal. Until 1936, the *Archiv für Dermatologie und Syphilis* was the most prestigious dermatological journal in the world. Because of its emphasis on basic research and profound clinicopathologic studies, the

ARCHIV FÜR DERMATOLOGIE UND SYPHILIS

KONGRESSORGAN DER DEUTSCHEN DERMATOLOGISCHEN GESELLSCHAFT

HERAUSGEGEBEN VON

L. ARZT	E. BRILL	W. FRIEBOES
WIEN	ROSTOCK	BERLIN
S. LOMHOLT	G. MIESCHER	K. ZIELER
KOPENHAGEN	ZÜRICH	WÜRZBURG

174. BAND

MIT 194 ABBILDUNGEN IM TEXT

BERLIN
VERLAG VON JULIUS SPRINGER
1936

FIG 69 TITLE PAGE OF THE *ARCHIV FÜR DERMATOLOGIE UND SYPHILIS* AFTER REMOVAL OF JEWISH EDITORS.

journal attracted authors from many foreign countries. Numerous diseases, such as Kaposi's sarcoma, lichen nitidus, Mucha-Habermann disease, acrodermatitis chronica atrophicans, and necrobiosis lipoidica, were described for the first time in the *Archiv für Dermatologie und Syphilis*. In contrast, after 1936, hardly any article of lasting import was published in that journal. The number of articles printed per year decreased from almost 150 in 1933 to 75 in 1939, and the percentage of foreign vis-à-vis German authors from 64.1 in the years 1933 to 1938 to 37.7 in the years 1939 to 1944.[22]

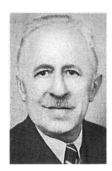

FIG 70
FRITZ CALLOMON
(1876–1964)

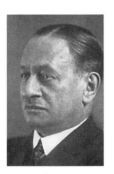

FIG 71
ERNST DELBANCO
(1869–1935)

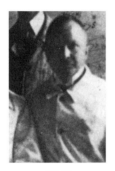

FIG 72
PAUL UNNA, JR.
(1883–1943)

Similar changes occurred in *Dermatologische Wochenschrift*, another highly regarded journal whose emphasis was more practical. It had been founded in 1882 by Paul Gerson Unna, Hans von Hebra, and Oscar Lassar. Among the diseases described first in this journal were epidermolysis bullosa, angioneurotic edema, scleroderma of Buschke, and Behçet's syndrome. Until 1933, three of the four editors of the *Dermatologische Wochenschrift* were of Jewish descent. One of them, Fritz Callomon (fig. 70), a former assistant of Albert Neisser, was well known for his textbook on nonvenereal diseases of the genitalia. Since 1920, Callomon had run a private practice of dermatology in Dessau, but in 1938 he was forced to give it up and move to Berlin. In March 1940, he emigrated to the United States, where he worked in Philadelphia and in Berkeley. He died in September 1964 at the age of eighty-eight. Another editor was Ernst Delbanco (fig. 71) from Hamburg, a disciple and one of the closest co-workers of Paul Gerson Unna. Delbanco was greatly respected for numerous original contributions, chiefly about infectious diseases and the histopathology of the skin. In 1898, he had been the first to describe the histopathologic findings in erysipeloid. After two nervous breakdowns, Delbanco committed suicide in 1935. The third editor of Jewish descent was Paul Unna, Jr. (fig. 72), the son of Paul Gerson Unna, who died during a bombing raid on Hamburg in 1943.

According to the new directives given by the Nazi party, Callomon, Delbanco, and Paul Unna, Jr., had to be removed from the editorial board of the *Dermatologische Wochenschrift*. Nevertheless, the publisher of the journal made an attempt to prevent, or at least to postpone, their dismissal. In a letter to Kurt Klare, he emphasized the merits of "Dr. Paul Unna, who has been decorated in the war and whose father, although a Jew, fought with distinction in the Prussian army in 1870. Another editor of the journal is Dr. Callomon-Dessau, who received the Iron Cross on White, Black Ribbon."[23]

His arguments were disregarded, and the three Jewish editors of the *Dermatologische Wochenschrift* were discharged within a year (figs. 73, 74). Only Johann Heinrich Rille, former chairman of the skin clinic in Leipzig, remained on the editorial board, the new members being Bodo Spiethoff, Egon Keining, Wilhelm Richter, and Josef Schumacher.

The names of the Jewish founders of these journals no longer appeared on the frontispiece. *The Dermatologische Wochenschrift* eliminated the name of Paul Gerson Unna; the *Archiv für Dermatologie und Syphilis* removed the names

DERMATOLOGISCHE WOCHENSCHRIFT

GEGRÜNDET VON P.G.UNNA

UNTER MITWIRKUNG VON

J. ALMKVIST-Stockholm, E.ARNING-Hamburg, L.ARZT-Wien, B. BERON-Sofia, S.BETTMANN-Heidelberg, H. BOAS-Kopenhagen, P. L. BOSELLINI-Rom, C. BRUHNS-Berlin, E. BRUUSGAARD-Oslo, A. BUSCHKE-Berlin, J. CAPPELLI-Florenz, M. F. ENGMAN-St.Louis, E. FINGER-Wien, W. FISCHER-Berlin, E. FREUND-Triest, W. FRIEBOES-Berlin, R. FRÜHWALD-Chemnitz, O. GANS-Frankfurt a. M., E. HOFFMANN-Bonn, J. JADASSOHN-Breslau, A. JORDAN-Moskau, W. KERL-Wien, E. KLAUSNER-Prag,V. KLINGMÜLLER-Kiel, W. KOLLE-Frankfurt a. M., A. KOLLMANN-Leipzig, L. KUMER-Innsbruck, H. P. LIE-Bergen, J. MAYR-München, E. MEIROWSKY-Köln, S. MENDES DA COSTA-Amsterdam, G. MESTSCHERSKY-Moskau, L. MO-BERG-Stockholm,V. MONTESANO-Rom, P. MULZER-Hamburg, O. NAST-Danzig, L. NIELSEN-Kopenhagen, P. NIKOLSKI-Rostow a. D., G. NOBL-Wien, M. OPPENHEIM-Wien, M. PELAGATTI-Parma, A. PERUTZ-Wien, G.PHOTINOS-Athen, F. PINKUS-Berlin, S.POLLITZER-NewYork, C.RASCH-Kopenhagen, E. RIECKE-Göttingen, H.RITTER-Hamburg, G.ROST-Freiburg i.Br., P.RUSCH-Wien, F. SAMBERGER-Prag, J.F.SCHAM-BERG-Philadelphia, W. SCHOLTZ-Königsberg i. Pr., W. SCHÖNFELD-Greifswald, K. SCHREINER-Graz, H. TH. SCHREUS - Düsseldorf, J. SCHUMACHER - Berlin, J. SELLEI - Budapest, A. STÜHMER - Münster, G. STÜMPKE-Hannover, L. TÖRÖK-Budapest, A. TRYB-Brünn, P. UHLENHUTH-Freiburg i. B., K. ULL-MANN-Wien, F. v. VERESS - Klausenburg, H. VÖRNER - Leipzig, J. WERTHER - Dresden, CH. J. WHITE-Boston, U.J. WILE- Ann Arbor, F. WINKLER - Wien, K. ZIELER-Würzburg, L. v. ZUMBUSCH - München

HERAUSGEGEBEN VON

J. H. RILLE   E. DELBANCO   F. CALLOMON   P. UNNA JUN.
LEIPZIG   HAMBURG   DESSAU   HAMBURG

SECHSUNDNEUNZIGSTER BAND

1933

JANUAR BIS JUNI (Nr. 1—26)

MIT 128 ABBILDUNGEN IM TEXT

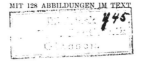

LEIPZIG / VERLAG VON LEOPOLD VOSS / 1933

FIG 73 TITLE PAGE OF THE *DERMATOLOGISCHE WOCHENSCHRIFT* BEFORE REMOVAL OF JEWISH EDITORS.

DERMATOLOGISCHE

WOCHENSCHRIFT

UNTER MITWIRKUNG VON

J. ALMKVIST-Stockholm, E. ARNING-Hamburg, L. ARZT-Wien, F. BERING-Bonn, B. BERON-Sofia, H. BOAS-Kopenhagen, P. L. BOSELLINI-Rom, E. H. BRILL-Rostock, J. CAPPELLI-Florenz, M. F. ENGMAN-St. Louis, W. FISCHER-Berlin, E. FREUND-Triest, W. FRIEBOES-Berlin, R. FRÜHWALD-Chemnitz, C. GROUVEN-Halle a. S., O. GRÜTZ-Bonn, L. HAUCK-Erlangen, E. HOFFMANN-Bonn, G. HOPF-Hamburg, J. JADASSOHN-Zürich, A. JESIONEK-Gießen, A. JORDAN-Moskau, W. KERL-Wien, E. KLAUSNER-Prag, V. KLINGMÜLLER-Kiel, A. KOLLMANN-Leipzig, L. KUMER-Innsbruck, H. P. LIE-Bergen, P. LINSER-Tübingen, J. MAYR-Münster i. W., G. MESTSCHERSKIJ-Moskau, L. MOBERG-Stockholm, C. MONCORPS-München, V. MONTE-SANO-Rom, P. MULZER-Hamburg, O. NAST-Danzig, P. NIKOLSKIJ-Rostow a. D., G. NOBL-Wien, M. OPPEN-HEIM-Wien, M. PELAGATTI-Parma, G. PHOTINOS-Athen, S. POLLITZER-New-York, C. RASCH-Kopenhagen, E. RIECKE-Göttingen, H. RITTER-Hamburg, A. RUETE-Marburg a. d. L., F. ŠAMBERGER-Prag, W. SCHOLTZ-Königsberg i. Pr., W. SCHÖNFELD-Heidelberg, K. SCHREINER-Graz, H. TH. SCHREUS-Düsseldorf, M. SCHUBERT-Frankfurt a. M., W. SCHULTZE-Jena, J. SELLEI-Budapest, A. STÜHMER-Freiburg i. B., G. STÜMPKE-Hannover, L. TÖRÖK-Budapest, P. UHLENHUTH-Freiburg i. B., K. ULL-MANN-Wien, F. v. VERESS-Klausenburg, H. VÖRNER-Leipzig, J. WERTHER-Dresden, CH. J. WHITE-Boston, U. J. WILE-Ann Arbor, F. WINKLER-Wien, K. ZIELER-Würzburg, L. v. ZUMBUSCH-München

HERAUSGEGEBEN VON

B. SPIETHOFF   E. KEINING   J. H. RILLE   W. RICHTER   J. SCHUMACHER
LEIPZIG   HAMBURG   LEIPZIG   BERLIN   BERLIN

EINHUNDERTSTER BAND

1935

JANUAR BIS JUNI (Nr. 1—26)

MIT 50 ABBILDUNGEN IM TEXT

LEIPZIG / VERLAG VON LEOPOLD VOSS / 1935

FIG 74 TITLE PAGE OF THE *DERMATOLOGISCHE WOCHENSCHRIFT* AFTER REMOVAL OF JEWISH EDITORS.

of its founders, Auspitz and Pick, and of its long-standing editor, Albert Neisser. During a period when even the poems of Heinrich Heine that appeared in German schoolbooks were attributed to an "unknown author," it is not surprising that there was no recognition of the accomplishments of Jewish physicians. Quoting Jewish scientists in scientific articles was no longer permitted. According to the Reich's Order for Academic Promotion of 1938, "It is not possible to prohibit entirely the quotation of Jewish authors in doctoral theses. However, Jewish authors may be quoted only rarely and briefly, even if no other literature is available. In individual cases, control of compliance to this rule must be the duty of the faculty. Principally, there are no reservations against quoting Jewish authors if this is done for the purpose of disproving or fighting their ideas. At any rate, the fact that Jewish literature has been employed in any work must be disclosed, and bibliography in regard to Jewish authors must be restricted to material that is deemed absolutely necessary."[24] At the skin clinic of Hamburg University, the bust of Paul Gerson Unna (fig. 75) was banished to the cellar of the hall of arts. In Hamburg, Unna Strasse was renamed, and in Frankfurt a new name was given to Paul Ehrlich Strasse. For a time, it was forbidden to mention in lectures the name of Emil von Behring, the winner of the first Nobel Prize in Medicine in 1901, because he had a Jewish wife.[25] That dermatology had been established as a medical specialty primarily by Jews was simply an embarrassing fact and one to be concealed.

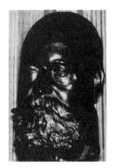

FIG 75
PAUL GERSON
UNNA (BUST FROM
1913).

THE REMOVAL OF JEWS FROM THE UNIVERSITIES

TO FURTHER ITS GOAL OF RIDDING THE MEDICAL PROFES-SION OF JEWS, THE NAZIS LOOKED BEYOND THE simple reform of professional organizations and medical societies. The removal of Jews from the governing and editorial boards of medical journals was a first step, to be followed by the total elimination, by any means possible, of all Jewish physicians from the practice of medicine in Germany.

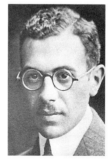

Even in the first days of Hitler's dictatorship, before any anti-Jewish legislation had been enacted, squadrons of storm troopers (the SA, or "Brownshirts") went into hospitals—even operating rooms—and arrested Jewish physicians at work. In open trucks, the prisoners were taken to the headquarters of the SA, where many were tortured and some beaten to death. The storm troopers, who were brutal hooligans, enjoyed humiliating respected citizens. Max Leffkowitz (fig. 76), an assistant medical director in the Department of Internal Medicine at the Moabit Hospital in Berlin, was made to crawl around on his hands and knees and bark like a dog. Later, he was forced to stand against a wall while storm troopers shot bullets around the contour of his body in the manner of circus knife-throwers. One month later, Leffkowitz emigrated to Palestine, where he became director of internal medicine at the Beilinson Hospital in Tel Aviv. He died there in 1971.[1]

The first victims of the new policy were prominent Jews and well-known political opponents of the Nazis, particularly those who were Jewish or of Jewish descent. Among all the German physicians of that time, only a few were Socialists or Communists; the Association of Socialistic Physicians, founded in 1924, had about fifteen hundred members in the entire German Reich, two hundred of whom lived in Berlin.[2] Many of those members were Jews and were at greater risk of being

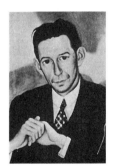

FIG 77
HANS HAUSTEIN
(1894–1933)

targeted. Max Leffkowitz was one, and Benno Chajes, a former member of the Prussian parliament and an authority in the field of occupational dermatoses, was another. In 1933, Chajes emigrated to Palestine, where he initiated the first private health insurance company. He died in 1939.[3]

Hans Haustein (fig. 77), a former assistant of Abraham Buschke and Georg Arndt, had a private practice for cutaneous and venereal diseases in the center of Berlin, where he treated prostitutes. He also hosted a salon in Berlin-Schöneberg that was known for its intellectual and erotic permissiveness and that became a gathering place for politicians and artists with socialist leanings, such as the composer Fred Raymond and the writer Lion Feuchtwanger. In 1933, after being arrested and tortured by the Gestapo, the secret police, Haustein apparently committed suicide with potassium cyanide. He had been responsible for the section about the epidemiology of venereal diseases in Jadassohn's *Handbuch*.[4]

Kurt Glaser, a practicing dermatologist in Chemnitz and a leading member of the Association of Socialistic Physicians, was taken into "protective custody" from March to September 1933 and, upon his release, lived five months in Augsburg under close observation of the Gestapo. In 1934, he managed to escape to Paris; when Paris was occupied by the Germans in 1940, he fled to the United States via Spain, Portugal, and Cuba. In the United States, he worked at the Skin and Cancer Unit of the New York University School of Medicine. After the war, Glaser returned to Germany to become president of the office for public health in Hamburg. He died in 1982 at the age of eighty-nine.[5]

Another dermatologist known for socialist leanings was Ernst Kromayer (fig. 78), who introduced dermabrasion into dermatologic therapy and invented the Kromayer lamp, a small water-cooled mercury-vapor lamp with a quartz window that produces ultraviolet radiation. Kromayer was the first professor of dermatology at the University of Halle. In 1904, he moved to Berlin, where, in a former factory build-

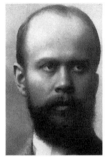

FIG 78
ERNST KROMAYER
(1862–1933)

ing, he opened a successful private skin clinic. Although Kromayer was wealthy and lived on an estate, he belonged to the circle that gathered around Rudolf Breitscheid, spokesman for foreign affairs of the Social Democratic Party and a member of the Reichstag. Breitscheid was later exterminated in the concentration camp at Buchenwald. Ernst Kromayer presumably avoided a similar fate by committing suicide on May 6, 1933.[6] According to one estimate, from January 1933 on, as many as 5 percent—several hundred—of all Jewish physicians living in Germany during the Nazi period committed suicide.[7]

Illegal acts against Jews at the beginning of Hitler's regime were said by the Nazis to be spontaneous outbreaks of anger by the German people for which Jews, as poisonous parasites of the nation, were themselves responsible. Actual harassment of Jews, however, was not perpetrated by the average German citizen but chiefly by goon squads of the SA. Brutalities against Jews also were not spontaneous acts, but were planned, initiated, and controlled by Nazi leaders. Many Germans recognized that these acts against Jews were wrong, but attempts to actually intervene on behalf of Jews were rare. In general, non-Jewish Germans, trying to maintain the illusion of a civilized life in a civilized state, tended to either ignore or underplay the increasing illegal encroachments on the rights of Jews, an attitude abetted by a subliminal form of anti-Semitism that was prevalent in Germany.

The most prominent example of officially sanctioned illegal terror by the Nazis occurred on April 1, 1933, the Day of the General Boycott of Jews (fig. 79). Days earlier, advertisements and newspaper notices had announced the precise time the boycott would begin, and at 10:00 A.M. on a Saturday, storm troopers positioned themselves in front of Jewish shops and harassed all those who tried to enter. The storm troopers "informed" passers-by about Jewish usury and unfair business practices and demanded, "Germans, protect yourselves, don't

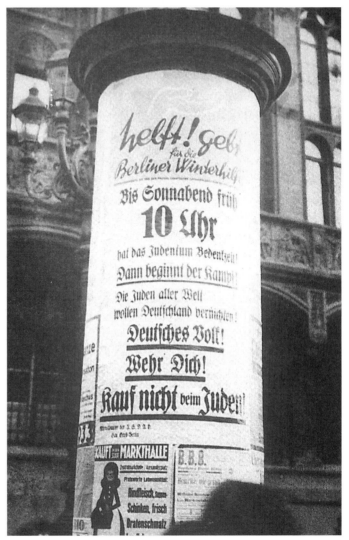

FIG 79 NOTICE ANNOUNCING THE DAY OF THE GENERAL
BOYCOTT OF JEWS: "UNTIL SATURDAY MORNING, 10 O'CLOCK, JEWRY
HAS TIME FOR REFLECTION! THEN STARTS THE FIGHT!"

buy from Jews" (fig. 80). People who patronized Jewish shops
were accused of being "traitors to their people" (fig. 81).

Outside doctors' offices, patients were warned about being
treated by Jewish physicians (fig. 82). Gynecologists and dermatologists especially were said to practice only for their own
sexual excitement. Jewish physicians and lawyers in public

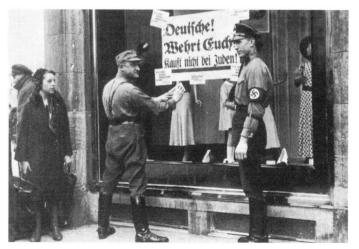

FIG 80 "GERMANS! STRIKE BACK! DON'T BUY FROM JEWS!"

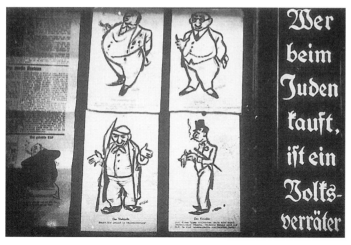

FIG 81 "WHO BUYS FROM THE JEW IS A TRAITOR."

service were laid off; some even were arrested. Throughout Germany, Jews were taken into "protective custody" because of the ostensible offense of usury.

The actions of the storm troopers reached such heinous proportions that even the ultraconservative German president, von Hindenburg, was offended by them. As a former general, Hindenburg intervened specifically on behalf of Jews who

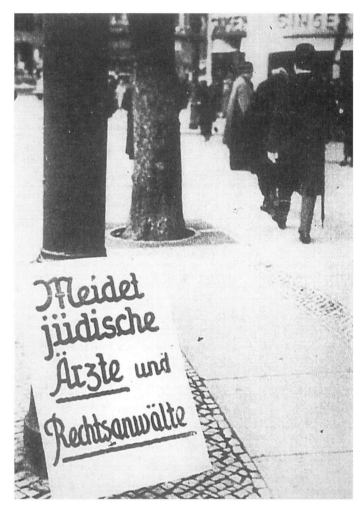

FIG 82 "AVOID JEWISH PHYSICIANS AND LAWYERS."

were veterans of the World War. In a letter to Hitler, dated April 4, 1933, he wrote these lines:

> *In the last few days, a series of incidents have been reported to me in which judges, lawyers, and civil servants of the judiciary, who had been wounded in the war and who had unblemished records of military service, have been forcibly removed from their positions and are planned to be dismissed permanently simply*

because they are of Jewish origin. For me personally, revering those who died in the war and grateful to those who survived and to the wounded who suffered, such treatment of Jewish war veterans in the civil service is altogether intolerable. . . . If they were worthy to fight and bleed for Germany, then they should also be considered worthy to continue serving their fatherland in their professions.[8]

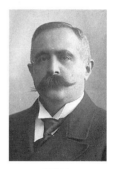

FIG 83
ABRAHAM BUSCHKE
(1868–1943)

On April 7, Hitler enacted the Law for the Restoration of Professional Civil Service, enabling the government to remove Jews and political opponents legally from civil service positions. In response to von Hindenburg's plea, the new law excluded veterans of the World War and officials who had been employed before April 1, 1914.

Less than a week later, newspapers published lists of university professors who had lost their positions and stated, "This, of course, is only a first, preliminary measure."[9] Within the next few months, most Jewish physicians who worked at public hospitals were fired. To continue providing medical services, hospital administrators were forced to replace those physicians with medical students. In Berlin, more than one-third of all positions for assistant physicians were filled by medical students who had not yet passed their examinations: twelve of forty-six at Urban Hospital, eighteen of thirty-eight at Moabit Hospital, thirty-one of fifty-two at Rudolf Virchow Hospital, and forty-seven of eighty-four at Charité Hospital. In 1933, mortality rates for patients at hospitals in Germany rose by about 16 percent.[10]

Among the Jewish physicians who lost their jobs as a consequence of Hitler's edict were many prominent dermatologists, including Abraham Buschke (fig. 83), director of the dermatology department at the Rudolf Virchow Hospital in Berlin, and his assistant, Ludwig Löwenstein. Both names are linked eponymically to the Buschke-Löwenstein tumor, a verrucous carcinoma on mucocutaneous and volar surfaces thought to be

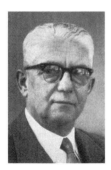

FIG 84

ERNST SKLARZ

(1894–1975)

caused by human papillomavirus. Buschke continued to work in Berlin at the Jewish hospital until he was deported to the concentration camp at Theresienstadt, where he died of malnutrition in 1943. Ludwig Löwenstein left for the United States, where he joined the Skin and Cancer Unit of the New York University School of Medicine.[11]

Ernst Sklarz (fig. 84), a former assistant of Abraham Buschke, was consultant dermatologist at the Municipal Hospital of Berlin-Neukölln and director of dermatology of the new Polyclinic at the Alexanderplatz. Because Sklarz was Jewish, he was dismissed in 1933 and, three years later, emigrated to Great Britain. His German medical degree was not accepted by British authorities, and Sklarz was required to resume the study of medicine at the University of Wales. In 1937, he passed the British qualification examination and within a year was appointed postgraduate lecturer in dermatology at Blackfriars Hospital for Diseases of the Skin. In 1953, Sklarz became consultant dermatologist at New Cross General Hospital in London, and when he retired in 1962, his contributions to dermatology in England were recognized by his appointment as honorary consultant to the Bermondsey and Southwark hospital group. Sklarz died on May 6, 1975.[12]

Franz Blumenthal (fig. 85), an observant Jew and member of a highly respected Jewish family in Berlin, was acting chairman of dermatology at the Charité Hospital after the death of Georg Arndt. In 1934, he received a call from the University of Michigan in Ann Arbor. To be excused from paying emigration tax, Blumenthal claimed that his activities in the United States would be in the interest of the German Reich. The judgment of the National Socialist Physicians' League was different: "There is no German interest in Mr. Blumenthal's lectures abroad but only in the chance to get rid of as many Jewish physicians as possible. However, it would have to be guaranteed that Mr. Blumenthal will under no circumstances return to Germany. Such a guarantee would be, in my judgment, that he

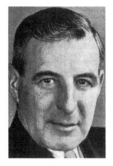

FIG 85

FRANZ

BLUMENTHAL

(1878–1971)

renounces his German citizenship or at least his German license to practice medicine."[13] Blumenthal was forced to pay emigration tax and, in the fall of 1934, left Germany for the United States. He joined the Department of Dermatology at the University of Michigan, which was directed by his friend Udo J. Wile. Blumenthal never returned to Germany. He died in Ann Arbor in 1971 at the age of ninety-three. Blumenthal recorded advances in dermatology in his textbooks on radiotherapy of the skin and contact allergy.[14]

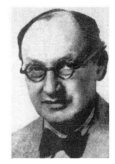

Ludwig Halberstaedter (fig. 86), professor of dermatology and radiology at the Charité, was stripped of his license to teach at a university in November 1933 and left for Palestine shortly thereafter. In Jerusalem, he became director of the Department of Radiotherapy at the Hadassah Hospital, which, under his direction, became a leading center in the Middle East. Halberstaedter also joined the faculty of the Hebrew University in Jerusalem. He died during a visit to New York in 1949. Halberstaedter discovered inclusion bodies in lesions caused by trachoma and, with Eugen Galewsky and Heinrich Finkelstein, wrote the first textbook on pediatric dermatology in 1922. Halberstaedter's co-authors also were Jewish. Finkelstein, who was director of the Municipal Pediatric Hospital of Berlin, emigrated to Chile in 1939 and died three years later. He introduced albumin milk for feeding infants and described acute hemorrhagic edema of the skin of the newborn, known today as Finkelstein's disease. Galewsky died in 1935.[15]

In Heidelberg, the Jewish lecturer of dermatology, Fritz Stern, was informed of his dismissal in a polite but terse way: "We take honor to transmit for your information the Ministerial Decree No. 7642. In execution of its provisions you are suspended as lecturer of the university until further notice."[16] Stern's chairman, Siegfried Bettmann (fig. 87), received a letter from the senate of the university in April 1933, in which he himself was notified that "all members of the Jewish race employed by the state of Baden have to be furloughed, irrespective of their religious affiliation . . . ."[17] Bettmann was a

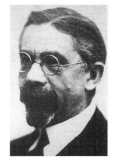

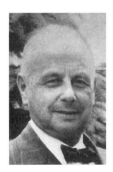

FIG 88
OSCAR GANS
(1888–1983)

professed Lutheran, but by ancestry he was Jewish.[18] Because of his age, his attainments, and his respect as chairman of the Department of Dermatology, he was granted permission to continue working as a dermatologist until 1935, when he emigrated to Switzerland. He died shortly thereafter. His son, a lawyer employed by the government, had been fired earlier, and committed suicide in 1934 after seeing storm troopers positioned in front of his father's medical office.[19]

Oscar Gans (fig. 88), chair of the dermatology department at the University of Frankfurt, was terminated on December 6, 1933 (see fig. 90). Gans was the most prominent dermatopathologist of his time, having published a two-volume revision of Unna's textbook *Histopathology of the Diseases of the Skin*, the first volume in 1925 and the second in 1928. After his dismissal as chair, Gans went to Bombay, where he engaged in private practice and conducted extensive studies on leprosy. To maintain the right to his pension, Gans designated his emigration as an "expedition for research." His pension continued to be paid into a German bank account on the condition that the monies be spent exclusively in Germany, but in November 1941, Gans' German citizenship was revoked and his bank account confiscated. In 1949, the University of Frankfurt recalled Gans to his previous position. Eleven years later, at the age of seventy-two, Gans retired to Comano near Lugano in Switzerland. He died in Comano in 1983 at the age of ninety-five.[20]

Gans' associate, Franz Herrmann (fig. 89), was Christian, but, because of his Jewish ancestry, was dismissed from his position at the skin clinic of Frankfurt in the fall of 1933. Until 1938, Herrmann worked in a private practice and unofficially continued to conduct experimental studies at the Institute of Biology at the University of Frankfurt. In November 1938, he left Germany, crossing the border by train disguised as a worker. He lived in London for two years, where he worked at the Royal Northern Hospital, and then moved to New York City. At New York University, he joined the staff of

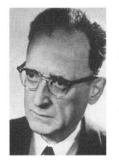

FIG 89
FRANZ HERRMANN
(1898–1977)

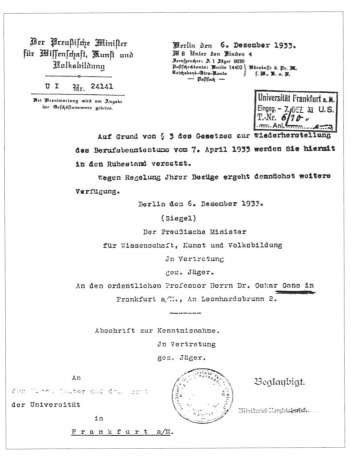

FIG 90 NOTE OF DISMISSAL TO OSCAR GANS.

the Skin and Cancer Unit and was put in charge of basic and laboratory research in dermatology. In the twenty-one years that followed, Herrmann published eighty-six original papers, most of them on the physiology of sweat and sebaceous glands. His ability and productivity were honored by the creation of a full professorship in experimental dermatology for him, the only such position in the United States then. In 1959, Herrmann was invited to return to Frankfurt as successor to his former teacher Oscar Gans. It was a difficult decision for him, but in 1961, Herrmann accepted and assumed the chair

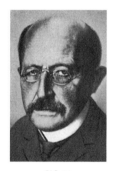

FIG 91
MAX PLANCK
(1858–1947)

of dermatology in Frankfurt. He retired in 1969 at the age of seventy-one and died in Wiesbaden eight years later. In his will, Herrmann established a foundation to provide financial assistance to young researchers in dermatology, specifying that they be Jewish.[21]

In Leipzig, the Jewish lecturer on dermatology, Ludwig Friedheim, was dismissed in 1933. In Nuremberg, Ernst Nathan, director of dermatology at the Municipal Hospital, met the same fate. Like many others, Nathan emigrated to New York, where he worked at the Skin and Cancer Unit of New York University. He died in 1981.[22]

The vast majority of German academics continued to tolerate quietly the dismissal of their Jewish colleagues. There were extraordinarily few efforts made to prevent the ousting of Jews, and those generally proved entirely ineffective. Max Planck (fig. 91), the winner of the Nobel Prize in Physics in 1918, raised the issue when he met Hitler in May 1933. Planck observed that "there are all kinds of Jews, some worthless to humanity, and some very valuable," and suggested that a measure of discrimination be used when considering dismissal of them. The editors of the *Danziger Ärzteblatt* protested discrimination against Jewish physicians in these words: "The German medical profession cannot remain silent when a great doctor is branded a Jew. . . . Even if Germany finds itself in a state of siege from world Jewry, we cannot deny the individual contributions of an Ehrlich or a Wassermann."[23]

In Düsseldorf, two professors, Ernst Edens and Paul Huebschmann, defended Jewish colleagues with such fervor that the Nazi gynecologist Friedrich Siegert wrote to Goebbels in April 1933 that the university was guilty of "systematic protection of its Jewish professors."[24] The efforts of Edens and Huebschmann were in vain, however. Among the Jewish professors dismissed at the University of Düsseldorf was the chair of pharmacology, Philipp Ellinger. Otto Krayer from Berlin, who was not Jewish, was asked to replace Ellinger, but he rejected the offer because he did not want to take advantage of the misfortune of a Jewish colleague. As a result, Krayer himself was dismissed and was forced to emigrate in 1934. The chair of pharmacology was given to a staunch Nazi, Otto Girndt.[25] In Marburg, the entire medical faculty intervened on behalf of pediatrician Ernst Freudenberg, who was about to be terminated because his wife was Jewish, but the Ministry of Education was not swayed and Freudenberg was dismissed.

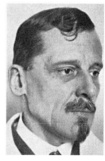

FIG 92
RICHARD SIEBECK
(1883–1965)

On April 5, 1933, Heidelberg's dean of medicine, Richard Siebeck (fig. 92), wrote a letter to the Ministry of Education in which he asserted that although it was necessary for academics to be "of German stock and German spirit," it was also evident that "German Jews take part in advances of science and that great medical personalities have emerged from their midst." Siebeck averred that "we feel obligated . . . to take the stand of true humanity, to raise our concern wherever there is danger that a responsible attitude is superseded by wholly emotional or instinctive powers. We have to emphasize how necessary it is to preserve a sense of justice."[26] Siebeck was supported by the rector of the University of Heidelberg, Willy Andreas, and their combined efforts made it possible for several Jewish professors—the chair of dermatology, Siegfried Bettmann, among them—to remain in their positions. To comply with the Law for the Restoration of Professional Civil Service, those professors were officially dismissed, but the edicts were suspended. The success of Siebeck and Andreas, however, was short-lived. On October 1, 1933, Andreas was replaced as rector of the university by an ardent Nazi, Wilhelm Groh, who soon forced out Siebeck as dean of the medical faculty and ensured that the spirit of the Law for the Restoration of Professional Civil Service at the University of Heidelberg was fully met.

To sustain the teaching program of the medical faculty, the rector of the University of Breslau asked the Ministry of Education for permission to postpone the dismissal of Jewish lecturers as had been demanded by the National Social-

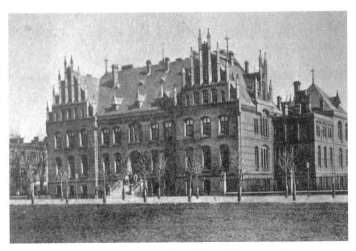

FIG 93 SKIN CLINIC AT THE UNIVERSITY OF BRESLAU.

ist Physicians' League. In making his case, the rector quoted a declaration by Aryan physicians at the university to the effect that "all of us who want to participate enthusiastically in the rebuilding of our fatherland share the view that too quick or precipitous proceedings, as demanded by the Physicians' League of Breslau, may have negative consequences for German science and especially for students. . . . We trust securely that the highest authorities will take necessary measures for the benefit of the German people and of academics, and believe that hasty individual actions can only hamper steady development designed to serve the benefit of the whole."[27]

The situation in Breslau proved particularly vexing to the Nazis because of the long tradition of Jewish contributions to the university. Many of Breslau's teachers of medicine were Jewish or of Jewish descent, and the skin clinic had been decorated, as a matter of pride, with Stars of David (figs. 93, 94). Nevertheless, the university's request went unacknowledged. Within a few months, the medical faculty lost some of the most highly regarded dermatologists in the world and, in the process, its own international standing.

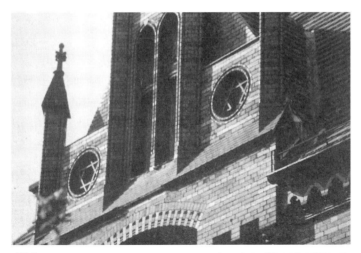

FIG 94 DETAIL OF THE SKIN CLINIC AT THE UNIVERSITY OF BRESLAU
SHOWING STARS OF DAVID.

The first to leave the University of Breslau was Rudolph
Leopold Mayer (fig. 95), a dermatologist highly respected for
his work on chemotherapy and allergic contact dermatitis. In
January 1933, news of Hitler's appointment as chancellor of
the German Reich reached Mayer on vacation in Czechoslovakia. Intuiting how life would change for Jews in Germany,
he called his chair, Max Jessner, and submitted his resignation. Jessner urged him to reconsider this decision and
reminded him that a Prussian civil servant must fulfill his
responsibilities and not act impulsively. But Mayer never
returned to Breslau. From Czechoslovakia he traveled to
France and, after a short stay in Paris, settled in Lyon. The
years in Lyon were the happiest of his life. As director of the
research laboratory of a large pharmaceutical company,
Mayer was engaged primarily in the synthesis of new types of
sulfonamides. Following the German occupation of large
areas of France, Mayer was forced to flee in 1942, this time to
Summit, New Jersey, where he became director of the micro-
biology laboratory of the Ciba Corporation. During his time
there, he developed pyribenzamine, one of the first antihista-
mines. Mayer died in Washington, D.C., in 1962.[28]

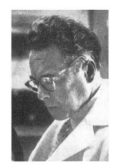

FIG 95
RUDOLPH LEOPOLD
MAYER
(1895–1962)

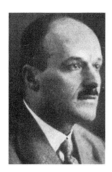

FIG 96
WALTER
FREUDENTHAL
(1893–1952)

The next lecturer in dermatology to leave the University of Breslau was Wilhelm Siegmund Frei. Since 1929, Frei had also served as director of the dermatology department of Berlin-Spandau Municipal Hospital. In the spring of 1933, he was dismissed from his position in Berlin, and in April 1934 was struck from the roster of teachers at the University of Breslau, effective retroactively to the date of enactment of the Law for the Restoration of Professional Civil Service. Frei left Germany for New York City, where he worked at Montefiore Hospital. He died in New York in January 1943 at age fifty-seven. Frei is famous for the innovative work that now bears his name—the Frei test for lymphogranuloma venereum.[29]

Walter Freudenthal (fig. 96) left the University of Breslau in 1934 for London, where, in the Department of Dermatology at University College Hospital Medical School, he was able to pursue his specialty of histopathology of the skin. As one of the most eminent dermatopathologists of his time, Freudenthal, in 1945, became the first holder of a readership in dermatologic histology at the University of London in 1945 and was able to attract to that institution many established dermatologists from England and abroad who sought to learn from him. Several names of diseases still in common usage were introduced by him—lichen amyloidosus, for example. In 1926, he had been the first to detail findings in solar keratosis and, in collaboration with Geoffrey Dowling, also provided the first description of what came to be known as Dowling-Degos disease, a reticulated pigmented anomaly of the flexures. Freudenthal died in London in 1952 at the age of fifty-eight.[30]

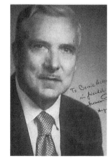

FIG 97
HERMANN PINKUS
(1905–1985)

Hermann Pinkus (fig. 97), the son of the celebrated dermatologist Felix Pinkus, was a young assistant in the Department of Dermatology in Breslau when he was dismissed in 1934 because of his Jewish heritage; his father was Jewish and his mother was Christian. Felix Pinkus stayed in Germany and maintained a private practice in Berlin, whereas Hermann Pinkus, who was Christian, went to the United States. He arrived as a refugee without money, work, or prospects. With the help of Marion Baldur Sulzberger, a powerful force in dermatology at the Skin and Cancer Unit of New York University, Pinkus eventually found a position as a research fellow at the University of Michigan in Ann Arbor, studying tissue cultures. After a fellowship in dermatopathology at Wayne County General Hospital under Franz Blumenthal, Pinkus opened a private dermatology practice and taught part-time in the Department of Dermatology at Wayne State University in Detroit, where, in 1960, he was made full professor and chair of that department. In addition, he operated a private dermatopathology laboratory in Monroe, Michigan, where he was later joined by Amir Mehregan.

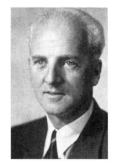

FIG 98
STEPHEN EPSTEIN
(1900–1973)

Hermann Pinkus was one of the leading dermatopathologists in the world and possibly the most reflective and imaginative of his time. *Pinkus' Guide to Dermatohistopathology*, now in its sixth edition, became an important resource. Pinkus made many contributions to the field: He identified the acrotrichium and the acrosyringium as distinct anatomic entities and was the first to recognize several neoplasms as distinctive, among them eccrine poroma, premalignant fibroepithelial tumor, and trichodiscoma. In 1957, Pinkus described and named alopecia mucinosa. He was president of the Society for Investigative Dermatology in 1958, president of the American Society of Dermatopathology in 1964, and vice president of the American Academy of Dermatology in 1970. Pinkus also was the first recipient of the prestigious Founder's Award of the American Society of Dermatopathology. He died in Monroe, Michigan, in 1985.[31]

Stephen Epstein (fig. 98) was chief of the mycological research department at the skin clinic of Breslau from 1929 to 1933 and chief of the sections of radiology and allergy from 1933 to 1935. In December 1935, he left Germany for the United States, where he founded the Department of Dermatology at the Marshfield Clinic in Marshfield, Wisconsin. In 1946, he was appointed associate professor of dermatology at the University of Minnesota. He wrote two books, *Allergic*

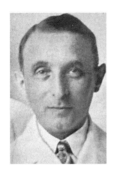

FIG 99
CURT ROSENTHAL
(1892–1937)

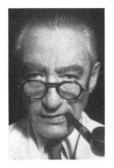

FIG 100
MAX JESSNER
(1887–1978)

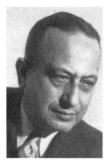

FIG 101
HANS BIBERSTEIN
(1889–1965)

Pruritus, published in 1952, and *An Atlas and Manual of Dermatology*, published in 1959. Epstein developed the concept of photoallergic dermatitis. In 1960 he was elected vice president of the Society for Investigative Dermatology. He retired in 1965 and died in Madison, Wisconsin, in 1973.[32]

Curt Rosenthal (fig. 99), a Jewish neurologist at the University of Breslau, was author of the first comprehensive account of Melkersson-Rosenthal syndrome, which consists, in its classic presentation, of a triad of facial paresis, scrotal tongue, and granulomatous cheilitis. In 1933, the chair of his department proposed Rosenthal for appointment to associate professor. For "racial reasons," this request was rejected by the Prussian Ministry of Education, and, even worse, Rosenthal's employment at the University of Breslau was terminated. In the same year, Rosenthal emigrated to Switzerland, where he struggled financially, working without adequate pay at the University of Bern's Department of Neurology and later at a private sanitarium. Unhappy with his professional situation, Rosenthal contacted the London-based Emergency Organization of German Scientists in Foreign Countries, whose purpose was to find positions for German scientists in exile. On his way to London, Rosenthal was hit by a car and died on April 4, 1937. His wife advised that, "this tragic event possibly happened only because my husband, due to the uncertainty of our living conditions and the fight for our existence, was, at that time, emotionally and physically not in good shape."[33]

The Hindenburg exemptions in the Law for the Restoration of Professional Civil Service meant that not every Jew was dismissed immediately. In Breslau, those exemptions applied to the chair of the Department of Dermatology, Max Jessner (fig. 100), and his associate, Hans Biberstein (fig. 101), both of whom had fought for Germany in World War I. The Nazis, however, were not deterred by legal restraints. It was, they believed, "imperative for the new development of the medical faculty in Breslau, which was almost entirely Jewified, that the last remnants of this Jewification vanish, even if those involved are war veterans. That necessity is derived from the extremely delicate questions of treatment that Germans and Aryans have to tolerate from non-Aryans in the therapy of cutaneous and venereal diseases."[34]

On May 17, 1934, one year after the enactment of the Law for the Restoration of Professional Civil Service and before von Hindenburg's death, the exemption for Jewish veterans of the World War was revoked. Jessner and Biberstein lost their right to teach and to test medical students; orderly operation of the department became impossible. In the fall of 1934, both were dismissed, reputedly at their own request, which was said by the authorities to be "in the interest of the University of Breslau and the reorganization of all university affairs."[35]

Biberstein, who was recognized for developing immunotherapy for viral warts, subsequently worked at the Jewish hospital in Breslau for five years, and then emigrated to the United States, where he became professor of dermatology at the Skin and Cancer Unit of the New York University School of Medicine and one of the most respected clinicians in that institution. He died of acute congestive heart failure in 1965.[36]

Max Jessner emigrated to Switzerland in 1935. Six years later, he moved to New York City, where he worked at the New York Postgraduate Medical School and later joined the teaching staff of the Skin and Cancer Unit of the New York University School of Medicine. He was appreciated for his early studies of thorium X, which led to the first therapeutic application of radioactive isotopes in medicine, and for his description, in 1953, of lymphocytic infiltration of the skin. After he retired, Jessner returned to Switzerland, where he died at the age of ninety-one.[37]

In addition to Jews, the Nazis also rid the universities of political opponents, former members of the Socialist and Communist parties, and people who did not quietly endure the activities and inequities of the new ruling party. Such was the case in Bonn for Erich Hoffmann and in Tübingen for Paul Linser (fig. 102), chair of dermatology, who had introduced sclerotherapy for varicose veins.[38] In September 1936,

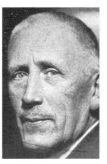

FIG 102
PAUL LINSER
(1871–1963)

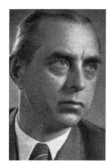

FIG 103
FRANZ KOCH
(1905–1956)

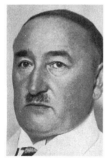

FIG 104
FRIEDRICH BERING
(1878–1950)

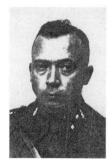

FIG 105
KARL HERMANN
VOHWINKEL
(BORN 1900)

Linser reached the official age for retirement of sixty-five years. Normally, the contracts of chairs of university departments were extended beyond that age, but Linser's was terminated because he was thought to have little sympathy for the Nazis. The leader of the National Socialist Lecturers' League at the University of Tübingen falsely accused Linser of having belonged to a Catholic fraternity and giving preference to members of that fraternity when positions in his clinic had to be filled. After his retirement, Linser wanted to accept invitations to give lectures in Turkey and France, but those trips were forbidden because he was considered to be "unsuited to officially represent German science on lecture trips abroad."[39] Linser died in 1963 at the age of ninety-one.

Linser's assistant, Franz Koch (fig. 103), also was considered by the Nazis to be "politically unreliable" and was dismissed in 1935. Koch was fortunate to find a new position six months later in the Department of Dermatology of the University of Cologne, whose director, Friedrich Bering (fig. 104), was a member of the Nazi party, chiefly for opportunistic reasons, and was not identified closely with the ideas of National Socialism. Nevertheless, Koch's academic career continued to be hampered. In 1944, he was at last appointed associate professor and, after the war, became director of the skin clinic in Wuppertal. He died in 1956.[40]

Another of Linser's assistants, Karl Hermann Vohwinkel (fig. 105), was less fortunate than Koch. Vohwinkel, who first identified keratoma hereditarium mutilans (Vohwinkel's syndrome), made no secret of his critical attitude toward the Nazis. He was dismissed in 1937 and had no chance of finding a position at another university. After his dismissal, Vohwinkel wanted to open a private practice but was denied placement on insurance-funds panels. The only job available to him was as a physician in the German army. Vohwinkel joined the medical corps at a garrison near Würzburg and tried to resume his teaching activities at the university there. The medical faculty of the University of Würzburg was receptive to that offer, but the leader of Tübingen's National Socialist Lecturers' League interfered, detailing the negative political attitude of Vohwinkel and discouraging his colleagues in Würzburg from appointing him to their teaching staff. As a consequence, Vohwinkel was denied any affiliation with the University of Würzburg. After the war, he opened a private practice in Stuttgart and only in 1947 was he appointed associate professor at the University of Tübingen.[41]

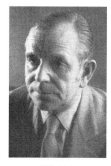

FIG 106
WILHELM SEVIN
(1900–1976)

At the new skin clinic of Stuttgart-Bad Cannstatt, the assistant medical director, Wilhelm Sevin (fig. 106), was dismissed in 1936 for political reasons. Sevin opened a private practice in Stuttgart, where he worked until the end of the war. In 1945, he was made director of the skin clinic in Stuttgart-Bad Cannstatt. He died in 1976.[42]

In Munich, Leopold Ritter von Zumbusch (fig. 107), who had created one of the most modern dermatology centers in Europe at the University of Munich and had been elected rector of that university, was targeted for dismissal. Von Zumbusch was famous worldwide in his own time, having described, in 1907, generalized pustular psoriasis, a condition that still bears his name. Living in Munich, von Zumbusch was familiar with the National Socialist movement from its earliest days. In the 1920s, he had attended a meeting of the NSDAP; had read Hitler's book, *Mein Kampf*; and had come to the conclusion that Hitler was a "lunatic." When the "lunatic" ascended to power, von Zumbusch found himself in a thorny situation. Overnight, it seemed, he was forced to deal with people he despised and who wanted to take control of the university for which he, as rector, was responsible. The new Bavarian minister of culture, Hans Schemm (fig. 108), for instance, told professors at the University of Munich in 1933 that "from now on, it is no longer important for you to find out if something is true but if it corresponds to the spirit of the National Socialist revolution."[43] Schemm also criticized the university for having failed in its task to serve the community. Von Zumbusch's response was sarcastic. In his letter to

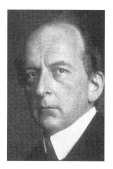

FIG 107
LEOPOLD RITTER
VON ZUMBUSCH
(1874–1940)

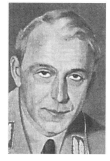

FIG 108
HANS SCHEMM
(1891–1935)

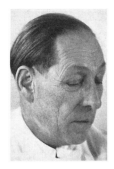

the minister, he suggested that Schemm was ignorant of the activities of the university because he was preoccupied with his own professional duties as an assistant orderly in a military hospital and as a teacher in an elementary school. Von Zumbusch also strongly protested the progressive curtailment of university independence and, as a consequence, was removed from his position as rector of the University of Munich in October 1933.

Still chair of the Department of Dermatology, von Zumbusch continued to resist interference by the new government. In contrast to most other chairs, he employed foreign physicians in his department and supported colleagues whom the Nazis considered "politically unreliable." Despite von Zumbusch's energetic protests, several members of his staff were dismissed.

Among those discharged was his assistant, Rudolf Maximilian Bohnstedt (fig. 109), whose thesis had just been accepted by the medical faculty of the University of Munich. Bohnstedt's academic promotion, however, was prevented by the National Socialist Lecturers' League for both political and racial reasons. On one hand, Bohnstedt was thought to be opposed to National Socialism, and his joining the SA on November 4, 1933, was not regarded as proof to the contrary. On the other hand, the Nazis had conducted inquiries into Bohnstedt's descent and had found out that one of his great-grandmothers was Jewish. In the distorted mentality of the Nazis, Bohnstedt was one-eighth Jewish. According to the Reich's Habilitation Order of 1934, Bohnstedt could still have been promoted, but he was unable to provide evidence that all of his other forebears were Aryan. Another reason for the decision of the National Socialist Lecturers' League to declare itself against Bohnstedt's promotion was "the un-German physical appearance of Mr. B."[44] As a consequence, Bohnstedt's contract at the University of Munich was not extended.

Bohnstedt left Munich in March 1935 and took over a private practice in Dresden. Nevertheless, he continued to apply for his academic promotion, arguing that "idealistic motives may play a role for the appointment of a lecturer. For bestowing a title, however, only legal aspects should be decisive in a constitutional state. The bestowal of the title Dr. habil. depends on Aryan descent. Legally, everybody is Aryan whose pairs of grandparents belonged to the Christian church from their birth. With me, those preconditions are fulfilled. Therefore, I do not see why I should not claim this title without further ado."[45]

Before long, Bohnstedt was compelled to realize that legal aspects were not decisive in Nazi Germany; his attempts to achieve academic promotion remained unsuccessful. Furthermore, he was denied placement on insurance-fund panels. As a consequence, his economic situation in Dresden was desperate. In 1939, he found better conditions in Berlin, where he worked in private practice until the end of the war. In 1948, Bohnstedt was appointed temporary chair of dermatology in Marburg and one year later assumed chairmanship at the University of Giessen, which he held until his retirement in 1969. Bohnstedt died in 1970.[46]

Nineteen thirty-five was not only Bohnstedt's last year at the University of Munich's skin clinic but von Zumbusch's as well. The Nazis had thought initially that they could induce von Zumbusch, like so many others, to cooperate with them, and when they realized he would not, they conspired to get rid of him. To this end, they smuggled a spy of the Gestapo, in the role of a patient, into the skin clinic. They also contacted assistant physicians with an eye on career advancement who willingly passed von Zumbusch's damaging political comments to the Gestapo. On April 2, 1935, von Zumbusch was summoned for questioning by Nazi officials and university administrators. He was accused of misdemeanors, some of which he had committed but many of which had been invented. Von Zumbusch was accused of having called Hitler a "stupid man," of having responded to his patients' cry in unison of "Heil Hitler" with the words "Don't roar so loud," and of having failed to enforce a university policy of employee participation in party rallies. Furthermore, he was

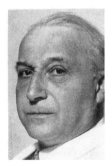

FIG 110
GEORG ALEXANDER
ROST
(1877–1970)

charged with corruption for such crimes as the use of clinic oint-ments to soften his own hands and the use of state-owned towels after having examined his private patients. Von Zumbusch was forced to resign his chairmanship in October 1935. He spent the next few years on his private estate at Lake Chiem, close to Munich, devoting his time not only to his family but also to the discreet support of colleagues who, like himself, were viewed by the government as subversives. He did not encourage former col-leagues to contact him; he did not want to drag others, by associ-ation, into his own problems. On March 31, 1940, von Zumbusch died from inoperable cancer of cardiac muscle. According to some sources, he committed suicide. Only one obituary was pub-lished in a German medical journal; it was written by his disci-ple, Carl Moncorps, chair of the Department of Dermatology in Münster. No mention was made of the circumstances that had led to von Zumbusch's banishment from university life. Never-theless, publication of the obituary was widely perceived as a sign of extraordinary courage on the part of Moncorps. Von Zum-busch's funeral was not attended by a single official of the Uni-versity of Munich. In his will, von Zumbusch requested that his tombstone carry his name alone, without academic titles, until it would again be an honor to be professor at a German university.[47]

Through slander and falsehood, the Nazis also removed the chair of dermatology in Freiburg, Georg Alexander Rost (fig. 110). Rost had been an active member of a democratic political party and was therefore regarded as "politically unreliable." The Ministry of Education was informed that Rost's hostile attitude had caused "considerable agitation among the stu-dents," and that it might be necessary to take him into "protec-tive custody." According to a report by the National Socialist Students' League, "Rost was a democrat and pacifist. . . . It is known that Rost has derided and mocked everything that was related to National Socialism."[48] It was also reported that Rost had asked two students who had attended a dermatology lec-ture to remove their party badges because the swastika might be offensive to patients. Furthermore, Rost had to vindicate himself for having purchased for his clinic, a few years earlier, the German flag of the Weimar Republic with the colors black, red, and gold. The National Socialists, like all right-wing parties of the Weimar Republic, hated that flag and tolerated only the old colors of the German monarchy—black, white, and red. Finally, Rost was accused by one of his own assistants of having sexually molested nurses, an accusation that, although refuted, seriously impaired his professional reputation.[49]

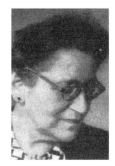

FIG 111
BERTA OTTENSTEIN
(1891–1956)

On August 7, 1933, Rost was dismissed as director of the skin clinic in Freiburg. Attempts to have this decision revoked were thwarted by the resistance of the National Socialist Students' League, whose leader characterized Rost "as a man who has supported the ideas of the Peace League and thereby has contributed, in the eyes of National Socialist students, not only to the suppression of the German people's military spirit, but also of the liberation movement of Adolf Hitler. . . . In the name of National Socialist students, I ask the leader of the university to reject any attempt at reinstatement of Professor Rost and to do everything possible to prevent his reinstatement as a teacher at a German university."[50]

A few months after his dismissal as chair of dermatology in Freiburg, Rost moved to Berlin, where he opened a private practice in dermatology. He also edited the *Zentralblatt für Haut- und Geschlechtskrankheiten*, succeeding its former Jewish editor, Oskar Spitz. The engagement of Rost by the Springer publishing company met with fierce resistance from the new editors of the *Archiv für Dermatologie und Syphilis*, Walter Frieboes, Ernst Heinrich Brill, and Karl Zieler. As a consequence, Rost's name was not allowed to appear on the frontispiece of the *Zentralblatt für Haut- und Geschlechtskrankheiten*; for eleven years, the editor of this journal was anonymous. After the war, Rost became director of dermatology at the Berlin-Spandau Municipal Hospital. He died on July 1, 1970, at the age of ninety-three.[51]

In addition to Rost, several other renowned members of the skin clinic of Freiburg were dismissed. Berta Ottenstein (fig. 111), the first female lecturer in dermatology in Ger-

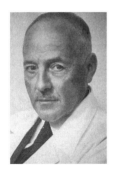

FIG 112
WILHELM LUTZ
(1888–1958)

many and the first and only woman member of the faculty of the University of Freiburg, was among them. Ottenstein, a learned chemist, had acquired a reputation for knowledge about the biochemistry of the skin through the publication of her numerous articles. As a Jew, she was forced to leave the University of Freiburg in March 1933. Rost, her chair, requested that the ministry have her dismissal revoked. Shortly afterward, however, he had to inform Dr. Ottenstein that "the Ministry of Culture and Education . . . is not able to rescind the termination. Hence, it is settled that our nice working group, from which many a worthwhile study has emerged, is finished once and for all. Of course, I shall still try to help you in your career. On that you can firmly rely."[52]

In order to find a new position for Ottenstein, Rost wrote to the chair of dermatology in Basel, Wilhelm Lutz (fig. 112), whose name is still invoked today because of his description in 1922 of epidermodysplasia verruciformis (Lewandowsky-Lutz disease), an inherited disorder characterized by widespread and persistent infection with human papillomavirus. Lutz replied promptly and politely, but evasively, alerting Rost to difficulties in getting a working permit in Switzerland and arguing that his clinic was too small and had no laboratory facilities that would satisfy Ottenstein. In short, he did not help. Through the efforts of Stephan Rothman, however, Ottenstein found a position at the skin clinic of Budapest under Lajos Nékám (fig. 113), who is known for his description of keratosis lichenoides chronica (Nékám's disease). Subsequently, she became director of the chemical laboratory of the skin clinic of the University of Istanbul under Hulusi Behçet, whose name is linked eponymically to Behçet's syndrome.[53] Beginning in 1945, Ottenstein worked at Harvard University, where she made important contributions to the elucidation of the pathogenesis of lipoidoses, especially Gaucher's disease. As reparation, she later was appointed professor of dermatology at the University of Freiburg. Berta Ottenstein died in 1956.[54]

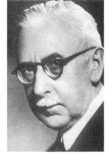

FIG 113
LAJOS NÉKÁM
(1868–1957)

A second Jewish lecturer in the skin clinic at Freiburg, Erich Uhlmann (fig. 114), was in charge of the Radiology Unit and had published a compendium on radiotherapy of the skin. Like Ottenstein, he was terminated in March 1933. Uhlmann, however, fulfilled the "Hindenburg clauses" of the Law for the Restoration of Professional Civil Service, having participated in battles against Communists in 1920. Therefore, he hoped to have his revocation reversed. The Ministry of Culture and Education acknowledged, in a letter to the senate of the University of Freiburg, that "a withdrawal of the license to teach is out of consideration. However, a regular termination of his contract as an assistant is possible."[55] Georg Alexander Rost tried to change the ministry's decision by calling Uhlmann "indispensable," but his effort was in vain. Astonishingly, Uhlmann, only a few weeks after Rost's petition on his behalf, contributed to the campaign against Rost by officially denouncing him to the dean of the medical faculty. Although the denunciation was welcomed by the Nazis, it did not alter Uhlmann's fate, and he was dismissed in July 1933. Like Ottenstein, he emigrated to Turkey, where he worked at the skin clinic of the University of Istanbul. In 1938, Uhlmann moved to Chicago to become director of the Department of Radiologic Therapy at Michael Reese Hospital. He died in Chicago of metastatic carcinoma to the spine and brain in September 1964.[56]

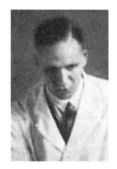

FIG 114
ERICH UHLMANN
(1901–1964)

Philipp Keller (fig. 115), Rost's assistant medical director, was dismissed for political reasons. As a former member of the Social Democratic party, he was suspended from his duties in the spring of 1933, and when the university considered the possibility of revoking his suspension a few weeks later, the National Socialist Students' League intervened: "According to section 3f of the Students' Constitution, the body of students is obligated to contribute to the maintenance of strict academic discipline. Therefore, the body of students of the University of Freiburg feels compelled to inform the Badian Ministry of Culture and Education that the body of students of the University of Freiburg is not able to guarantee an orderly course

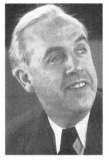

FIG 115
PHILIPP KELLER
(1891–1973)

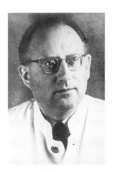

of the lectures of Dr. Keller. The announcement of the revocation of Dr. Keller's suspension would doubtlessly cause great consternation among students which could easily lead to a violation of academic discipline."[57] As a consequence of such overt threats, Keller was forced to leave the skin clinic of the University of Freiburg in 1933 and soon opened a private practice of dermatology in Aachen. After the war, Keller became director of the skin clinic of Aachen and was elected president of the German Society for the Fight Against Venereal Diseases. He died at the age of eighty-two in 1973.[58]

Alfred Marchionini (fig. 116), who studied aspects of the skin surface and introduced the concept of an "acid mantle" of the skin, was considered by the Nazis to be unreliable for two reasons: He had been a member of the Social Democratic party and his wife was of Jewish descent—her grandmother, a practicing Lutheran, had been born Jewish. Marchionini's appointment as associate professor, which had been requested by the medical faculty of the University of Freiburg in December 1932, was never granted. Because he was the only lecturer in dermatology left at the university, he was allowed to continue his work there, but his chances for an academic career were all but destroyed. When Alfred Stühmer succeeded Georg Alexander Rost as chair at Freiburg, he asked the rector of the university, the philosopher Martin Heidegger (fig. 117), about Marchionini's prospects. As Marchionini's future chair, Stühmer argued he would have to take on "the entire responsibility for his [Marchionini's] further academic career." Heidegger, at the time a staunch Nazi supporter, responded on February 21, 1934, by stating that "Mrs. Marchionini has a non-Aryan grandmother. As far as I know, there is no chance of his receiving a chair because of this fact" (fig. 118).[59] Nevertheless, Marchionini was disqualified only partially by the Nazis. According to a letter of the Reich's Ministry of Sciences and Education, Marchionini, "because of the not purely Aryan descent of his wife, will not be acceptable for a permanent position at a university within the confines of

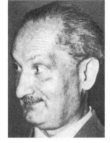

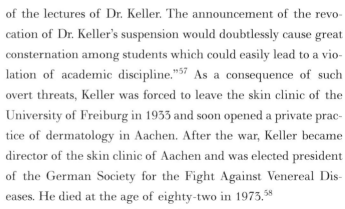

Abschrift!   Formblatt 2.

Anzeige über Verheiratung.

Am 19. Februar 1931 ~~beabsichtige~~ habe ich mit ~~dem~~ der Dr. med.

Marie Mathilde Marchionini

geborenen S o e t b e e r   evangelischer Konfession

die Ehe geschlossen. ~~zu schließen.~~

Nähere Angaben über die Abstammung meine r Ehefrau , ~~Ehemannes~~

Eltern:	
Name des Vaters	Dr. med. Soetbeer
Vornamen	Franz
Stand und Beruf	a.o. Univ. Professor, Facharzt f. innere Krankheiten
Geburtsort, -tag, -monat und -jahr	Altona/Elbe 6. I. 1870
Sterbeort, -tag, -monat und -jahr	./.
Konfession (auch frühere Konfession)	evangelisch
verheiratet { in Hannover . am 2. XII. 1898	
Geburtsname der Mutter . .	Schrader
Vornamen	Emmi, Anna, Ottilie
Geburtsort, -tag, -monat und -jahr	Siegen/Westfalen 20. X. 1871
Sterbeort, -tag, -monat und -jahr	./.
Konfession (auch frühere Konfession)	evangelisch
Großeltern:	
Name des Großvaters (väterlicherseits)	Soetbeer
Vornamen	John, Friedrich , Wilhelm
Stand und Beruf	Kaufmann in Hamburg
Geburtsort, -tag, -monat und -jahr	Altona/Elbe 12. II. 1836
Sterbeort, -tag, -monat und -jahr	Altona/Elbe 8. III. 1928
Konfession (auch frühere Konfession)	ev.-luth.
Geburtsname der Großmutter (väterlicherseits.)	Heymann
Vornamen	Mathilde
Geburtsort, -tag, -monat und -jahr	Altona/Elbe 9. II. 1840
Sterbeort, -tag, -monat und -jahr	Altona/Elbe 4. II. 1903
Konfession (auch frühere Konfession)	evang. (früher israelit.)

II Nr. 65, Anzeige über die Verheiratung eines Beamten.
(Berlin 1936).

FIG 118 THE END OF A CAREER: MARCHIONINI'S CERTIFICATE OF
MARRIAGE REVEALED A JEWISH GRANDMOTHER AMONG
THE FOREBEARS OF HIS WIFE (SEE BOTTOM OF PAGE).

the German Reich. However, as a respected scientist he could have a lasting, positive effect on German causes as professor at a foreign university."[60] When the National Socialist Students' League became aware of the fact that Marchionini's wife had a Jewish grandmother, the pressure on Marchionini increased. Attempts to secure for him the chair of dermatology in Prague were unsuccessful. In 1938, however, the University of Ankara made an offer to Marchionini, and with the permis-

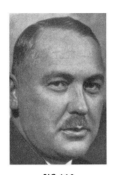

FIG 119
SIEGFRIED
THANNHAUSER
(1885–1962)

sion of the Reich's government, he became director of dermatology in Ankara. Marchionini stayed in Turkey for ten years. After his return to Germany in 1948, he became chairman of the Department of Dermatology in Hamburg and soon thereafter in Munich, where he achieved international recognition for his efforts to bring German dermatology back into the family of world medicine.[61]

By 1936, 458 physicians—twenty-three of whom were dermatologists—had been ousted from German universities for racial or political reasons, and the largest number of university chairs dismissed came from departments of dermatology. In the first three years of the National Socialist regime, about thirty Jewish chairs in all branches of medicine were removed, including such renowned figures as Siegfried Thannhauser (fig. 119), professor of internal medicine and dean designate of the University of Freiburg, who is still recalled for his work on lipidoses; Martin Hahn and Carl Prausnitz, professors of hygienics in Berlin and Breslau; physiologists Rudolf Höber, Hans Winterstein, and Bruno Kisch; ophthalmologist Alfred Bielschowsky; and gynecologist Ludwig Fränkel, to mention only a few. Among the associate professors were pediatrician Stefan Engel, radiologist Franz Groedel, surgeons Rudolf Nissen and Eduard Melchior, and internists Rachel Hirsch and Georg Klemperer. By 1939, 45 percent of all academic positions at the universities had been filled by new appointees.[62]

The revolution at the universities brought about by the Nazis affected not only faculty but students, too. The National Socialist Students' League, which was more active and radical than its counterpart, the National Socialist Lecturers' League, disrupted so many lectures that many Jewish professors had to stop teaching even before they were dismissed.

Nazi students were also active propagandists on behalf of new anti-Semitic regulations. All over Germany, local student organizations of the party demanded a numerus clausus for Jews—a restriction in the number of Jews allowed to attend a

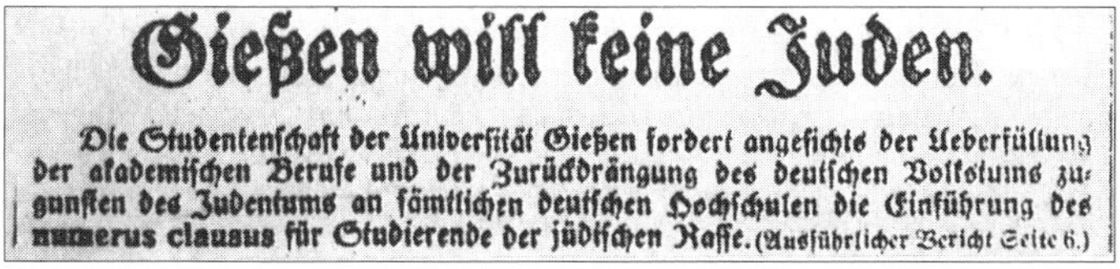

Gießen will keine Juden.

Die Studentenschaft der Universität Gießen fordert angesichts der Ueberfüllung der akademischen Berufe und der Zurückdrängung des deutschen Volkstums zugunsten des Judentums an sämtlichen deutschen Hochschulen die Einführung des numerus clausus für Studierende der jüdischen Rasse. (Ausführlicher Bericht Seite 6.)

FIG 120 "GIESSEN DOES NOT WANT JEWS."

university. In Giessen, for example, the Nazi Students' League proclaimed in leaflets and newspapers, "Giessen does not want Jews" (fig. 120).[63] Students' demands were aimed at medicine in particular, not only because of the well-known inclination of Jews to practice medicine, but also because of an overall increase in the number of medical students during the last years of the Weimar Republic. From the summer term of 1926 to the winter term of 1932–1933, the percentage of medical students within the universities had risen from 13.0 to 26.2.[64] In the Nazi view, Jewish students had come to occupy places meant for Aryans, an intolerable situation that they meant to correct. On April 25, 1933, shortly after enactment of the Law for the Restoration of Professional Civil Service, a numerus clausus was established limiting the percentage of Jews at the universities to reflect the percentage of Jews in the general population. The true objective, however, was total exclusion of Jews from higher education and from university life in Germany.

Life for Jewish students and those of Jewish descent changed dramatically. They were suddenly excluded, provoked, and otherwise discriminated against by professors in examinations. Overnight, it seemed, famous scientists who had previously ridiculed the Nazis now glorified the Führer— for example, Robert Feulgen (fig. 121), known for the development of the Feulgen stain, a method for demonstrating chromatin and deoxyribonucleic acid. Feulgen, who was professor of physiological chemistry at the University of Giessen, declared loudly and proudly that he would "throw everybody out of the lecture who does not support the Führer totally,"[65]

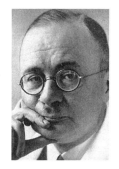

FIG 121
ROBERT FEULGEN
(1884–1955)

91

knowing full well that Jewish students in the audience would not dare to say a word. Feulgen was an opportunist. At the beginning he was opposed to Nazism, but when the future for the Nazis burned bright, he joined eight Nazi organizations. After the war, he was classified by the American military government as a "hanger-on" and was sentenced to a penalty of a mere two thousand Reichsmarks.[66]

Jewish students suffered more than just humiliation. Some were attacked physically and forced to turn in their student identification cards. Jewish students who received financial assistance were treated with open hostility by Aryan students, who hoped to redirect those funds to themselves. Even before any government or university regulation had been put into effect, Aryan students insisted that Jews study separately, and at several universities, Jewish students were not even allowed to enter the campus. At the University of Freiburg, Jewish students were ordered in 1933 to exchange their normal students' identification cards, which were brown, for yellow ones that were given exclusively to Jews.[67] In February 1933, the medical faculty of the University of Munich announced, "The Jewish students of medicine are advised, in their own best interest and in the interest of maintenance of peace and order in the lecture halls, to take their seats only after the lectures have begun. The first rows are reserved for other medical students. In case this well-meant advice is not heeded, we will be forced to resort to stricter measures."[68]

In Giessen, a newly matriculated Jewish student received a letter from Gerhard Pfahler, rector of the university, that read, "Nothing stands in the way of pursuit of your studies in Giessen. Nevertheless, I consider it my duty to call to your attention that especially at our small university with its accordingly small, tightly knit study groups, your participation as a non-Aryan might be much more difficult than at a middle-sized or large university."[69]

A decree issued on October 20, 1933, stated that non-Aryan students of medicine and dentistry were to be excluded from "national duties." That these national duties were prerequisites for admission to examinations meant that most Jewish students were unable to complete their studies. Graduates who wanted to submit their dissertations to receive a doctor of medicine degree were informed that they would be denied diplomas. In 1934, these regulations were relaxed somewhat; Jewish medical candidates who made clear their intention to move abroad and renounce their German citizenship would be eligible to receive a doctorate. German Jewish students found themselves in a quandary. As long as they remained in the Reich, it was legally impossible for them to lose their citizenship, yet in it they could not receive their degree. If they wished to emigrate to take jobs abroad, they had to have their doctorates in hand as a prerequisite for a post, yet inside the borders of Germany this was impossible.[70] In response to this situation, the University of Basel offered to accept the dissertations of Jewish graduates of German medical schools. If the dissertations were found to be satisfactory, the students would be officially promoted. Rudolf Baer (fig. 122), who, thirty years later, became chairman of the Department of Dermatology at the New York University School of Medicine, accepted this offer. In 1934, after having passed the examination in Basel, he emigrated to the United States. Born in Strasbourg—which had been German before World War I and French after it—Baer was allowed to enter the United States under the French contingent for immigration.[71] At that time, the German quota for immigration had already been filled, and many Germans had to wait for years before receiving permission to immigrate to the United States.

Baer was one of the last Jewish medical students to graduate in Germany. By the end of 1934, the number of Jewish medical students in Germany had dropped from more than two thousand to just two hundred sixty-three. Less than one year later, Jewish students had been excluded completely from matriculation and from sitting for examinations.[72]

Radical changes at the universities, however, were not the only blows against Jewish or "politically unreliable" physicians in Germany. A decree issued by the German Ministry of

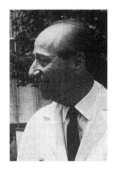

FIG 122
RUDOLF BAER
(1910–1997)

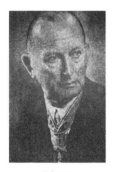

FIG 123
KARL HAEDENKAMP
(1889–1955)

Labor on April 22, 1933, was perhaps more damaging. According to the edict, "the practice of insurance-panel doctors of non-Aryan descent and doctors who have been active in Communistic causes is now terminated. New admissions of such physicians to practice in the scope of health insurance will not happen any more."[73]

The decree had been formulated with considerable help from Karl Haedenkamp (fig. 123), the former executive director of the Hartmannbund, who had been assigned administratively to the ministry. When the decree was announced in several medical journals, Haedenkamp's public comment was: "The legally binding licensing regulations now are precisely formulated with the intention to eliminate non-Aryan physicians." Haedenkamp also explained that "the new regulations about the eligibility to work in private practice and to treat insured patients derive primarily from the intention to implement an employment enhancing strategy within the medical profession itself."[74]

Because the ousting of undesired colleagues was seen as an "employment enhancing strategy" to overcome the unemployment of physicians, professional organizations were eager to compile lists of colleagues to whom the decree applied. They often did that in an offhand way, particularly when it came to accusations of Communist activity. Many insurance-panel doctors who were excluded by their own professional organizations were reaccepted by the Ministry of Labor. (Of 1,377 appeals submitted by professional organizations in the first months, only 550 were accepted.) In addition, the decree did not apply to Jewish insurance-panel doctors who had seen front-line duty in World War I or who had established their practices before August 1, 1914. These "Hindenburg clauses" for exemption, adopted from the Law for the Restoration of Professional Civil Service, applied to many more insurance-panel doctors than to physicians in the civil service, because insurance-panel doctors tended to be older than their colleagues in hospitals and in other public institutions. In some cities, including Munich and Stuttgart, relatively few Jewish

Praxis abgemeldet:

Dr. Max van Wien
Dr. Martha Gernichowski
Dr. Albert Reißner
Dr. Siegfried Levinger
Dr. Ludwig Haydn
Dr. Dionis Heinle
Dr. Wladimir Eliasberg
Dr. Eugen Doernberger
Dr. Hans Luxenburger
Dr. Heinrich Seitz
Dr. David Roßnitz
Dr. Eugen Koenigsberger
San. Rat. Franz Kleinschrod

FIG 124 LIST OF MEDICAL PRACTICES CLOSED BY THE NAZIS.

doctors were affected. By 1935, more than half of the doctors on the insurance panel in Berlin were Jewish.[75] Nevertheless, the lists of excluded physicians were long; by early 1934, more than two thousand physicians were forced to cease work within the scope of health insurance and lost their means of economic survival (fig. 124).

The situation continued to deteriorate. A decree issued on August 10, 1933, by the Reich's leader of physicians, Gerhard Wagner, forbade any cooperation between Aryan and non-Aryan physicians, including referrals, substitutions, and joint practices (which at that time were common). Karl Linser (fig. 125), an Aryan who became chair of dermatology in Leipzig after the war, practiced with Eugen Galewsky (fig. 126), who was Jewish, in Dresden. In response to the decree, Linser and Galewsky informed their patients in a newspaper advertisement that the dissolution of their practice had been undertaken in an amiable way. Because of this statement, Karl Linser was put under arrest for one day.[76]

When Hitler assumed power in January 1933, Galewsky was sixty-eight years old and one of the most prominent dermatologists in Germany. His practice had been established in 1891 (after an assistantship with Albert Neisser in Breslau) and was therefore unaffected by the new regulations concern-

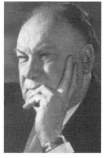

FIG 125
KARL LINSER
(1895–1976)

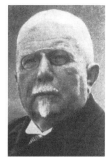

FIG 126
EUGEN GALEWSKY
(1864–1935)

ing Jewish insurance-panel doctors. As a highly esteemed specialist, credited with having introduced Cignolin (anthralin) for the treatment of psoriasis in 1916, Galewsky saw many private patients and enjoyed relative independence from public health insurance constraints. Although he continued to work in Dresden until his death in 1935, the last two years of his life saw him defamed as a "liquor Jew" because his father had once operated a liquor factory.[77]

The situation of most of Galewsky's younger colleagues was less favorable. New governmental regulations meant that they lost most of their poorer patients, who were unable to pay bills without the aid of insurance. The number of private patients these physicians saw also declined steadily because Aryan patients were forbidden by their employers and governmental institutions from visiting Jewish physicians. Medical certificates would be honored only if they had been issued by Aryan physicians. Patients who insisted on seeing Jewish doctors were subject to threat by storm troopers, like the one referred to in the following letter written by a special agent of the Highest SA Command in Nuremberg:

> I came to know that you are under medical treatment of a Jew. But Germans attend only German physicians. The Jew is not a German. It shall also serve for your information that you receive your public benefits from the German people and not from the Jewish people, who only enjoy hospitality in Germany. I hope that this instruction will suffice to enable you to act as a German in the future. I shall conscientiously oversee the success or failure of my admonition and warning. In the case of nonobservance, we will have to deal with this affair in a different manner. Heil Hitler! [78]

As patients were forced more and more to heed such thinly veiled threats, Jewish physicians were forced out of practice. Even non-Jewish physicians who had Jewish-sounding names

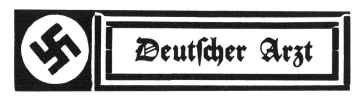

FIG 127 "GERMAN PHYSICIAN."

found themselves in trouble. Dr. Seeliger, an ophthalmologist in Munich, placed ads in newspapers in an attempt to make clear to his patients his purely Aryan lineage. Aryan descent was also indicated by a sign hung at the entrance of a medical practice that displayed the swastika and the words "Deutscher Arzt" (fig. 127).

THE NEW LEADERS OF GERMAN DERMATOLOGY

THE MAJORITY OF GERMAN PHYSICIANS IN THE MID-1930S ACCEPTED THE NEW POLITICAL REALITIES WITHOUT RELUC-tance. Many embraced National Socialism, and nearly half were actually members of the NSDAP, despite the fact that the party, in trying to preserve its elitist character, was not even open to enrollment between 1934 and 1936, all of 1938, and during the years 1942 to 1945. A formidable number of German physicians also belonged to Nazi organizations other than the party. Between 1933 and 1935, membership in the National Socialist Physicians' League rose from 2,786 to 14,500 and continued to increase until almost one-third of all German physicians belonged. Twenty-six percent of all male physicians were members of the storm troops (the SA or "Brownshirts") and seven percent were members of the defense corps (the SS or "Blackshirts").[1] The number of physicians in these organizations far exceeded that of any other single profession. For instance, eleven percent of teachers belonged to the SA and only 0.4 percent to the SS.[2]

How can the extraordinary acceptance of Nazi policies by physicians be explained? One important factor was the influence of home and schools. Many physicians were raised by conserva-tive parents and indoctrinated by teachers who helped create a climate of nationalism and militarism. After the chaotic years of the Weimar Republic, many authority figures welcomed the restoration of an autocratic regime, and the physicians-to-be were particularly receptive to authoritarianism. After all, one reason they had succeeded at home and school was because they were obedient to authority and rarely challenged it.

The trying social and economic circumstances of young Ger-man physicians at the time heightened the appeal of Nazism. Every medical school graduate was required to spend three years as an assistant physician in a hospital, earning just enough money to exist. Most assistant physicians could not even afford apartments and were housed instead in small rooms in the hospital, for which rent was automatically deducted from their pay. These stressful conditions prevented young doctors, who generally did not obtain their medical licenses until age twenty-seven, from marrying and starting families. Even if they wanted to or had the means to do so, their contracts stipulated immediate dismissal if they married against the will of the chair of their departments. A surplus of physicians that resulted in substantial unemployment for doctors compounded the situation. A residency at a university was difficult to obtain, and the establishment of a private practice was even more difficult because insurance-fund panels permitted only one new doctor for every six hundred patients. The sum of these factors meant that young physicians were highly receptive to change and welcomed with enthusiasm the promise of new opportunities.

Those who became the "movers and shakers" among Nazi physicians were recent graduates of medical school who, in the last years of the Weimar Republic, had found themselves excluded professionally by their older, well-established colleagues. After the Nazis' rise to power and the dismissal of Jews from medical service, Nazi physicians found their opportunities greatly enhanced (fig. 128). Young German physicians who had joined the SA before January 30, 1933, were eligible for immediate placement on insurance-fund panels. Allegiance to the Nazis was well rewarded, and those who could boast Old Fighter laurels were favored by the German Panel Fund Physicians' Union. Registrants whose support of National Socialism was not so evident were nearly always bypassed.

At the universities, the situation was similar. Before Hitler's rise to power, young scientists had to endure humble living conditions and an uncertain future. Teaching positions were difficult to find, and the chances for advancement were small. According to statistics published in 1932, only one of seven lecturers in medical schools could expect an offer of a full-time, tenured post. After the elimination of Jews from the

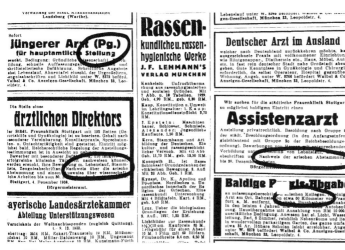

FIG 128 ADVERTISEMENT FOR PHYSICIANS IN THE *MÜNCHENER MEDIZINISCHE WOCHENSCHRIFT* IN 1933: A PRECONDITION FOR APPLICATION WAS PROOF OF ARYAN DESCENT AND SOMETIMES EVEN MEMBERSHIP IN THE NAZI PARTY. ("PG." = "PARTEIGENOSSE.")

universities, the future suddenly looked brighter, especially for younger faculty members who were active in the party.[3]

These circumstances set the stage for a bizarre scenario of unbridled opportunism. Within a matter of weeks, German physicians rapidly pursued Nazi party membership. In teaching clinics and university departments, assistant physicians and lecturers seeking professional advancement suddenly began to flaunt their formal affiliation with the Nazis, a behavior that only weeks earlier might have caused them considerable embarrassment. Although the white smock remained standard garb for physicians in hospitals, the party badge, a symbol of loyalty, was often displayed on it. In their offices, doctors more and more often dressed in SA or SS uniforms. Aspiring physicians enrolled not only in the party but also in the SS, realizing its usefulness as a step toward ensuring professional success. At the University of Tübingen, the medical faculty's entire corps of assistants joined the storm troops in May 1933, and at a Christmas celebration the same year, enthusiastic assistant physicians in Berlin glorified Hitler by comparing him to the ancient god Wotan (figs. 129, 130).[4]

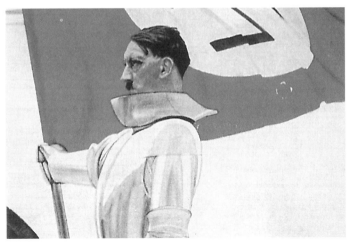

FIG 129 GLORIFICATION OF HITLER: HITLER IN ANCIENT ARMOR.

Scrupulous care was taken to avoid any hint of political dis-
loyalty, and previous ties to organizations—political, cultural,
or religious—not aligned with National Socialism had to be
concealed. Failure to do so could result in loss of appointment
or immediate dismissal, as was the case with Georg Alexander
Rost, Philipp Keller, Rudolf Maximilian Bohnstedt, and many
other dermatologists.

Karl Hoede, an assistant to Zieler in the Department of
Dermatology at the University of Würzburg, was to be terminated solely because of his membership in a Freemason's
lodge until 1933. In all other respects, Hoede fulfilled the conditions for an academic career in National Socialist Germany.
He had fought for Germany in the first World War and, in the
early years of the Weimar Republic, had been a member of
the nationalist Volunteer Corps and of the Stahlhelm, a right-
wing organization of World War I veterans. In 1920, Hoede
had participated actively in the Kapp putsch directed against
the democratic constitution of the Weimar Republic. After
Hitler's assumption of power, Hoede again joined the
Stahlhelm, which was incorporated into the SA on February 1,
1934. One year later, he was excluded from the SA because of
his former membership in a Freemason's lodge. For the same

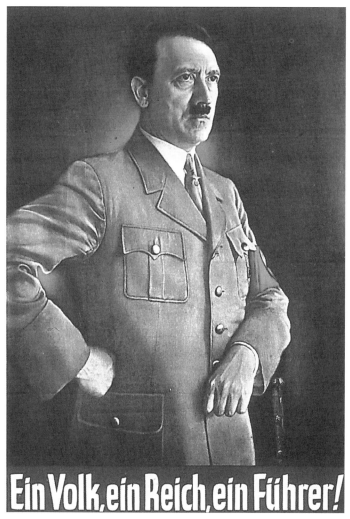

Ein Volk, ein Reich, ein Führer!

FIG 130 GLORIFICATION OF HITLER: "ONE PEOPLE,
ONE REICH, ONE FÜHRER!"

reason, he was prevented from becoming a member of the
Nazi party in 1936. When Hoede's contract at the University
of Würzburg expired in 1936, the Bavarian Ministry of Education and Culture stated, without equivocation, that "with
regard to lecturer Hoede's membership in a lodge, a prolon-
gation of Hoede's contract as an assistant for two years is out
of the question. To avoid hardships, the employment of Dr.
Hoede as an assistant may be extended, with approval by the

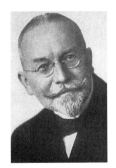

FIG 131
KARL ZIELER
(1874–1945)

Reich's minister, until June 30, 1937. By then, at the latest, he must be terminated."[5]

Hoede, however, had influential Nazi friends who considered him to be superbly suited—scientifically and politically—for an academic career. The leader of the National Socialist Lecturers' League asserted, "Ideologically, Dr. Hoede seems to fulfill all requirements."[6] Hoede's department chair, Karl Zieler (fig. 131), wrote several appeals to the Reich's minister, contending that Hoede had joined the lodge only because of a family tradition and had never been a very active member. He emphasized Hoede's contributions to various organizations of the party, including lectures for the Office of Race Politics and participation as a member in the Genetic Health Courts. According to Zieler, Hoede "lives National Socialism." As a consequence of those appeals, doubts about Hoede began to wane. Upon special permission by the deputy of the Führer, Rudolf Hess, Hoede (fig. 132) was allowed to stay at the University of Würzburg and, in 1940, succeeded Zieler as chair of dermatology. In 1942, he was granted membership in the party and two years later became dean of the medical faculty. After the war, Hoede was dismissed by the military government and went into private dermatology practice in Würzburg. He died in 1973.[7]

The Nazis were also suspicious of universities because they considered them bastions of democratic ideas and ideals. Even though most academics were cooperative and docile, the Nazis remained dissatisfied with the political composition of the faculties. They stated unambiguously that "National Socialism denies the current professorship the right and claim to the political and ideological guidance of the nation [until] complete spiritual and ideological change at the universities" could be achieved.[8] Although the exact nature of that claim was not made clear, there was a vague concept of an ideal National Socialist university, where different faculties would be unified on the basis of race and nation, and all fields of science would be imbued with the thinking of the people.

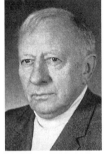

FIG 132
KARL HOEDE
(1897–1973)

Like all other public institutions, the universities were integrated into the hierarchy of National Socialist administration, one that was based entirely on order and obedience. The rectors of universities and deans of faculties were given much more power by the Nazis; they no longer were elected and monitored democratically but were responsible only to the superiors who appointed them—to wit, the dean to the rector of the university and the rector to the Reich's governor. The role of rectors and deans was mostly a political one—namely, to be political leaders of the universities and propagandists for National Socialist thinking. Several dermatologists eventually assumed those functions: Ernst Heinrich Brill and Friedrich Bering were rectors of the universities of Rostock and Cologne; Julius Dörffel and Josef Vonkennel were vice rectors of the universities of Halle and Kiel; and Friedrich Bering in Cologne, Walter Scholtz in Königsberg, Walther Krantz in Göttingen, Alfred Stühmer in Freiburg, Josef Hämel in Halle, Heinrich Adolf Gottron in Breslau, and Karl Hoede in Würzburg were deans of their medical faculties.[9]

Even the installation of rabid Nazis as rectors, vice rectors, and deans was considered by the Nazi leadership to be insufficient. To create the National Socialist university, a new generation of academics—one raised from grade school through university on Nazi ideology—was required. Soon after Hitler's assumption of power, students who fit the bill were promoted. Attempts at habilitation, the prerequisite for becoming a lecturer at a university, had to be approved by the Ministries of Education and Culture before being considered by the faculties. Before their promotion, all candidates for a teaching position were required to attend a military sports or labor camp followed by several months in political training camp, during which they were indoctrinated in Nazism. Furthermore, the Nazis relied on fellow members of the party who already held leading academic positions to help create the National Socialist university. Karl Zieler, chairman of dermatology in Würzburg and new president of the German Dermatological Society, was one of them.

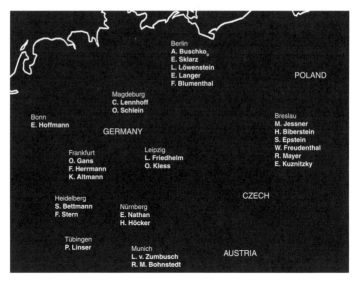

FIG 133 PROFESSORS AND LECTURERS IN DERMATOLOGY
DISMISSED FROM GERMAN UNIVERSITIES.

The rest of the task was accomplished by the gradual dissolution of existing faculties through dismissal, retirement, or
death. As a rule, professors who had reached retirement age
were denied the traditional right to continue teaching. Exceptions were made for professors known "to guarantee that . . .
their political attitude does not jeopardize the National Socialist education of academic youth."[10] The same guarantee was a
requirement for promotion as well. The retirement or death
of a department chair inevitably led to passive politicization of
faculties. This included many departments of dermatology,
such as in Leipzig, where the Nazi Bodo Spiethoff succeeded
Johann Heinrich Rille, and in Giessen, where Walther
Schultze succeeded Albert Jesionek (figs. 133, 134).

A more obvious form of politicization was the replacement
of faculty who had been dismissed for political or racial reasons. Within a few months of the Nazis' rise to power, dozens
of new professors had to be appointed; in dermatology alone,
seven chairs were vacated when those who held them were
dismissed (at the universities of Bonn, Breslau, Frankfurt,
Freiburg, Heidelberg, Munich, and Tübingen).

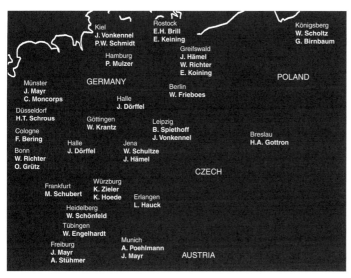

FIG 134 "NEW LEADERS" IN GERMAN DERMATOLOGY.

Many of those who were relieved—Gans, Hoffmann, Jessner, and von Zumbusch—are still esteemed by dermatologists worldwide for their contributions to the field. In contrast, those who replaced them, except for Heinrich Adolf Gottron, are forgotten (fig. 135). This disparity can be explained by the criteria applied to chairs who were to be appointed. Ability, competence, and professional promise were of little or no import, whereas vigorous support for the new National Socialist state was of major concern. The Nazis overrode the traditional system of appointment of chairs that was based on the opinions of the chairs of other departments. Instead, they developed a network of party organizations within and around the universities, among them the National Socialist Physicians' League, the National Socialist Students' League, and the National Socialist Lecturers' League, all of which attempted to influence faculty decisions in favor of fellow party members.

According to a decree by the Prussian Ministry of Science, Culture, and the People's Education issued in the summer of 1933, faculties were no longer allowed to offer their own lists of candidates for chairmanships but were obliged instead to vote

City	Old Chair	New Chair	Year	Reason
Bonn	E. Hoffmann	W. Richter	1934	P
		O. Grütz	1934	
Breslau	M. Jessner	H.A. Gottron	1934	R
Frankfurt	O. Gans	M. Schubert	1933	R
Freiburg	G.A. Rost	J. Mayr	1933	P
		A. Stühmer	1934	
Heidelberg	S. Bettmann	W. Schönfeld	1935	R
München	L.R. v. Zumbusch	A. Poehlmann	1935	P
		J. Mayr	1937	
Tübingen	P. Linser	W. Engelhardt	1935	P

FIG 135 OLD AND NEW CHAIRS OF DERMATOLOGY IN GERMANY, 1933–1937. (R = RACIAL REASONS [JEWISH]; P = POLITICAL REASONS.)

on candidates offered by the ministry. In November of that year, Rudolf Hess "requested" that all medical faculties consult Gerhard Wagner, the "leader" of all German physicians, before acting on any new appointments. The faculties did not always obey this request, and Wagner established the post of "confidants of the NSDAP at the medical faculty." Among those confidants were several dermatologists—namely, Ernst Heinrich Brill from Rostock, Walther Schultze from Giessen, and Martin Schubert from Marburg and Frankfurt, who was confidant of the NSDAP at the medical faculties of both universities. Chosen as chief confidant was one of Wagner's oldest and most loyal Nazi compatriots, Franz Wirz, extraordinary professor of dermatology at the University of Munich. In July 1934, Rudolf Hess founded the party's own Commission on Higher Education, which soon became controlled by Wagner and Wirz.[11] Although the commission's mandate was to manage all university faculties, Wagner and Wirz's major concerns were the medical faculties and the appointment of the party's own candidates to positions within them. In the autumn of 1934, Wirz proudly reported, "Within a short period of time, thirty-four appointments have been declared according to the suggestions of the Commission on Higher Education."[12]

The political reliability of a candidate for a chair of medicine was sometimes difficult to assess.[13] A professor who had joined the Nazi party after its assumption of power might have done so merely out of opportunism and prudence rather than loyalty. Therefore these highly subjective and arbitrary judgments, which were part of every candidate's personnel file, were often dictated by personal preference. The fact that the judges and their decisions remained secret further amplified a sense of powerlessness felt by apolitical physicians who wanted a university career.

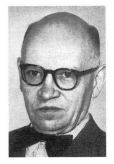

FIG 136
EGON KEINING
(1892–1971)

Candidates who believed they had been rejected on personal or political grounds often reacted by emphasizing their affiliations with Nazi organizations, stressing the authenticity of their conviction to the ideas of National Socialism and reiterating their allegiance to Nazism. Such was the case for Karl Hoede in Würzburg and for Egon Keining in Hamburg. Keining (fig. 136), assistant medical director of the Department of Dermatology, had joined the Nazi party in May 1933, regularly attended regional meetings of the party, and gave lectures at them. Yet when he was to be evaluated as a candidate for the chair of dermatology in Königsberg in 1936, the leader of Hamburg's National Socialist Lecturers' League designated him a "not exactly political nature"; Ernst Heinrich Brill, the chair of dermatology in Rostock, criticized him on the grounds that he had never served as a soldier, and both Alfred Ruete, chair of dermatology in Marburg, and Ruete's former assistant, Martin Schubert, cast aspersions on his character. In this instance, Keining came to know about the conspirators and their assertions, and he decided to bring legal proceedings against Ruete and Schubert.[14] In the meantime, he was passed over for the chair of dermatology at the University of Königsberg, which was given to a committed Nazi, Georg Birnbaum from Dortmund. After refuting all accusations, Keining was given the chance to prove himself as temporary chair of dermatology at the University of Rostock. In October 1944, he was made chair of dermatology in Greifswald and after the war became chair of dermatology in

Mainz. Keining is noteworthy for his work in clinical dermatology; for his description of the thickened, rough, hyperkeratotic cuticle of nails in patients with dermatomyositis, known also as the Keining sign; and for a popular textbook on dermatology, written with his pupil, Otto Braun-Falco, and published in 1961. Keining died at age eighty in 1971.[15]

The subjectivity of political assessments of faculty was not the only problem that hampered the efforts by Gerhard Wagner and Franz Wirz to gain control of the universities for the Nazis. Another was the fact that the role of the Commission on Higher Education had not been clearly defined. In principle, the universities and the ministries of education were responsible for commenting on the scientific qualification of a candidate for a new professorship, whereas party organizations were empowered to render judgments about political suitability for such a position. Decisions about scientific competency and political allegiance became inextricably intertwined as each side tried to expand its influence at the expense of the other. The ministries of education, although directed by the Nazis, tended to follow less radical political guidelines than those advocated by Wagner and Wirz, and conflict often arose between them. Such conflict between the ministry and party organizations is illustrated by negotiations that took place over the appointment of a new chair of dermatology to the University of Leipzig.

In the early 1930s, the Skin Clinic of the University of Leipzig was one of the most important dermatology centers in Germany (fig. 137). The list of candidates to succeed Johann Heinrich Rille as chair was compiled by the medical faculty of the university. Originally, it included Bruno Bloch from Zürich, who, among other contributions, had first recognized the melanocyte for what it was and had elucidated the mechanism of formation of melanin; Otto Kren from Vienna; Leo Kumer from Innsbruck; and Alfred Stühmer, Walther Schönfeld, Paul Mulzer, and Hermann Werner Siemens from various cities in Germany. Because of the agitation and intervention of high-

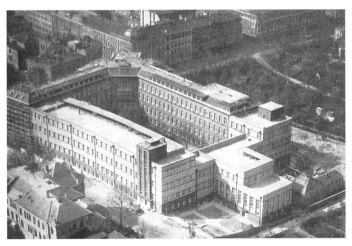

FIG 137 THE NEW SKIN CLINIC OF THE UNIVERSITY OF LEIPZIG, OPENED IN 1931. THE ENTIRE BUILDING WAS DEDICATED TO DERMATOLOGY.

ranking Nazis, the Prussian Ministry of Education added another name to the list—that of Bodo Spiethoff.

Spiethoff (fig. 138) had belonged to the NSDAP since January 1931. Not only was he involved prominently in restructuring the German Society for the Fight Against Venereal Diseases, he also belonged to the expert committee of the German Ministry of the Interior, which was devoted to the politics of population and race. In spite of these political merits, Spiethoff's nomination was disregarded by the ministry and the medical faculty. On the basis of scientific merit, both institutions agreed instead on Hermann Werner Siemens (fig. 139) as the new chair of dermatology and informed him of their decision.[16]

Scientifically, Siemens's work was considered more substantive and held greater promise than Spiethoff's. He was known for his studies on the genetic background of skin disease, as made manifest in his thesis "On the Importance of Genetics for the Development of Nevi." In 1925, Siemens had described dystrophic epidermolysis bullosa (known eponymically as the Hallopeau-Siemens type of the disease). Politically, Siemens was thought to be sympathetic to the Nazi cause, and his interest in genetics and racial hygiene was

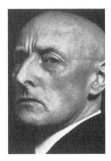

FIG 138
BODO SPIETHOFF
(1875–1948)

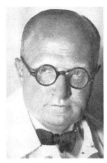

FIG 139
HERMANN WERNER
SIEMENS
(1891–1969)

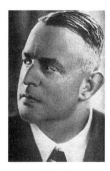

FIG 140
ERNST HEINRICH
BRILL
(1892–1945)

judged to be evidence of this. In 1916, Siemens had published a monograph, *Racial Hygiene and Population Policy: Foundations of Genetics.* Two years later, in an article titled "The Proletarization of Our Future Generations: A Danger of Non-Racial Hygienic Population Policy," he warned that unless the rising tide of inferior human beings was stemmed, "the best of human heredity will be swamped with a mess of inferior types."[17]

Still, Siemens was criticized by the Nazis for not directing enough attention to the racial aspects of genetics. Furthermore, he was not a party member, and unlike Spiethoff, he did not have old buddies among the leaders of the party and state. Although the decision of the ministry in favor of Siemens had already been announced, the Commission on Higher Education went into action. Gerhard Wagner and his colleagues forced the appointment of Spiethoff as chair of dermatology in Leipzig. On April 1, 1934, Spiethoff succeeded Johann Heinrich Rille. He remained director of the skin clinic of Leipzig until 1942, when he retired early for health reasons. He died in 1948. Siemens, who had prepared himself for relocation to Leipzig, received a short note that read: "A leading office outside our ministry, whose approval had to be obtained and from whose decision we cannot diverge, has declared itself against your appointment."[18]

In similar fashion, the party also took good care of other loyal followers. In October 1933, Ernst Heinrich Brill (fig. 140), a former student of Spiethoff, was appointed chair of the Department of Dermatology at the University of Rostock. He was a member of the Nazi party, the storm troops, and the Death's Head Units of the SS and was a district leader of the National Socialist Lecturers' League. Scientifically, however, his record was considerably less impressive. After reviewing the documents of the two candidates for the chair of dermatology, Brill and Julius Mayr from Munich, the medical faculty of Rostock came to the conclusion that "on the basis of study of their scientific publications and on the basis of com-

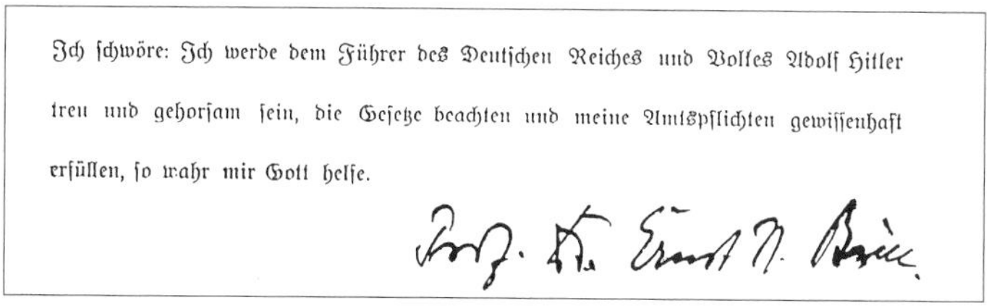

Ich schwöre: Ich werde dem Führer des Deutschen Reiches und Volkes Adolf Hitler treu und gehorsam sein, die Gesetze beachten und meine Amtspflichten gewissenhaft erfüllen, so wahr mir Gott helfe.

Prof. Dr. Ernst H. Brill

FIG 141 OATH OF OFFICE OF ERNST HEINRICH BRILL.

ments of representatives of their specialty, the faculty cannot undertake the responsibility to recommend either of the two gentlemen to the ministry."[19]

Brill, however, could rely on Spiethoff, who recommended him as a "man fighting for Hitler within the student body and popular among national-thinking students." To ensure Brill's appointment, Spiethoff contacted Hans Reiter, a leading Nazi physician and close adviser to the University of Rostock's rector, who also used his influence on Brill's behalf. Finally, these concerted efforts proved successful, and Brill was given the chair. On October 12, 1934, he took the oath of office that had to be taken by all civil servants of the German Reich, including Jews: "I swear: I shall be loyal and obedient to the Führer of the German Reich and People, Adolf Hitler, shall observe the laws, and shall fulfill my duties of office conscientiously, so help me God" (fig. 141). Three years later, Brill became rector of the university. He committed suicide in 1945.

Julius Mayr (fig. 142), Brill's competitor for the chair of dermatology in Rostock, also had been a member of the NSDAP since 1933. When the Nazis assumed power, he was an assistant in von Zumbusch's department in Munich. A few months later, however, after the dismissal of Georg Alexander Rost, he became temporary chairman of the skin clinic in Freiburg. When Alfred Stühmer was called from Münster to Freiburg to fill Rost's chair, Mayr succeeded Stühmer in Münster.

According to his personnel file, Mayr was recommended to the university as "an honest, open, nationally thinking, true German man." His character was classified as "excellent" and

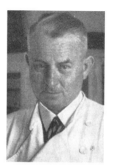

FIG 142
JULIUS MAYR
(1888–1965)

113

Prof. Dr. med. Julius Mayr
Direktor der Dermatolog. Klinik u. Poliklinik
der Universität München

München 15, den   28.VIII.1939
Frauenlobstraße 9
Fernruf 5792·181/482/483/477

3 1. AUG 1939

An den Verwaltungsausschuss der Universität München.

Betreff : Zugehörigkeit von Beamten zur N.S.D.A.P.;
        Tätigkeit als politischer Leiter.

Ich habe war in Münster (Westfalen Nord) Gauamtsleiter (Amt
N.S-D.Dozentenbund = Gaudozentenbundsführer) in der Zeit von
II.1936 – Nov.1937.

FIG 143 LETTER BY JULIUS MAYR CONFIRMING THAT
HE WAS ACTIVE AS A POLITICAL LEADER.

"beyond reproach." This estimation, however, was not shared by everybody. Because of Mayr's reputation as an ardent Nazi, all but one of Stühmer's former assistants resigned their positions rather than work with Mayr. From February 1936 to November 1937, Mayr was leader of the National Socialist Lecturers' League in Münster (fig. 143). In November 1937, he was called to Munich to succeed von Zumbusch.

Julius Mayr remained chair of the Department of Dermatology at the University of Munich until the collapse of the Third Reich in 1945. After his dismissal by the military government, he presented several statutory declarations by colleagues affirming that he had been a strict opponent of the Nazis and that he had been "unable to conceal his anti-Nazi attitude." On the basis of these statements, further proceedings against Mayr were dropped, but he never reassumed his academic career. Mayr died in 1965 at the age of seventy-seven.[20]

After von Zumbusch's removal as chair of dermatology in Munich in 1935, his position had been temporarily filled by his assistant, August Poehlmann (fig. 144). Poehlmann had been a member of the SS since 1933, yet according to the leader of the National Socialist Lecturers' League in

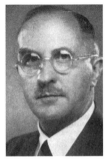

FIG 144
AUGUST
POEHLMANN
(1882–1954)

Munich, Otto Hettche, he had "only slowly adjusted himself to the Third Reich."[21] In regard to scientific ability, character, and ideological-political attitude, Hettche considered Poehlmann to be unsuitable for a full professorship. In 1938, Poehlmann left the Department of Dermatology at the University of Munich to become director of the dermatology unit at the Munich-Schwabing Municipal Hospital. He died in 1954.[22]

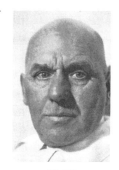

The National Socialist Lecturers' League, founded in 1928, represented all teachers at universities who were affiliated with the party. The organization was highly engaged and powerful in the internal affairs of universities, monitored the political attitude of employees, and carried out disciplinary measures against colleagues who did not act in strict compliance with government regulations. On occasion, the National Socialist Lecturers' League was also able to influence the appointment of department chairs, such as in Göttingen, where a new chair of dermatology was sought upon the retirement of Erhard Riecke (fig. 145) in March 1935.

Initially, the medical faculty of the University of Göttingen listed as possible successors to Riecke the names of Walther Schönfeld, Heinrich Adolf Gottron, and Egon Keining. The National Socialist Lecturers' League managed to push through the appointment of Walther Krantz (fig. 146) from Cologne, a man of lower stature and reputation than the other candidates. Krantz did not belong to the party but, as a member of the Stahlhelm, was incorporated into the SA in 1934. Furthermore, he was cozy with the leader of Göttingen's National Socialist Lecturers' League, anatomist Werner Blume. These connections alone assured the ascendancy of his career: Only four months after his appointment as director of the skin clinic, Krantz was promoted to vice dean. In 1937, he became dean of the medical faculty of the University of Göttingen.

Under Krantz's stewardship, the skin clinic of the University of Göttingen deteriorated, and Krantz himself soon referred to it as an "expanse of rubble." After Krantz had been fired at the

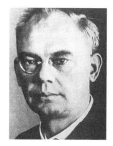

end of the war, the registrar of the university wrote to the new minister of culture: "Had Professor Krantz not been dismissed by order of the military government, I would have filed a claim to institute proceedings against him for culpable negligence of the duties assigned to a director of a clinic."[23]

In Jena, Josef Hämel, a student of Karl Zieler, was appointed chair of dermatology in 1935, despite unimpressive reports about his scientific merits. The chair of dermatology in Cologne, Friedrich Bering, stated, "Until now, Hämel has not proven that he is capable of grasping his own ideas and elaborating on them in a scientific way," whereas Alfred Stühmer, chair of dermatology in Freiburg, advised that Hämel was too young and that there were older candidates whose scientific work was "at least of equal value."[24] Politically, however, Hämel fulfilled the preconditions for the position, having joined the Nazi party on May 1 and the SA on November 23, 1933, for "idealistic reasons," according to his own testimony.[25] This helped to secure his career. In April 1935, Hämel was appointed chair of dermatology in Greifswald. A few months later, he assumed the same position in Jena and on July 1, 1939, he was appointed dean of the medical faculty of the University of Jena.

By then, however, Hämel's fervor about Nazism had cooled. Because he could not leave the party without facing major consequences, he decided to try to diminish the influence of the Nazis from within the party. As dean of the medical faculty, he succeeded in pushing through the appointment of professors who did not belong to the party. In 1944, he was removed from the office of dean for having concealed a political offense—the smashing by students of a bust of Adolf Hitler. This conduct caused Hämel to spend several weeks in custody. After his release, he was to be sent to the front for disciplinary reasons, but the progressively unfavorable course of the war and his indispensability in Jena prevented him from that fate. Hämel resumed his duties in Jena in 1945, and in the last months of the Third Reich, he hid a man who was half Jewish from the Gestapo. In December 1945, Hämel was dismissed as chair of the Department of Dermatology by the Soviet military government, but fourteen months later, after a more thorough examination of his behavior during the Nazi regime, he was reinstated. From 1952 to 1959, Hämel was rector of the University of Jena. Having learned from the past, he tried to mute the growing influence of the Socialist party at the university. When he realized the futility of this effort, he escaped to the West, three years before the Berlin Wall was built. His flight caused great excitement and was widely discussed in newspapers, radio, and television. In 1960, Hämel succeeded Walther Schönfeld as chairman of dermatology in Heidelberg, and in 1961 was elected dean of the medical faculty of the University of Heidelberg. He died in 1969.[26]

Walther Schultze (fig. 147), an assistant of Albert Jesionek in Giessen, had joined the NSDAP on November 9, 1931; he used to boast that the number in his party membership book was lower than 1,000,000, evidence of his early support of the Nazis.[27] In 1934, Schultze succeeded Spiethoff as chair of dermatology in Jena. A few months later, after Jesionek's retirement, Schultze was appointed chair of the Department of Dermatology in Giessen.

The original list of candidates to succeed Jesionek included Walther Schultze, Heinrich Adolf Gottron, and Paul Wilhelm Schmidt, all of whom were members of the Nazi party. The university made the usual inquiries about the scientific merit and political suitability of each candidate. In regard to Schmidt (fig. 148), an associate professor at the skin clinic of the University of Freiburg, the "strictly confidential" judgment made by the leader of the students of medicine at that university was devastating: "As a teacher, Prof. Schmidt is incapable of keeping the students together in a disciplined fashion and to be a leader of them. In regard to his character, it is—as we have heard—dubious. Politically, he is absolutely indifferent."[28]

According to Gerhard Pfahler (fig. 149), rector of the University of Giessen from 1934 to 1937, Walther Schultze had been "involved prominently in the penetration of the revolu-

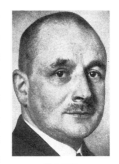

FIG 147
WALTHER
SCHULTZE
(1893–1970)

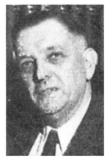

FIG 148
PAUL WILHELM
SCHMIDT
(1896–1950)

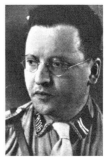

FIG 149
GERHARD PFAHLER
(BORN 1897)

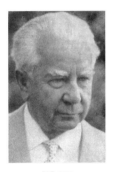

FIG 150
WILLY
ENGELHARDT
(1895–1977)

tion into the realm of the university so that further inquiries were unnecessary." Pfahler—who, like most university rectors, thought of himself as a political leader and usually wore a Nazi uniform—stated in a letter to the ministry that he had not yet collected enough information about Gottron. In regard to Schmidt, Pfahler was certain that he "does not correspond to the course of university politics that I have followed for new appointments within the medical faculty. Therefore, I want to ask the Reich's Minister of Culture to offer the chair to Professor Schultze; otherwise to Mr. Gottron, but Mr. Schmidt should not be considered."[29]

Pfahler's arguments prevailed, Schultze was nominated, and, in the summer of 1935, he succeeded his teacher, Albert Jesionek, as chair. Schmidt did not receive a chair of dermatology until 1943, when he was appointed director of the skin clinic in Kiel. He died only seven years later, at the age of fifty-three.[30] Gottron, also passed over for the chairmanship in Giessen, received a call to the University of Breslau in 1935.

In addition to his duties as chair of dermatology, Schultze was active in the National Socialist Lecturers' League and was its leader in 1936 and 1937. Six of the seven leaders of Giessen's National Socialist Lecturers' League between 1933 and 1945 were physicians—incontrovertible evidence of the dominant role physicians played in assisting National Socialism to achieve its aims at the universities.[31] Under the direction of Schultze, every physician at the skin clinic of the University of Giessen belonged to the NSDAP. In 1945, Schultze was dismissed by the American military government from his position as chair of dermatology. He died in 1970.[32]

Another former assistant of Jesionek, Willy Engelhardt (fig. 150), had left Giessen in 1930 to become assistant medical director of the Department of Dermatology in Düsseldorf. Engelhardt joined the Nazi party on April 1, 1933, the SA in November 1933, and the National Socialist Physicians' League in July 1934. He also was deputy leader of the National Socialist Lecturers' League in Düsseldorf.[33] In 1934, Engelhardt was appointed extraordinary professor and, two years later, chair of dermatology at the University of Tübingen. Engelhardt was dismissed by the military government in 1945 but continued to work in private practice in Rottweil, where he died in 1977.[34]

At the University of Frankfurt, a successor was sought to replace Oscar Gans, who had been thrown out as chair of dermatology in December 1933. The medical faculty considered six candidates, including thirty-eight-year-old Martin Schubert (fig. 151), an assistant to Alfred Ruete in Marburg. Schubert was by far the youngest candidate, and his scientific contributions were meager at best. Nevertheless, he was selected for the position because, as the dean of the medical faculty wrote, he had "proved himself as an inspiring, vivid teacher, who is able to impart to the students, by practical teaching and personal ideas, medical knowledge in the spirit of the National Socialist ideology."[35]

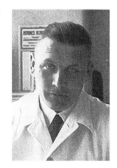

FIG 151
MARTIN SCHUBERT
(1896–1964)

Schubert had joined the NSDAP as early as February 1932. He was also a high-ranking member of the SA and of several other Nazi organizations. At the universities of Marburg and Frankfurt, Schubert was made confidant of the NSDAP at the medical faculties and, in 1938 and 1939, he became deputy leader of the National Socialist Lecturers' League in Frankfurt. After the fall of the Nazi regime, Schubert was dismissed by the military government, his home was seized, and he was denied the right to work as a physician, a measure that was eventually revoked. In one of the denazification trial tribunals instituted by the military governments all over Germany for the purpose of assessing involvement of German citizens in the Nazi movement, Schubert was considered to be only slightly incriminated and therefore was given an ordinary pension. He never resumed his academic career and died in Cologne in 1964.[36]

The chair of dermatology in Halle, Carl Grouven (fig. 152), a longtime member of the Stahlhelm, died in 1936. Among the candidates to succeed him were Carl Moncorps, associate professor at the University of Munich, and Egon Keining. Neither man was especially active in the National Socialist move-

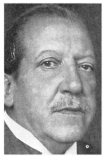

FIG 152
CARL GROUVEN
(1872–1936)

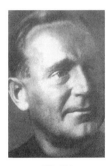

FIG 153
JULIUS DÖRFFEL
(1900–1953)

ment, so the ministry selected thirty-seven-year-old Julius Dörffel (fig. 153), an associate of Walter Scholtz in Königsberg. Dörffel had little scientific reputation, but his political credentials were impeccable and assured him a career in National Socialist Germany. He had been a member of the Nazi party since February 1933. In April, he had joined the SA, and by October he had acquired a high rank in the National Socialist Lecturers' League. When asked about Dörffel's qualifications, the leader of the National Socialist Lecturers' League at the University of Königsberg, Lothar Loeffler, a renowned party activist and specialist in racial hygiene, stated unambiguously:

> *Scientifically, Dörffel is generally said to be good. . . . He has a dependable character and an honest nature. He is one of the younger academic teachers on whom one can rely in any regard. Politically, he is also absolutely unobjectionable. . . . He has devoted himself fully to the duties of the SA and, as my commissioner for the medical faculty, contributes regularly and reliably to the activities of the Lecturers' League. . . . Based on my own knowledge about the rising generation of dermatologists, I consider D. to be the one who, under any circumstances, has to be mentioned first when it comes to the appointment of a chairman.*[37]

In 1937, Dörffel succeeded Grouven as chairman of dermatology in Halle, and two years later was appointed vice rector of the university. During the war, Dörffel was medical officer in an SA brigade, responsible for managing cutaneous disorders of hard laborers from foreign countries who had been brought to work in central Germany. After the war, he was dismissed by the Soviet military government and opened a private practice in dermatology in Heidelberg. He died in a car accident in 1953.[38]

Josef Vonkennel (fig. 154) had been a member of the NSDAP since April 1933, and in the days of the Weimar Republic had been arrested for agitation against Jews. When the Nazis

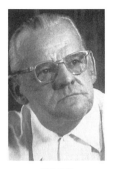

FIG 154
JOSEF VONKENNEL
(1897–1963)

assumed power, he was an assistant in the skin clinic of Munich-Schwabing. He had never worked in a university department. Nevertheless, Vonkennel was considered to be superbly suited for the "fight for the National Socialist university" and, in 1934, was given the chair of dermatology at the University of Kiel, where he proved capable. In 1937, he succeeded Spiethoff as chair of dermatology in Leipzig. Vonkennel was a prominent member of the SS and the consulting dermatologist of the armed SS squadrons. After the war, he continued his academic career as chair of dermatology in Cologne.[39]

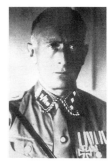

FIG 155
WILHELM RICHTER
(1892–1944)

It was splendid connections to the highest members of the party, rather than scientific merit, that made the career of Wilhelm Richter (fig. 155). In 1933, Richter was the director of a small private skin clinic in Berlin. Previous attempts to gain affiliation with the university had been thwarted by the objections of several leading German dermatologists who criticized his scientific work. When Rudolf Hess interceded on his behalf, Richter was appointed extraordinary professor, and his clinic was given the status of a university hospital. In February 1934, Richter temporarily assumed the chair of dermatology at the University of Bonn, succeeding Erich Hoffmann. The only lasting effect that he had there was the purchase of a bust of Adolf Hitler that, from then on, decorated the entrance of the clinic. In September 1934, Richter returned to Berlin as an ordinary professor. A few months later, he was appointed chair of dermatology at the University of Greifswald, became director of the section of "war medicine" of the Reich's Office of Research in 1937, and from October 1939 on was the highest medical officer of the district of Warsaw, where he was responsible for medical matters in the ghetto. He died at the front in March 1944. As noted in the obituary notice of his family, "a life that was dedicated to Führer and fatherland found its heroic end."[40]

Despite the new political realities and priorities that dictated university policy, medical faculties occasionally succeeded in appointing a chair who was a distinguished scientist

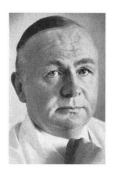

FIG 156
WALTHER
SCHÖNFELD
(1888–1977)

and not simply a Nazi supporter. Such was the case in Heidelberg, where Walther Schönfeld (fig. 156) succeeded Siegfried Bettmann as chair of the Department of Dermatology. Schönfeld was a member of the National Socialist Physicians' League, but he did not belong to the NSDAP or any other Nazi organizations. After the war, he was among the few chairs of dermatology who retained their titles without having been interrogated by the military government.[41] He retired in 1959 and died in 1977 at the age of eighty-eight. Schönfeld was the author of several textbooks and of a monograph on the history of dermatology and venereology.[42]

At the University of Münster, Carl Moncorps was appointed chair of the Department of Dermatology, despite the fact that his political attitude was criticized harshly by influential members of the party. According to Walther Schultze, the chair of dermatology in Giessen, Moncorps "belongs to the type of scientist who, in the past, has had a profoundly negative influence on German universities. . . . Unfortunately, I have no evidence that he is active as a National Socialist."[43] Nevertheless, on the basis of his scientific achievements, Moncorps was given the chair.

In Freiburg, a new chair for the Department of Dermatology was sought after the dismissal of Georg Alexander Rost. The ministry strongly supported the nomination of Gerhard Wagner's choice, Franz Wirz. In the official call to nominate candidates for the vacant chair, Freiburg's medical faculty was specifically asked by the ministry to declare its position on the appointment of Wirz. Of dermatologists from various departments in Germany who were asked for their opinion, not one recommended Wirz, including his own chair, von Zumbusch. The faculty disregarded the ministry's candidate and nominated Walther Schönfeld and Alfred Stühmer.

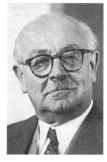

FIG 157
ALFRED STÜHMER
(1885–1957)

On April 1, 1934, Alfred Stühmer (fig. 157) was appointed chair of dermatology at the University of Freiburg. That a university was able to override a ministry's proposal was extraordinary in itself. It helped that Stühmer, though not a member of the party, was known as a conservative nationalist and was a former member of the Stahlhelm. Furthermore, Freiburg's medical faculty had presented an additional, embarrassing argument against Wirz—his previous marriage to a sister of the Jewish chair of internal medicine at the University of Freiburg, Siegfried Thannhauser.[44] Despite his excellent connections, Wirz never occupied a chair of dermatology. Instead, he stayed in the headquarters of the NSDAP in Munich. As a close collaborator of Gerhard Wagner and Leonardo Conti and leader of the party's university section, Wirz had great influence on the affairs of all German universities for many years.

Of course, even the men who were responsible for the new policy at the universities, such as Wirz and Wagner, had to be aware of the fact that the use of political rather than scientific criteria for university appointments would impair the quality of work done there, but few academics voiced their concerns. Erich Hoffmann was one who did. He wrote many letters to the Reich's Ministry of Education about the inevitable result of its policy and sought to mobilize his colleagues in an attempt to save the traditional system of appointing department chairs. Leopold von Zumbusch made the following declaration in a letter to the government: "Because of my age and academic experience, I consider it to be my duty to emphasize that German science will lose, irrevocably, its worldwide recognition if appointments are based on criteria by which mediocrities are nominated to protect and preserve it. It also will be detrimental to the German people if bad professors educate bad physicians."[45]

His predictions were borne out. Germany's universities soon became populated by countless medical "pseudoscholars" who attempted to compensate for their ineptitude by taking shortcuts in their science in order to collect easy rewards. Some new professors were so incompetent that they had to be removed. Kurt Strauss, a surgeon and good friend of Leonardo Conti, was described by his former assistant—the Nobel Prize winner Werner Forssmann—as a butcher who flirted with litigation, an habitué of wild parties, and a womanizer.[46] As a rule, the worse a man was as a scholar, the better he was as a Nazi.

It was inevitable that medical students would notice the declining quality of their professors, and before long they stopped attending lectures given by the most incompetent ones. The situation was aggravated further by the fact that whatever solid medical teaching remained was squeezed into a few hours, while absurd subjects like "biology of race" were given much more time. Following directives from Gerhard Wagner, the number of compulsory lectures in the minor specialties of medicine was reduced by thirty percent.[47] The progressive curtailment of legitimate medical education was concurrent with increasing Nazi preoccupation with student participation in party activities such as parades and demonstrations. For Walter Lever, the author of the textbook *Histopathology of the Skin* (which, from 1949 on, appeared in seven editions over a period of more than forty years), this focus of the Nazis was one factor that prompted him to emigrate to the United States, according to his widow, Gundula Schaumburg-Lever, who claimed that Walter Lever had left Germany "because he wanted to have an academic career and he did not think he could do this in Nazi Germany. When he was an intern in Cologne and studied in the library, he was told to go out and march for Hitler instead of reading."[48]

There was also a marked decline in the abilities and interests of medical students. Ferdinand Sauerbruch, the famous surgeon who developed, among other innovations, the iron lung and open chest surgery, characterized the "intellectual state" of medical students as appalling. They "are picked because of the low number of their membership card," he wrote, "and preference is given to those with fathers in the party and mothers in the National Socialist Womanhood. Five times weekly they have to attend marching and combat exercises and lectures on the theory of race. Next morning they sleep through class, if they show up at all."[49]

These factors combined resulted in a substantial decline in the quality of German medicine, which had already suffered greatly because of the mass exodus of Jewish scholars, many of them brilliant. Even in the first years of the National Socialist regime, the decline was evident when Aryan patients stopped consulting physicians newly appointed to insurance-fund panels. During the war, the consequences of a much-flawed medical education system were visited on the German army. Wounded soldiers were often treated by badly trained physicians who were knowledgeable about current theories of race but were unable to perform even the most basic surgical procedures properly. After the fall of the Third Reich, it took decades for medicine in Germany to recover from the Nazis. It may never recover fully.

NEW MANNERS, MORALS, AND SUBJECTS IN MEDICINE

THE REPLACEMENT OF ACADEMICS BY POLITICAL APPOINTEES SYMPATHETIC TO THE NAZIS SOON CAUSED A DRAMATIC change in the manners and language of medicine in Germany. When an article about phototherapy by Walther Schultze, chair of dermatology at the University of Giessen, was subjected to academic criticism by Leopold Freund, a Jewish physician from Vienna who had introduced Grenz ray therapy for the treatment of cutaneous disorders, Schultze responded by attacking the journal's editor for having published Freund's letter: "It is entirely clear that one risks being attacked when publishing scientific papers, but one still is not pleased by attacks by crafty Jews who are unable to separate science from business, and in Germany one should not give these persons an opportunity for polemics in scientific papers. . . . I really see no need to have my scientific reputation tarnished by a Viennese Jew."[1]

Like most aspects of life in Germany at the time, medical specialties were soon organized in strict accordance with the "leadership principle." In short, the principle stated that the individual was a mere cog; what mattered was the group and its adherence to the directives of its leader. This principle, incompatible with critical scientific endeavor, was exemplified by the way the German Dermatological Society prepared for the Ninth International Congress of Dermatology, to be held in Budapest in September 1935. Months before the congress was convened, all possible delegates were assessed with respect to their political reliability and suitability to represent the German state. The chair of the German Dermatological Society, Karl Zieler of Würzburg, compiled meticulous lists classifying the participation of certain dermatologists as "mandatory," "acceptable," or "undesirable." The first group, in addition to the new leaders of German dermatology such as Brill, Schumacher, and Spiethoff, included the names of two Jewish dermatologists, Paul Unna, Jr., and Abraham Buschke,[2] because, in Zieler's words, "It would cause unnecessary noise throughout the world if there were no Jews at all among the German participants."[3] Included in the last group was Alfred Marchionini, who, though highly respected, was persona non grata because his wife was of distant Jewish descent.

In compiling his lists, Zieler tried to prevent any circumstance that could prove to be discomforting during the congress. In a letter to the German congress office, he explained:

> *In my view, the men marked by a cross in pencil as prominent German scientists must travel to the international congress in Budapest unconditionally. . . . Mr. Benedek, list C, deserves special consideration. Admittedly, he does not belong to our sphere of responsibility but, as far as I know, he is Hungarian, possibly Jewish, probably naturalized in Germany. Special consideration must also be given to Prof. Moro [Heidelberg] who supposedly is Aryan, but descended from a family that has immigrated from the east. He is reputed to have scientific capacity; however, it must be taken into account that his former Jewish assistant medical director is now head of a clinic in Budapest. This relationship might lead to unpleasant incidents.[4]*

In several instances, Zieler vacillated and shifted names of colleagues from one group to the other. The participation of Karl Hermann Vohwinkel, for example, was originally considered to be "mandatory" because Vohwinkel was scheduled to give a lecture in Budapest. The leader of the National Socialist Lecturers' League at the University of Tübingen intervened, however, asserting that Vohwinkel "tends to criticism and gives little credit to the Third Reich and even to the deeds of the Führer. Furthermore, his attitude toward the Jewish question is extremely doubtful."[5] In response to these opinions, Zieler excluded Vohwinkel from the German delegation.

Alois Memmesheimer (fig. 158), chair of dermatology in Essen and, after the war, president of the German Dermatological Society, was originally classified as "acceptable." Subsequently, Zieler changed his mind and advised that Memmesheimer be excluded from the German delegation. The reason was that Memmesheimer had been arrested and jailed on Christmas Eve in 1933, having been accused of slandering a district leader of the party. Although Memmesheimer was later acquitted, his political attitude was in doubt, and he was deemed unreliable.[6]

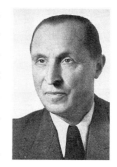

FIG 158
ALOIS
MEMMESHEIMER
(1894–1973)

In similar fashion, Erich Hoffmann's participation in the congress was originally considered important because Hoffmann was the only German who had been invited to give a special lecture of thirty minutes. Furthermore, Hoffmann had donated books of several thousand Marks' value to the German Dermatological Society and, in response, had more or less been promised that he would be allowed to participate.[7] However, in view of Hoffmann's political attitude, the need for his presence in Budapest was reassessed, and he was designated "undesirable." To prevent Hoffmann from traveling, Zieler worked closely with Franz Wirz. In a letter to Wirz, he complained:

The most unpleasant circumstance is Hoffmann's person and his whopping self-complacency. I fully agree with your judgment about his lecture. It is soft-soap, empty gossip, intended only for casting proper light on Hoffmann himself. But what can we do? The lecture or at least its print can no longer be prevented. Doubtlessly, the reputation of German science will not be improved by it and by Hoffmann's appearance. If one allows him to give the lecture, he may work off his complexes. If one prohibits the lecture, he will do harm by his general attitude in Budapest. Hence, we can only prevent him from leaving the country. This would be highly welcome. But is this possible?[8]

Wirz used Zieler's characterization of Hoffmann and of the lecture that Hoffmann had prepared for the congress in Budapest to convince the leader of the German Congress Office to deny Hoffmann a visa for foreign travel. On July 27, he wrote:

> *I hold the opinion that Hoffmann has to be kept away from Budapest under any circumstance. . . . I wish to give only the following reasons: Professor Hoffmann has been removed from his chair in Bonn because of political unreliability. 1.) He has attacked the movement and the Führer in word and deed. 2.) On his last trip to Dutch India, Hoffmann has represented Germany in the most disgraceful way. . . . Professor Schultze, formerly Giessen, now Jena, has heard by chance from a reliable German who traveled with Hoffmann on the ship that he behaved in such an arrogant way that all Germans dissociated themselves from him. . . . It has to be apprehended that slips, such as those quoted here only as an example, cannot be prevented and that Hoffmann will damage the German reputation seriously. Because of all these factors, I ask you to arrange that Hoffmann be denied the visa for travel abroad.*[9]

In any case, Hoffmann had already decided that he would not participate in a congress as a member of a group that claimed to represent German dermatology but that, in fact, was led by a younger colleague who had never even been elected by the society.[10]

The "younger colleague" to whom Hoffmann referred was Karl Zieler, who had been appointed leader of the German delegation by the Reich's and Prussian Ministry of Science and Education. Zieler, a vehement anti-Semite, had been a member of a right-wing nationalistic party from 1919 to 1933 and had refused to take an oath of office sworn on the constitution of the Weimar Republic. Even before the assumption of power by the

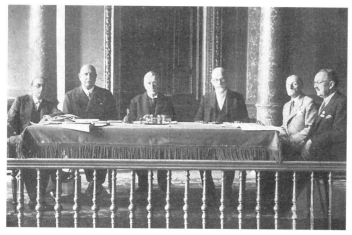

FIG 159 SEMINAR AT THE INTERNATIONAL CONGRESS
OF DERMATOLOGY IN BUDAPEST. BODO SPIETHOFF IS
SECOND FROM THE RIGHT.

Nazis, he flaunted the swastika on his lapel. Later he became a member of the SA and the Nazi party. As leader of the German delegation to Budapest, Zieler attempted to keep his group united, instructed the delegation members to avoid unauthorized discussion of politics in Germany, and told members precisely how to behave. Although he could not have been ignorant of the obvious decline in German dermatology, he steadfastly refused to acknowledge the problem. Instead, he emphasized the number of German delegates serving as faculty at the congress and their favorable seating assignments at official meetings. Zieler tried to compensate for incompetence by showing strength in numbers, a kind of charade that appeared as ridiculous then as it is today. Zieler's most important objective, however, was not achieved. Many German dermatologists whom he had sought to exclude—most of whom were Jewish—came to Budapest anyway through personal invitation from the Hungarian organization committee. The failure to exclude "undesirable elements" from the congress was highly embarrassing to Zieler, and he complained about it bitterly in his official report concerning the congress (figs. 159, 160).

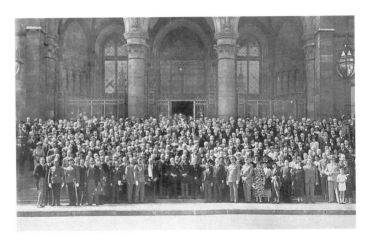

FIG 160 AMONG THE APPROXIMATELY 1000 PARTICIPANTS IN THE
INTERNATIONAL CONGRESS OF DERMATOLOGY IN BUDAPEST IN 1935,
THERE WERE MORE THAN 100 DERMATOLOGISTS FROM GERMANY.

When asked to discuss the failures that occurred in
Budapest, the German congress office in Berlin explained the
matter in a letter to the Reich's and Prussian Ministry of Science and Education thus:

> *The most important grievance was that the Hungarian
> travel agency invited German dermatologists indiscrim-
> inately and directly through a circular, alerting them to
> the fact that all the costs for this trip could be paid in
> Reichsmarks within the confines of Germany.... This is,
> indubitably, an infringement of the rights of the Hun-
> garian travel agency and at the same time also improper
> use of the special credit of the Hungarian government.
> All those abuses and grievances should become impossi-
> ble next year when the intended basic reform of the pass-
> port regulations is carried out. For coming congresses, we
> will have to work towards a decision that the composition
> of the delegations remains within the competence of the
> different national groups so that, in the future, invitations
> to international congresses will not be sent out indiscrim-
> inately by the particular international congress offices,*

but by the national groups. Through such a regulation
it will also become impossible for foreign countries to
more or less determine through invitations who will
represent, as a German speaker, German science at con-
gresses abroad.[11]

In actuality, the regulations governing the attendance of
German physicians at international congresses were soon
made stricter. From then on, every potential attendee had to
be approved by the appropriate ministry and by the German
congress office in Berlin. Physicians who applied for permission to attend international meetings needed both good reasons and good connections. Without them, they were denied
visas and the foreign currency necessary to travel abroad.

But good reasons and good connections were not always
enough if the organizers of international meetings were
judged by the Nazis to be "suspicious." For example, Professor
Weber, a cardiologist at the University of Giessen, was denied
permission to give a lecture at the 1936 Cours International de
Haute Culture Médicale in Brussels solely because the secretary of the congress' consulting board—L.W. Tomarkin from
the University of Athens—was Jewish. Weber asked the chair
of dermatology of the University of Giessen, Walther
Schultze, to intervene on his behalf, arguing that "at the present time, it is not possible to find an international scientific
congress in which Jews will not appear in considerable numbers." Schultze sent Weber's petition to Gerhard Wagner and
assured the Reich's leader of physicians that Weber was "a
man of an absolutely national attitude." Nevertheless, Wagner's office denied permission, stating, "Tomarkin is a Jew, a
former communist, and a man who organizes courses only in
order to enhance his own business."[12]

In 1938, Alfred Stühmer, chair of the Department of Dermatology of the University of Freiburg, was invited to attend
a meeting of the Dermatological Society of Strasbourg. He and
Erich Hoffmann were also asked to join a committee to honor

the University of Strasbourg's chair of dermatology, Lucien Marie Pautrier. Stühmer applied for permission to travel to Strasbourg, which is only about fifty miles from Freiburg. In making his case, he described the French dermatologist hosts as "not at all chauvinistic or hostile to Germans." They were not afraid of Germany, Stühmer said, but of "revolutionary activities" occurring in France. Furthermore, the French were full of "admiration for the calm and order in our country." Pautrier, specifically, was characterized as "absolutely friendly toward Germany." In February 1938, Stühmer and Hoffmann received permission to join the honorary committee, but later that year the permission was revoked. The minister informed them that "belated, sincere objections have arisen in regard to Professor Pautrier." He included a report by the Reich's embassy in Lisbon, according to which Pautrier, three years before, had alluded to anti-German tendencies of French citizens in a lecture about Strasbourg and Alsace.[13]

In March 1939, the chair of the German Dermatological Society, Karl Zieler, asked the Reich's Ministry of Research for instructions on the attendance of German dermatologists at the annual meeting of the Italian Dermatological Society in Bologna. Zieler's problem was that the chair of the Italian Dermatological Society had asked specifically for Erich Hoffmann and Georg Alexander Rost to attend, both of whom were honorary members of that society. In his letter to the ministry, Zieler explained:

> *Prof. Rost is impossible because he has been dismissed from his chair in Freiburg for political reasons in 1933 [although with a pension]. The issue of Prof. Hoffmann is more difficult because he has received permission to travel abroad several times in the past years. As I have reported previously, he has not advanced the German cause on those trips. The Reich's Propaganda Ministry, however, declared that it did not want to interfere. At any rate, it would be highly embarrassing to those who wish to*

attend the meeting of the Italian Dermatological Society in Bologna to meet Prof. Hoffmann there because we would have to expect misbehavior. The purpose of my inquiry is the following: Is there a possibility of an application by me to form a German delegation if only personal invitations are issued? If participants at the Italian meeting were subordinated to me as leader of the delegation in general and in political questions, this would also apply to the professor emeritus of Bonn, Erich Hoffmann. This circumstance alone would presumably be sufficient to prevent him from travelling. Thereby, a trouble-free course that we all wish would be ensured."[14]

In contrast to what had happened at the Ninth International Congress of Dermatology in Budapest four years before, Zieler achieved his objective this time: Neither Hoffmann nor Rost participated in the meeting in Bologna.

In short, the longer the Nazis maintained power, the more complex it became for German scientists to attend congresses in foreign countries. Even those who did receive permission to travel abroad were instructed to contact the local representatives of the German Reich and the NSDAP immediately upon their arrival. After their return to Germany, they were required to write a detailed report about their experience, which had to be submitted in triplicate to the rector of the university.

These regulations ensured nearly complete surveillance of all activity by academics. Furthermore, the attendees of international scientific congresses were turned into spies; their reports were used as sources for political information. Some reports were very rich in that regard. For instance, one by Paul Mulzer, chair of dermatology in Hamburg, after a 1941 trip to a meeting in Budapest stated the following:

We were accommodated at the Elisabeth Sanitarium that is excellently directed by Prof. Dr. Schmidt. Unfor-

tunately, there were a large number of Jews in that san-
itarium who continue to behave in the usual ostentatious
and arrogant way, as they generally do in the former
spas at the Balaton. In private conversation, the popula-
tion rejects the Jews, complains about them, and calls
them the sources of the most ugly anti-German rumors
(which they really are!), but they are there and terror-
ize the people. Some examples: On three high Jewish
holidays, almost all shops were closed because most of
them are in Jewish hands. Neither visitors nor local res-
idents could buy anything on those days. . . . My wife
wanted to buy a comb in a hairdresser's shop. She was
informed that the combs she wished to buy were no
longer available because the English had destroyed all
factories in Germany, including all comb factories. The
Jews had said so. . . . One hates the Jews and wants to get
rid of them but believes that this is impossible for Hun-
gary, partially because high and highest circles of the
society have family bonds with Jewish clans and
because Jews hold positions in public life that cannot be
substituted by Hungarians. I put an end to such discus-
sions by saying that Hungary should not believe that it
would become a sort of national reservation park for
Jews in the new Germany. As already stated, the wish
to get rid of the Jews is universal but one doubts that it
is possible. However, as long as this is not the case and
the Jewish question is not resolved completely, Hungary
will never be a dependable and true ally.[15]

Mulzer's attempts to direct the attention of the German
authorities to the "Jewish question" in Hungary were successful. Almost immediately, connections with Hungarians were
impeded, and Mulzer himself was denied acceptance of an
honorary membership in the Hungarian Dermatological Society because that society was suspected of being "Jewified." At
the same time, the Hungarian government was pressed to

adopt Germany's anti-Jewish legislation, and after the German occupation of Hungary in 1944, more than 450,000 Jews were killed—70 percent of Hungary's Jewish population.[16]

As official regulations and rules of behavior continued to change in German medicine, so did areas of research and the daily activities of physicians. Nazi ideology led to a shift in ethics and principles of morality in medicine, whose highest objective was no longer the health of individual patients but the health of the German people. Medical care for a seriously ill patient could be interpreted as unethical by the Nazis because it interfered with the natural "healthy" process of selection and counterselection. Soon after the Nazis assumed power, Walter Schultze (fig. 161), a physician and Bavaria's new commissioner for health, stated publicly that the time-honored practice of caring for the weak would have to be abandoned "in favor of dedication to those who were racially intact and congenitally sound." He added that "this policy has already begun in our present concentration camps."[17] Schultze—not to be confused with the chair of the Department of Dermatology at the University of Giessen of the same name—was appointed professor of people's health at the University of Munich in 1934 and Reich's leader of lecturers in 1935. His claim to fame in the Nazi party was that, as a surgeon and first SA staff physician, he had treated Hitler's wrenched shoulder during the unsuccessful putsch of November 1923. Because of his involvement during the Nazi period in the killing of at least 380 disabled patients, he was sentenced by a German court to four years in prison in 1960. He died in 1979 at the age of eighty-five.

The new concept of medicine explained by Walter Schultze was at the core of National Socialist policy and was evident in the earliest writings of the movement's founders. In *Mein Kampf* (fig. 162), written during 1924 and 1925, Hitler addressed problems unique to medicine, particularly the fight against venereal diseases. He simplistically proposed to fight syphilis by putting an end to the "prostitution of

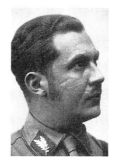

FIG 161
WALTER SCHULTZE
(1894–1979)

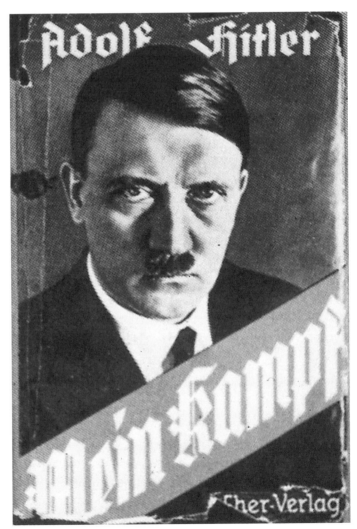

FIG 162 *MEIN KAMPF*, THE "BIBLE" OF NATIONAL SOCIALISM.

love " and referred to the use of Salvarsan—the first effective chemotherapeutic agent in medicine, which had been developed by the Jewish Nobel laureate Paul Ehrlich—as "the crafty application of a questionable drug."[18] That this drug could be used effectively meant nothing to Hitler, because the individuals who had contracted syphilis were hardly human beings in his eyes and were just a health risk to the nation.

Dermatologists were pleased by Hitler's interest in venereal diseases and tried to use it to improve the status of their specialty at German universities.[19] According to Bodo Spiethoff, venereal diseases especially had to be fought because they impaired fitness for military service and led to the birth of "inferior human beings who are a burden to the public. . . . Especially youth of high racial value are at risk of impotency and inability of parturition because of venereal diseases."[20] In an editorial on the occasion of his appointment as leader of the German Society for the Fight Against Venereal Diseases, Spiethoff emphasized:

> *The state, born by the national revolution, is conscious of the fact that not only hygienic but also important national and ethical aspects are linked to the fight against venereal diseases. For that purpose, the state has to count on unconditional obedience of the German Society for the Fight Against Venereal Diseases. I consider it my duty to secure that collaboration, in investing the activities of the German Society for the Fight Against Venereal Diseases with the ethos of our new national state, and in eliminating any non-German thinking and feeling. In the fight against venereal diseases, everybody should be guided by the idea that, in the words of our Führer, Adolf Hitler, the fight against this plague is not only one task, but the main task of the nation.[21]*

Together with this editorial, Hitler's remarks on syphilis were reprinted, without any qualifying comment, in the *Communications of the German Society for the Fight Against Venereal Diseases* and were presented as the model for how German medicine would be practiced in the future. The only German dermatologist who protested the publication in a medical journal of Hitler's ignorant remarks was, once again, Erich Hoffmann. His protest, however, was regarded only as evidence, in the words of Bodo Spiethoff, that "Mr. Hoffmann has an inwardly alien attitude to our Führer and National Socialism."[22]

As a consequence of the Nazis' distorted view of the human condition, persons with venereal diseases were treated like criminals rather than as patients. Walther Krantz, the new chair of dermatology in Göttingen, called them "mainly antisocial, inferior mentally, defective in character, and psychopaths."[23] In Stadtroda, near Jena, the dermatologist Walther Schultze, who, at that time, was still the director of the skin clinic in Jena, opened a ward for venereal disease patients. Those "antisocial individuals" were confined compulsorily and released only after evidence of good conduct. Further degradation came in the form of enforced labor. In Schultze's view, "the therapy of work is essential. By manual work, the incarcerated subjects shall contribute to reduce the burden of the public to a minimum. By severe physical strain, we want to put those with an aversion to work on another track, to discipline them, and also to achieve a deterrent effect on others."[24]

The Third Reich regarded individuals as organic parts of a racially defined people's community. They were considered worthy only if they played their part in the commonweal by being strong and productive, functioning like healthy cells in a healthy body. Disabled persons were defamed as parasites of the nation, and published statistics demonstrated what were perceived to be unreasonably high costs to the state of caring for them. For example, the yearly cost to the Prussian state to care for blind or deaf pupils was 1,500 Reichsmarks, compared to 125 Reichsmarks for unimpaired children. Statistics, pamphlets, and posters informed German citizens of how much they suffered from the terrible burden of caring for persons with hereditary diseases (figs. 163, 165). Even schoolbooks told, in distorted terms, of the prohibitive cost of caring for and rehabilitating the chronically sick and permanently crippled. One of the problems posed to high school students in a widely used mathematics textbook asked how many new housing units could be built and how many marriage-

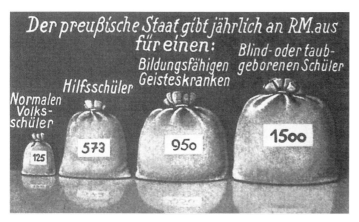

Der preußische Staat gibt jährlich an RM.aus
für einen:
Normalen Volks- schüler
Hilfsschüler
Bildungsfähigen Geisteskranken
Blind- oder taub- geborenen Schüler
125
573
950
1500

FIG 163 NAZI POSTER COMPARING THE YEARLY EXPENDITURES OF THE PRUSSIAN STATE FOR "NORMAL, BACKWARD, MENTALLY DISABLED, AND BLIND OR DEAF PUPILS."

allowance loans could be given to newlywed couples for the amount of money it cost the state to care for "the crippled, the criminal, and the insane."[25]

These exercises in propaganda were undertaken by the Nazis to pave the way for legislative measures designed to restrict the rights of disabled people. The first measure taken was a law on the enforcement of sterilization. The Nazis argued that existing principles of health care and social welfare encouraged reproduction of people with little value who would soon outnumber the nation's valuable citizens. To maintain the health of the nation, it was therefore mandatory that the reproduction of "inferior human beings" be restricted.

These ideas were not new. They had been advanced in the late nineteenth century by Francis Galton (fig. 164), a cousin of Charles Darwin, who sought to enhance the genetic quality of the human race by restricting the birth rate of the "unfit" and encouraging the reproduction of the "fit." Within a short time, Galton's proposals—promulgated under the terms "eugenics" and "racial hygiene"—gained popularity, especially in Germany, where a philosophy based on inequality of human beings found a firm foothold in a nation without a democratic tradition.

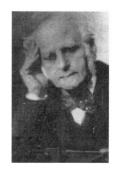

FIG 164
FRANCIS GALTON
(1822–1911)

141

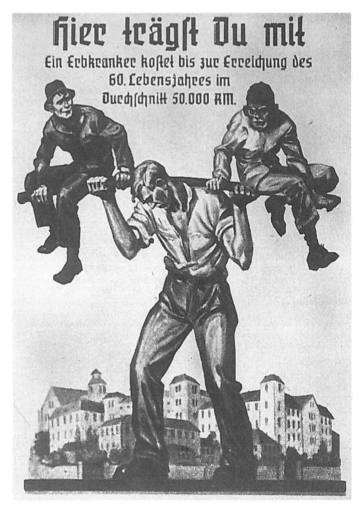

FIG 165 NAZI POSTER DEMONSTRATING THE BURDEN PERSONS WITH
HEREDITARY DISEASES REPRESENT FOR THE PUBLIC.

In the last years of the Weimar Republic, the issue of eugenics was addressed in public forums often. In addition to "positive eugenics," such as financial support for healthy couples who tried to start a family, there was a strong call for measures of "negative eugenics" directed against citizens who suffered from chronic diseases. The theory of eugenic sterilization found wide public support, and legislative measures on eugenics were under preparation by the Prussian government.[26]

Germany was not the first country to consider eugenic sterilizations. In 1907, the state of Indiana in the United States had
passed a law allowing compulsory sterilization of the mentally
ill and of the criminally insane. By the late 1920s, 28 states of
the United States and one province in Canada had enacted legislation that resulted in the sterilization of some 15,000 men and
women before the year 1930 arrived. For the Nazis, the laws of
the United States served as a model and were quoted frequently
in support of their own policy.[27]

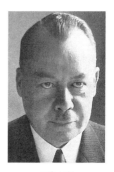

In contrast to other German parties, the Nazis were advocates
of compulsory measures and insisted on the need to banish false
sentimentality. According to Hitler, compulsory sterilization for
hereditary diseases was "the most humane act for mankind."[28]
Hitler's strong stand in favor of compulsory sterilization
attracted many physicians, especially gynecologists, psychia-
trists, and public health experts. One example is Hans Reiter
(fig. 166), for whom Reiter's disease is named. Reiter was a
fanatic anti-Semite and one of the main proponents of racial
hygiene. Since 1919, as an adjunct professor in Rostock, he had
taught hygienics with a strong racist emphasis. He was an avid
disciple of Hitler, had joined the Nazi party early on, and in 1932
claimed a deputy's seat for the NSDAP in the parliament of the
state of Mecklenburg. In the same year, he was a member of the
first group of professors to sign an oath of allegiance to Hitler.

After the Nazis' assumption of power, Reiter had a meteoric
career. In 1933, he was appointed honorary professor of
hygiene at the University of Berlin; the following year, at the
behest of the minister of internal affairs, he directed the Fed-
eration of Scientific Societies, which by then had taken over
all functions of the defunct National Health Office. In 1935,
Reiter was appointed president of the Robert Koch Institute
for Infectious Diseases, and until 1945 he represented Germany at the International Health Organization in Paris.[29] As
one of the leading figures in German medicine, Reiter was
instrumental in countless decisions that involved medical
ethics, including the institution of medical experiments on

internees of concentration camps. An example of that research is a series of studies on a vaccine against epidemic typhus for which prisoners at the concentration camp at Buchenwald were infected with *Rickettsia prowazekii*. Some of them had been vaccinated before being infected, whereas others had not been given the vaccine and served as a control group. More than 250 prisoners succumbed to the disease.[30] In 1945, Reiter was interned in an American camp where, according to his own testimony, he was "treated very decently" and asked to put his experiences in public health on paper. After his release, Reiter continued to practice medicine in Kassel, where he died in 1969 at the age of eighty-eight.[31]

Although a bill on eugenic sterilization had been formulated in the last years of the Weimar Republic, some changes still had to be made before it could pass into law. Most notable was the patient's consent clause, which had been included in the original version submitted to the Prussian parliament. In the final draft written by the Nazis, this clause was omitted. The Law for the Prevention of Genetically Diseased Offspring, promulgated on July 14, 1933, provided the legal basis for enforced sterilization by instructing that the mutilating operation "must be performed even against the will of the person to be sterilized. The attending surgeon must request any necessary assistance from the police authority. If other measures are insufficient, it is permissible to use direct force." Insurance companies and "the one who has been sterilized" were to be billed for the operation.[32]

The Law for the Prevention of Genetically Diseased Offspring, however, was only the foundation on which the tower of racial hygiene was to be built. Initially, only a few indications for sterilization were mentioned specifically—congenital mental retardation, congenital blindness, congenital deafness, and severe malformations—yet soon the list of diseases lengthened. In a 1934 official comment on the Law for the Prevention of Genetically Diseased Offspring, the authors emphasized that "the law is merely a remarkable start, and

Gesetz zur Verhütung erbkranken Nachwuchses

vom 14. Juli 1933

mit Auszug aus dem Gesetz gegen gefährliche Gewohnheitsverbrecher
und über Maßregeln der Sicherung und Besserung vom 24. Nov. 1933

Bearbeitet und erläutert von

Dr. med. Arthur Gütt
Ministerialdirektor
im Reichsministerium des Innern

Dr. med. Ernst Rüdin
o. ö. Professor für Psychiatrie an der Universität und Direktor
des Kaiser Wilhelm-Instituts für Genealogie und Demographie
der Deutschen Forschungsanstalt für Psychiatrie in München

Dr. jur. Falk Ruttke
Geschäftsführer des Reichsausschusses für Volksgesundheitsdienst
beim Reichsministerium des Innern

Mit Beiträgen:

Die Eingriffe zur Unfruchtbarmachung des Mannes
und zur Entmannung
von Geheimrat Prof. Dr. med. Erich Lexer, München

Die Eingriffe zur Unfruchtbarmachung der Frau
von Geheimrat Prof. Dr. med. Albert Döberlein, München

Mit 15 zum Teil farbigen Abbildungen

J. F. Lehmanns Verlag / München 1934

FIG 167 TITLE PAGE OF AN INTERPRETATIVE COMMENT ON THE LAW FOR THE PREVENTION OF HEREDITARILY DISEASED OFFSPRING. IN MARCH 1934, THE REICH'S PHYSICIANS LEADER, GERHARD WAGNER, REQUIRED THAT ALL PHYSICIANS PURCHASE THIS BOOK AT THE SPECIAL PRICE OF 5 REICHSMARKS.

that supplements to it will always be possible as scientific knowledge evolves" (fig. 167).[35]

Practitioners of every medical specialty were asked to assist and contribute to the ever-widening reach of the law, among them Karl Hoede, an assistant of Zieler at the Department of

Dermatology of the University of Würzburg. Throughout his professional life, Hoede had been interested in the genetic aspects of cutaneous diseases, especially psoriasis. When the Nazis assumed power, he continued to pursue this interest, particularly with regard to the new requirements of eugenics, and asked colleagues for their support. At the Seventeenth Congress of the German Dermatological Society held in Berlin in October 1934, Hoede gave a lecture titled, "The Dermatologist and Genetic Care," which began with these words: "At all times and among all peoples, the direction of scientific research has been profoundly influenced by political aims, as long as the leading men of different peoples succeeded in setting forward healthy political aims, and as long as the scientists had remained, or had ever been in regard to their blood, true children of their people, children of their country who knew what the people's body needed. In this respect, until last year, the conditions necessary for collaboration of dermatologists in Germany were worse than in any other field of medicine."[34] After this brief and not so subtle reference to the past Jewification of German dermatology, Hoede turned to the "drastic and effective measures" the Nazis had since instituted to restore the health of the people. "Skin diseases," he said, "have hitherto not been taken into account in the Law for the Prevention of Genetically Diseased Offspring. . . . To achieve clarity and to survey skin diseases in that regard, the traditional morphologic and histologic classifications are insufficient. After all, all skin diseases are more or less dependent on genetic influences. The crucial question is whether a condition is predominantly, substantially, or only partially caused by genetic factors."[35]

These considerations led Hoede to propose a new classification of skin diseases. In his view, any skin disease that was predominantly caused by genetic factors had to be included in the Law for the Prevention of Genetically Diseased Offspring. This included xeroderma pigmentosum, hydroa vacciniforme, epidermolysis bullosa hereditaria, and congenital hyperker-

atoses, including palmoplantar keratodermas. Another disease
mentioned in this context was neurofibromatosis of von Recklinghausen. The diseases characterized by a "substantial"
influence of genetic factors included acroasphyxia, adenoma
sebaceum, certain types of "eczemas," and above all psoriasis.
"From the standpoint of genetic care," Hoede declared, "one
cannot help a patient with psoriasis . . . any better than a
patient with hemophilia who is ordered never to injure himself to prevent bleeding." Hoede did not demand enforced sterilization for patients with psoriasis but insisted that "a decision
is badly needed to clarify in which patients with cutaneous diseases 'marriage is not in the best interest of the people.'" He
concluded, obtusely, that "all physicians should participate in
studies about hereditary factors. . . . In my view, the main task
of the next years for German physicians is collaboration in taking stock of the German people in matters of genobiology.
Only in that way will it be possible to overcome the troublesome, initially necessary determination and collection of singular signs of genetic burden and to find, at last, the type and
extension of the existing genetic lines of the people."[36]

Hoede and others considered the "genetic mapping" of the
entire German population to be a scientific foundation on
which future decisions about selection and counterselection
could be based. In practice, however, decisions about enforced
sterilization were arbitrary and, in most instances, made without any pretension to scientific credibility. The decision about
whether a person should be sterilized was based on the
"expert opinions" of medical officers whose education and
conscientiousness varied greatly. Very few were really experts
or specialists; about half were young, inexperienced assistants.
Patients considered for sterilization were usually examined
only once, and the report about them generally contained only
brief remarks by physicians about social behavior and conduct
in school. No serious attempt was made to take a patient's history, to conduct a thorough examination, or to discuss symptoms or signs of the purported disease. Because most diseases

specified by the law—among them schizophrenia, epilepsy, and Huntington's chorea—were not definitely known to be inherited, comments such as "heredity is definite but cannot be proven" were often found in the reports.

Enforced sterilization was not restricted to patients with supposedly inherited diseases. In accordance with official comments on the Law for the Prevention of Genetically Diseased Offspring, sterilization also was performed on persons considered to be socially inferior, among them alcoholics, prostitutes, and criminals. The threat of enforced sterilization was commonly used to coerce cooperative behavior.

Requests to perform enforced sterilization were considered by special genetic health courts. The hearings, to which patients were often dragged by the police, usually took place in district court buildings outside the scrutiny of the public and lasted, on average, about five minutes. In most instances, the decision had already been made before the hearing convened and on the basis of information in the files. Relatively few requests for sterilization were rejected, because the accuser and the judge were often the same person. In the first two years of the courts' existence, patients had the right to lodge a complaint based on a counter-report by an expert consultant of their own choice. In 1936, this right was withdrawn by Gerhard Wagner.[37]

According to data from the Reich's Ministry of Justice, some 240,000 enforced sterilizations were requested between 1934 and 1936; about 200,000 were carried out, whereas only about 10 percent of requests were denied. Altogether, approximately 360,000 patients were sterilized—almost 1 percent of the German population between eighteen and forty years of age. Sterilizations took place in hospitals scattered across Germany that were specifically authorized to perform the procedure. New surgical techniques were developed to guarantee that fertilization would never again be possible. Mortality associated with these operations was higher than generally believed. About 5,000 patients, mostly women, died because of the procedure.[38]

Enforced sterilization was only a first step in the realization of the Nazi goal of racial hygiene. The mass murder of mentally disabled patients, euphemistically called euthanasia, was the next. The direct order for euthanasia was given by Hitler on September 1, 1939, the same day that World War II began when he ordered the invasion of Poland. An organization was soon established to expedite the program, and all state institutions were required to report to the government those patients who had been ill for five or more years and who were unable to work. Data on the patients had to be provided on questionnaires, including name, race, marital status, nationality, frequency of visits and by whom, the person who bore financial responsibility, and so forth. Decisions as to which patients would be killed were based entirely on this kind of scant information and were made by "expert" consultants who never actually saw the patients. The consultants were paid for the number of questionnaires assessed. For 500 questionnaires, they got 100 Reichsmarks per month, and this amount could be increased to 400 Reichsmarks per month if more than 3,500 questionnaires were appraised. That one consultant assessed 2,109 questionnaires in only two weeks illustrates the indifference with which decisions were made. The Charitable Transport Company for the Sick carried patients to killing centers where they were gassed and their corpses burned. The Charitable Foundation for Institutional Care then collected fees to cover the cost of the killing from relatives of the victim, who were not told the real reason for the charges. The cause of death was falsified in death certificates.[39]

Despite the Nazis' attempts to cover up the euthanasia program, its dimensions were too great to be hidden from the public. In the obituary sections of newspapers, the names of killing centers were mentioned with increasing frequency, until publication of those obituaries was forbidden. In certain towns, citizens began to recognize the vehicles in which patients were transported to liquidation institutions and came to know the reasons for the heavy smoke billowing from the

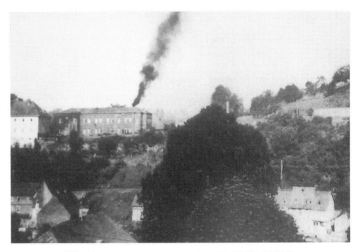

FIG 168 THE EUTHANASIA CENTER IN HADAMAR, CLOSE TO LIMBURG, IN 1941. SMOKE CAN BE SEEN BILLOWING FROM CREMATORIA.

buildings (fig. 168). Children on the streets called out, "They are taking some more people to be gassed," and rumors soon spread that homes for the aged were to be cleaned out next. Increasing public unrest and the protests of the church finally induced the Nazis to halt the euthanasia program officially in August 1941. By that time, at least 70,000 patients had been killed. It was calculated that the removal of these patients from the wards saved hospital expenses of "245,955.50 Reichsmarks per day," or "88,543,980.00 Reichsmarks per year." After 1941, the killing of patients continued unofficially as "wild euthanasia" until the end of the war and, occasionally, even beyond it.[40]

Just as enforced sterilization was a prelude to the killing of the chronically ill, euthanasia was only the beginning of an extermination of far greater magnitude. According to National Socialist ideology, the wholesale killing of Jews also qualified as euthanasia, because being Jewish in itself was a disease. In his blatant plan for the future, *Mein Kampf*, Hitler referred to Jews as "bacilli," ever ready to "poison the blood of the national body." He lamented the fact that Jewish "poison was able to penetrate the bloodstream of our people unhindered and do its work, and the state did not possess the power to control the disease."

Taking their cue as usual from Hitler, Leonardo Conti, the Reich's Leader of Health, stated that Jews could only survive "parasitically inside the people," and Rudolf Ramm, a medical officer on Conti's staff, wrote that Jews put the German people at risk through "the contagion of poisonous ideas and the destruction of germinating life." Auschwitz physician/killer Fritz Klein explained to a female inmate doctor that because he was a doctor, he wanted "to preserve life." It was "out of the respect for human life" that he would "remove a gangrenous appendix from a diseased body. The Jew is the gangrenous appendix in the body of mankind" (see fig. 170).[41]

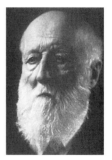

FIG 169
GEORG STICKER
(1860–1960)

Georg Sticker (fig. 169), professor of the history of medicine at the University of Würzburg, wrote the following in 1933 in the prestigious *Münchener Medizinische Wochenschrift*:

> *The German people . . . has often been close . . . to giving away its house, stove, and right of homeland to parasitic rabble that hardly has a right to live. At last it feels that its own existence means duty, and that destiny demands from everybody willing to live to maintain himself. A Führer has arisen with a strong will who speaks out on what we have to want and ought to do, unconcerned of the whimpering of a false, hypocritical humanity. If the German people, says Adolf Hitler, wants to recover and continue to live, it has to recognize the duties of the national racial state and must not have ears for the weaklings who cry and bemoan interferences in the holy rights of men.[42]*

Sticker had been the first to teach dermatology at the University of Giessen and was author of the chapter on the history of venereal diseases in Jadassohn's *Handbuch* and of monographs on the history of plague, cholera, and leprosy. Sticker also described and named erythema infectiosum.

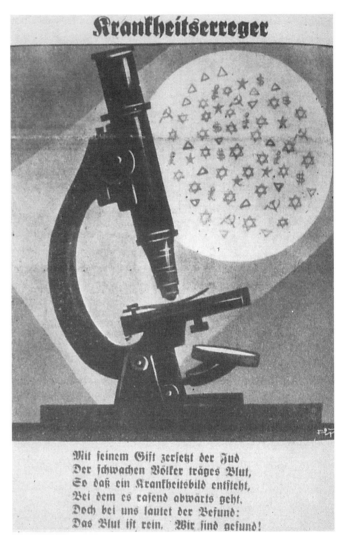

FIG 170 "INFECTIOUS GERMS": CARTOON FROM THE ANTI-SEMITIC
JOURNAL *DER STÜRMER*. THE POEM AT THE BOTTOM READS: "WITH
HIS POISON, THE JEW UNDERMINES THE SLUGGISH BLOOD OF WEAK
PEOPLES SO THAT A DISEASE ARISES THAT CAUSES DETERIORATION
RAPIDLY. WITH US, HOWEVER, THE DIAGNOSIS IS DIFFERENT: THE
BLOOD IS PURE. WE ARE HEALTHY!"

In short, the wholesale killing of Jews was prepared spiritu-
ally not only by leading Nazis but also by established leaders
of medicine, such as Georg Sticker. For them, Adolf Hitler
was the "physician of the German people," and the annihila-

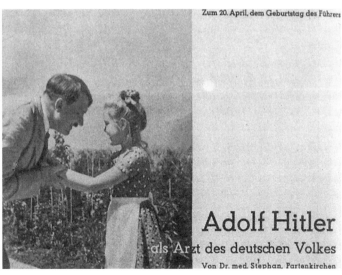

Zum 20. April, dem Geburtstag des Führers

Adolf Hitler
als Arzt des deutschen Volkes
Von Dr. med. Stephan, Partenkirchen

FIG 171 "ADOLF HITLER AS PHYSICIAN OF THE GERMAN PEOPLE."

tion of Jews was "killing in the name of healing," a realization of principles of racial hygiene inherent in that so-called
medical discipline (fig. 171).

Principles of racial hygiene had been discussed in German
medical circles before Hitler's ascension to power. In the late
nineteenth century, an optimistic vision of a better mankind,
based on principles of Darwinism, induced many physicians to
demand measures to stimulate the reproduction of healthy citizens. Racial hygiene was considered to be an integral part of
preventive medicine that sought to eliminate diseases before
their development. Other purposes of preventive medicine
were better working conditions and free health care for workers and their families. Physicians with socialist leanings who
practiced in the industrial suburbs of major cities became proponents of social hygiene. They sought to counter the industrial society's detrimental effects on the health of the working
class, including poverty that inhibited the growth of children,
led to alcoholism, and fostered occupational diseases. Because
of the high incidence of venereal diseases in rapidly growing
industrial centers, dermatovenereologists were prominently

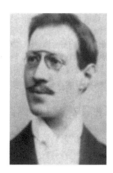

FIG 172
IWAN BLOCH
(1872–1922)

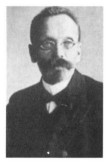

FIG 173
ALFRED BLASCHKO
(1858–1922)

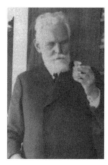

FIG 174
ALFRED PLOETZ
(1860–1940)

involved in that movement. Most of them were Jewish: for example, Iwan Bloch (fig. 172), a disciple of Paul Gerson Unna, who was a pioneer in sexual medicine, and Alfred Blaschko (fig. 173), who in 1901 called attention to a system of lines in the human skin along which many linear epidermal nevi and even some inflammatory diseases course. Those lines are now known eponymically for him.

As a medical student in the mid-1870s, Blaschko belonged to a circle that gathered around the revisionist politician, Eduard Bernstein. In 1877, Blaschko and his fellow students, Hermann Lisso and Ignaz Zadek, founded a secret socialist society in the anatomical dissection rooms of the University of Berlin. After Bismarck's ban on socialist parties had been lifted, those political parties campaigned for a municipal health policy in Berlin. In 1902, Blaschko was one of the founders and the first secretary of the German Society for the Fight Against Venereal Diseases and soon became involved in educational and legislative measures to prevent those maladies. As a leading representative of social hygiene, Blaschko was consulted by the founder of racial hygiene, Alfred Ploetz (fig. 174), who sought to amalgamate the different currents of preventive medicine. Social hygiene and racial hygiene were claimed to be different aspects of the same discipline. When the German Society of Racial Hygiene was founded in 1905, Blaschko was among its earliest members. Other renowned members and sponsors of the German Society of Racial Hygiene were Alois Alzheimer, Ludwig Aschoff, Alfred Grotjahn, Otto Lubarsch, and Julius Wagner-Jauregg, to mention but a few.[43] In 1920, Blaschko was one of the authors of a pamphlet about health education that was distributed to all those who intended to marry. It emphasized the value of health to the individual, the importance of health for the breeding of promising future generations, and the "holy duty" of marrying a healthy partner to avoid eugenic perils.[44]

The strong link to social hygiene helped establish racial hygiene at German universities. In the 1920s and early 1930s, teachers of medicine with anthropological leanings began to give instruction in racial hygiene. Early on, the teaching of racial hygiene was not done in a systematic fashion. Established medical schools were reluctant to accept racial hygiene as a subject worthy of serious medical study, and few degrees in racial hygiene were ever granted. With the rise of the Nazis, however, the status of racial hygiene changed almost overnight. Hitler, backed by Rudolf Hess and Gerhard Wagner, endorsed the institutionalization of racist-eugenic organizations and pledged support for them by the party or state. On July 14, 1933, Max Planck, the president of the prestigious Kaiser Wilhelm Society, wrote these lines to the minister of the interior: "Herr Reichsminister, I am honoured to most humbly inform you that the Kaiser Wilhelm Society for the Advancement of Sciences is willing to systematically serve the Reich in all aspects pertinent to research on racial hygiene."[45] Within a matter of months, medical faculty positions in racial science were established, and in 1933, Hitler appointed Fritz Lenz (fig. 175) to the first full chair of racial hygiene at the highly visible University of Berlin. Throughout German universities, this appointment was followed by the establishment of many more faculty positions, generally at the level of full professor, devoted to the "science of race."

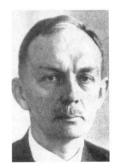

FIG 175
FRITZ LENZ
(1887–1976)

In an attempt to give the Nazi philosophy of race the appearance of true science, studies were designed to demonstrate a relationship between race and distinct types of behavior, such as antisocial behavior and criminality (figs. 176, 177). Identifying race-specific attributes of Jews was a popular field of "scientific" research. According to the findings in one study, Jews were more afraid of disease, more dependent on physicians, and more often affected by diabetes, blindness, deafness, and neural and mental disorders than non-Jews. Jews were found to have committed fewer violent crimes but showed a greater tendency to defamation, deceit, and forgery of documents. "Racial scientists" hoped to establish new criteria for differentiating one race from another. Alfred Böttcher, professor of medicine in Hannover, even recommended the applica-

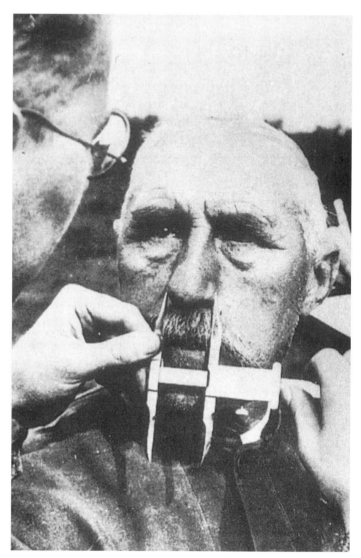

FIG 176 "BASIC RESEARCH" IN RACIAL HYGIENE:
A "SCIENTIFIC" EXAMINATION OF NOSE WIDTH.

tion of racial science to the practical goal of "making the blood
of the Jew become apparent in a test tube."[46]

Medical studies on racial factors were undertaken not only by
newly appointed professors of racial hygiene but also by practitioners of other medical specialties. Those who hoped for swift
academic promotion ingratiated themselves with the new polit-

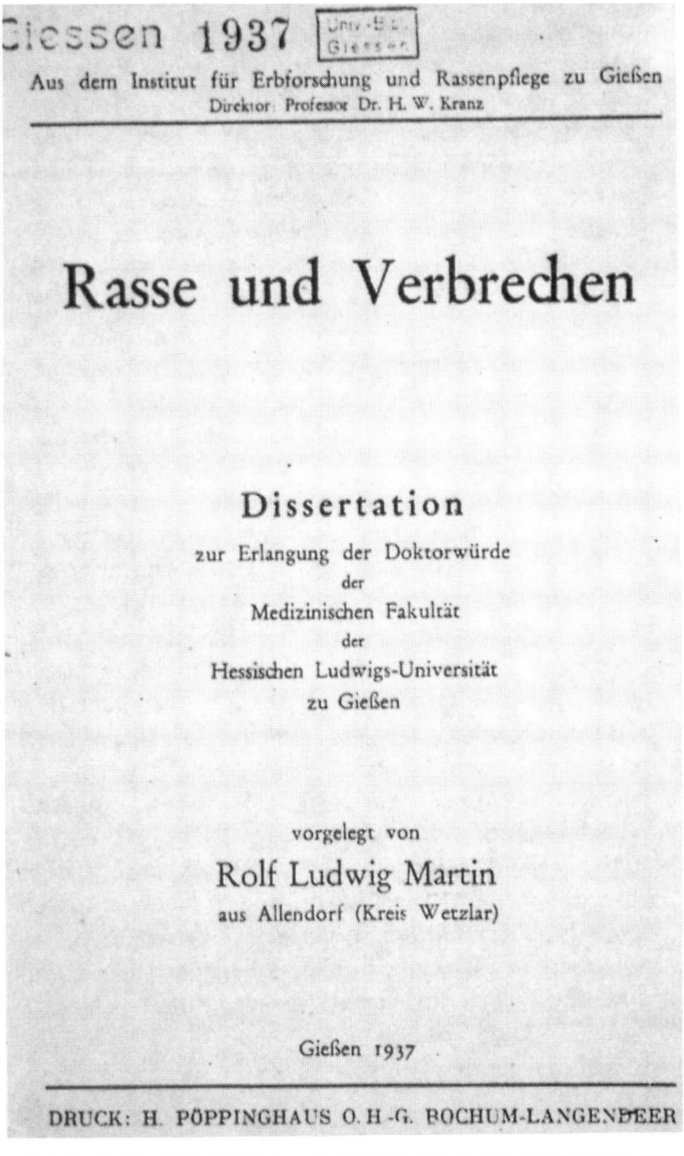

Giessen 1937 [Univ.-B. Giessen]

Aus dem Institut für Erbforschung und Rassenpflege zu Gießen
Direktor Professor Dr. H. W. Kranz

Rasse und Verbrechen

Dissertation

zur Erlangung der Doktorwürde

der

Medizinischen Fakultät

der

Hessischen Ludwigs-Universität

zu Gießen

vorgelegt von

Rolf Ludwig Martin

aus Allendorf (Kreis Wetzlar)

Gießen 1937

DRUCK: H. PÖPPINGHAUS O. H.-G. BOCHUM-LANGENDREER

FIG 177 "RACE AND CRIME," M.D. THESIS FROM THE INSTITUTE FOR
GENETIC RESEARCH AND PRESERVATION OF RACE, GIESSEN, 1937.

ical leadership by incorporating into their lectures and articles
as many aspects of race as possible. Heinrich Adolf Gottron, an
assistant professor of dermatology at the Charité Hospital in
Berlin, was a prolific contributor to books and journals devoted
to racial hygiene. In 1934, Gottron published an article titled

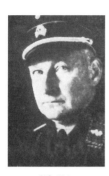

FIG 178
WILHELM KLEIN
(BORN 1887)

"Constitution and Skin Diseases," in which he discussed distinct racial odors. In 1935, when he was appointed chair of dermatology in Breslau, he demanded that the growing knowledge about the genetic foundation of diseases be put to practical purposes, "especially for the activities of physicians in regard to the prevention of hereditarily diseased offspring. . . . It is the task of us doctors to utilize the newly acquired knowledge of genetics for the reconstruction of our people in accordance with the guidelines of our leadership."[47]

Karl Zieler pointed out that the fundamentals of racial hygiene were essential "to work against the deterioration of the overall genetic heritage of our people in regard to health and race."[48]

Opportunism did not always present itself in obvious fashion. Established academic professors asked to contribute chapters to new textbooks on racial hygiene were not expected to be overtly racist; a few hints here and there were sufficient. The desired effect was achieved by integrating often moderate articles into a clearly National Socialist context. This strategy is illustrated in the 1934 textbook *Constitutional and Genetic Biology in the Practice of Medicine* by Walther Jaensch, professor of constitutional medicine at the University of Berlin. Among the contributors to it were prominent proponents of racial hygiene, such as Fritz Lenz, new director of the Institute of Racial Hygiene at the University of Berlin, and leading medical officials of the Nazi party, like Wilhelm Klein (fig. 178), medical adviser of Berlin, who was responsible for the dismissal, torture, and killing of many Jewish physicians. Their chapters, which appeared in the "general" section of the book, were "The Importance of Racial Hygiene for the German People," "The Office of Racial Policies of the NSDAP," and "Health Care in the Third Reich." Those chapters taught students that the natural process of selection and counterselection had to be supported by the state, that mixing human races was bound to result in progressive deterioration of the state, and that opposition to the Law for the Prevention

KONSTITUTIONS- UND ERBBIOLOGIE

IN DER PRAXIS DER MEDIZIN

Herausgegeben von

WALTHER JAENSCH

1 9 3 4

JOHANN AMBROSIUS BARTH·VERLAG·LEIPZIG

FIG 179 TITLE PAGE OF THE TEXTBOOK *CONSTITUTIONAL AND GENETIC BIOLOGY IN THE PRACTICE OF MEDICINE.*

of Genetically Diseased Offspring came perilously close to high treason (figs. 179, 180).

The chapters in the second, "special" part of Jaensch's textbook were of more solid medical content and were written by established pedagogues of medicine who did not shrink from closing ranks with unbridled racists such as Lenz and Klein. Among the more than twenty contributors were three dermatologists: Walter Frieboes, chair of dermatology at the Charité

Inhaltsverzeichnis

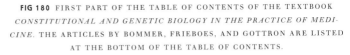

FIG 180 FIRST PART OF THE TABLE OF CONTENTS OF THE TEXTBOOK
*CONSTITUTIONAL AND GENETIC BIOLOGY IN THE PRACTICE OF MEDI-
CINE.* THE ARTICLES BY BOMMER, FRIEBOES, AND GOTTRON ARE LISTED
AT THE BOTTOM OF THE TABLE OF CONTENTS.

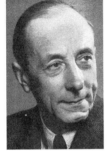

FIG 181
SIGWALD BOMMER
(1893–1963)

Hospital in Berlin; Sigwald Bommer (fig. 181), the future chair
of dermatology at the University of Greifswald; and Heinrich
Adolf Gottron, the future chair of dermatology at the University of Breslau. Their articles addressed dietary management
and genetic elements of cutaneous diseases and were relatively
free of racist notions. Nevertheless, without contributions from
them, the book would not have come to fruition.[49]

Fanaticism and opportunism soon established racial hygiene as an independent medical specialty, and in the process German medical students became imbued with Nazi racial doctrines. In Frankfurt, for instance, Otmar Freiherr von Verschuer, the mentor of Auschwitz killer physician Josef Mengele, was in charge of training medical students in "racial care" and of instructing them in the laws of the regime pertinent to the subject. Techniques for examination of potential marriage partners in regard to "conjugal fitness" (inadvertently humorously termed "congenital pathology") were as integral to the Frankfurt curriculum as were "hereditary diagnosis," "hereditary prognosis," and "sterilization assessment." In "racial science," miscegenation—especially involving Aryans and Jews—and racial differences were included in the course of medical study. In 1936, racial hygiene became a compulsory subject on examinations for medical students.[50]

In addition to racial hygiene, German medicine was "enriched" by another new discipline, "natural health science," also referred to as "new German healing." The new discipline exhibited a decided aversion to conventional specialized medicine with its often impersonal modes of treatment, a bias that was already becoming apparent during the years of the Weimar Republic. In reaction to this perception of allopathic medicine, the number of "healers" and hack physicians in Germany had increased greatly. Nazi doctrine held that official medicine was Jewified medicine and that medications given by Jewish doctors suppressed natural healing and had but a single purpose—to profit Jewish stockholders in the pharmaceutical industry (fig. 182). The Nazis did not think in terms of mechanisms of disease or disturbances of particular organs but advocated "holistic" medicine in which the entire human being would be restored by living in a natural way.

The principles of natural health science, as in racial hygiene, were rooted firmly in National Socialist ideology. Just as individuals were significant only as parts of a racially defined community, so, too, organs of the human body were important only in the context of the whole being. Specialization by physicians

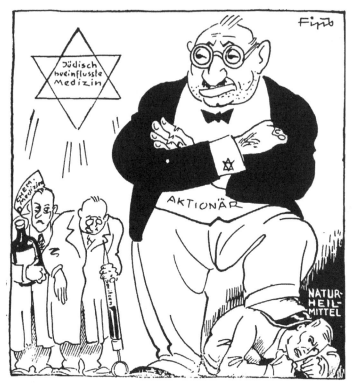

FIG 182 "JEWIFIED MEDICINE" IN THE EYES OF THE NAZIS. THE
JEWISH STOCKHOLDER (MIDDLE) CONTROLS HIS SLAVES IN OFFICIAL
MEDICINE (LEFT) WHILE AT THE SAME TIME SUPPRESSING
"NATURAL" HEALTH TREATMENT (RIGHT).

was discouraged. The National Socialist ideal of the German
doctor was a general practitioner who, in making house calls,
would attend the needs of the smallest cell in the community—
the family—and serve as a sort of biological block warden and
monitor on behalf of the party for the health of the nation. In
the Nazi paradigm, the general practitioner was diligent and
humble, living a stressful but honest life in the country, close to
nature and far away from erosive influences of modern civiliza-
tion: materialism, air pollution, and Jews.[51]

Proximity to nature and to hardy peasants, whom the Nazis
mythicized as still possessing the unspoiled qualities of their
Germanic forebears, was central to "new German healing."
Health was not a gift, they believed, but a duty every German

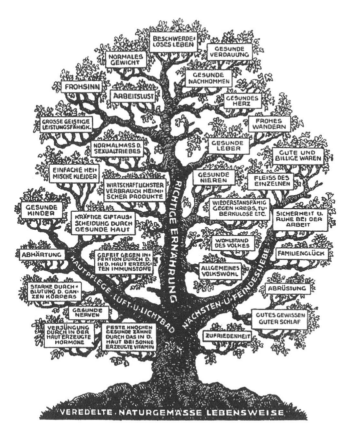

FIG 183 PROPAGANDA OF THE NATURAL HEALTH MOVEMENT: THE
TREE OF AN "ENNOBLED NATURAL FORM OF LIVING." THE TWIGS
ARE "SIMPLE DOMESTIC CLOTHING," "HARDENING," "HAPPY
HIKING," "SAFE AND QUIET WORK," ETC.

owed the fatherland and one that could be fulfilled best by living a simple and natural life; by devoting oneself to work, family, and development of a happy mind; by exposure to sun, wind,
and the gifts of the German soil; and by eating natural foods and
wearing domestically produced clothes (figs. 183, 185). Popular
ideas about health (which ranged from homeopathy to astrol-
ogy) combined with the new Nazi prescriptions for living to create a form of medicine with a uniquely German character.

Many prominent members of the Nazi party supported
these ideas. Julius Streicher (fig. 184), one of the earliest Nazi

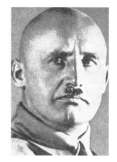

FIG 184
JULIUS STREICHER
(1885–1946)

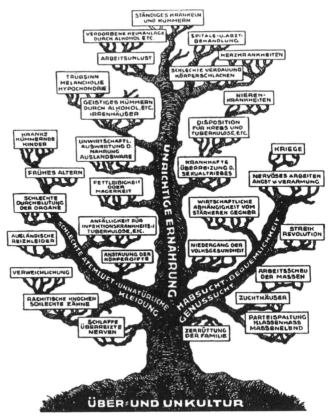

FIG 185 PROPAGANDA OF THE NATURAL HEALTH MOVEMENT: THE
TREE OF"EXAGGERATED AND NONCULTURE." THE TWIGS ARE
"FOREIGN IRRITATING CLOTHES," "EFFEMINACY," "MELANCHOLY,"
"STRIKE AND REVOLUTION," ETC.

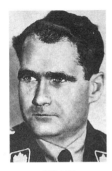

FIG 186
RUDOLF HESS
(1894–1987)

leaders, a virulent anti-Semite and editor of the notoriously
vicious anti-Jewish periodical *Der Stürmer*, was a proponent
of a national health movement based on the ideology of blood
and soil. The deputy of the Führer, Rudolf Hess (fig. 186),
consulted healers himself, and with his protégé, Gerhard
Wagner, tried to establish natural health science firmly at the
universities. Institutes for natural forms of living and healing
and for biological medicine were soon founded at the universities of Berlin and Jena, where natural health science became
part of the examinations given to medical students. In 1934,

Hess's name was attached to a large clinic for natural health science in Dresden that was designed to become the leading center for empirical research in natural forms of treatment.

In lieu of specific therapy based on precise diagnoses, the objective of natural health science was "to combine environmental stimuli of physical and dietetic nature, specially arranged in regard to intensity, quantity, and duration, in a system of treatment that enables the organism to restore its inner order."[52]

According to a letter from a young physician who temporarily worked at the Rudolf Hess Hospital, all patients received some kind of "biological" diet, all types of disease were treated by baths in water of increasing temperature, and nonspecific measures alone were used for diseases as dissimilar as appendicitis and highly contagious syphilis.[53]

An ignorant, uncritical view of illness by the proponents of new German healing is exemplified by a lecture titled "Clairvoyance—Telepathy—Divining Rod—Death Rays" (fig. 187). Sponsored by the National Socialist Physicians' League of Berlin, the "famous researcher," Dr. Gubich, spoke to an audience that included, as stated in the announcement, leading officials of the Nazi party.

The responses of representatives of official medicine to natural health science were varied; some dismissed new German

NSD-Aerztebund Gau Groß-Berlin

Einladung!

Der Gau Groß-Berlin des NSD.-Aerztebundes veranstaltet am Dienstag, den 8. Mai, abends 8.15 Uhr, einen Vortrag über

„Hellsehen – Telepathie – Wünschelrute – Todesstrahlen"

Der Vortrag wird gehalten von dem bekannten Forscher Gubisch-Dresden.

Ort der Veranstaltung: Bach-Saal, Berlin W 35, Lützowstraße 76.

(Tel. Nr. B 1, 0159)

Wir laden die deutsche Aerzteschaft Berlins hierzu ergebenst ein. Leitende Persönlichkeiten der NSDAP. und der Staatsführung haben ihr Erscheinen in Aussicht gestellt.

Heil Hitler!

Dr. von Stuckrad,
stellvertr. Gauobmann des NSD.-Aerztebundes
Gau Groß-Berlin.

Zur Unkostendeckung wird ein Eintrittsgeld von 0,50 RM. erhoben.
Karten sind zu haben im Vorverkauf ab 25. 4. 1934 im NSD.-Aerztebund, Berlin W 9, Voßstraße 11 (A 1, 0029) und an der Abendkasse.

FIG 187 "CLAIRVOYANCE—TELEPATHY—DIVINING ROD—DEATH RAYS."

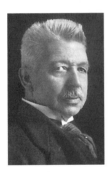

FIG 188
LUDWIG ASCHOFF
(1866–1942)

healing publicly and vocally. In 1934, Ludwig Aschoff (fig. 188), the great Freiburg pathologist who identified Aschoff's bodies in rheumatic myocarditis and elucidated the transmission of electrical impulses in the heart, declared in open opposition to the Nazis that there was no such thing as a "nationally delimited medicine," that diseases were "not contingent on individual cultural or political circles," and that medicine was, like no other discipline, dependent on the "cooperation of peoples."[54]

In other instances, opposition to the Nazis' woolly concept of medicine arose when an individual's own scientific reputation could be tarnished. This was the case with Max Borst, chair of pathology at the University of Munich, whose name is connected with the Borst-Jadassohn phenomenon.[55] In 1936, Borst (fig. 189) was nominated to be leader of the German delegation to the International Congress of Pathology in Brussels. One potential member of his delegation was the Nuremberg physician Dr. von Brehmer, who propagated the idea that human cancer could be detected by an "alkaline shift" in the blood. Von Brehmer also suggested that this metabolic abnormality could be corrected by blood transfusions, but to achieve a "cancer cure," the blood donors had to be Aryan. By this time, von Brehmer had already transfused numerous cancer patients and wanted very much to present his findings in Brussels. Toward this end, he sought and received endorsement by the SS, which supported all kinds of unproven, mystical ideas.

To protect his own reputation and that of his colleagues, Borst did everything possible to deny von Brehmer the opportunity to make a presentation before the congress that would be embarrassing to German medicine and to Borst himself. Borst even wrote a lecture about cancer that he sought to deliver to Hitler, but an invitation to Borst from the Reich's chancellery in Berlin never arrived. Borst and his colleagues decided, therefore, that they would not attend the Brussels meeting if von Brehmer was included in the delegation. At the last minute, the authorities retreated, and the German delegation went to Brussels without von Brehmer. Even in a seem-

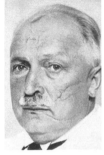

FIG 189
MAX BORST
(1869–1946)

ingly minor matter such as this one, it is apparent that the bluff of the Nazis could be called if only a single voice was raised trenchantly enough.[56]

The von Brehmer incident demonstrates that opposition to the Nazis not only was possible but could be successful. Voicing opposition required courage, however, and most physicians— like the rest of the population—did not have it; they remained silent as they went through their schooling and after it. Leading German physicians made little use of their privilege to resist the Nazis, even when the quality of medicine was at stake. All too many of them paid lip service to the Nazis by adopting the terminology of new German healing and by supporting the usefulness of a "new approach" to medicine. Heinrich Adolf Gottron, in his article in 1934 on constitution and skin diseases, towed the party line when he stated, "Dermatology also is ready now to try to understand the development of diseases by observation of the organism as a whole."[57] Max Borst likewise spoke publicly about the necessity for science and scholarship to serve "the people" in a time of need and stressed the call of Nazi physicians to practice medicine based on the unity of organs.[58]

At the opening ceremony of the Seventeenth Congress of the German Dermatological Society on October 8, 1934, Ernst Heinrich Brill, speaking as the official deputy of Gerhard Wagner, rejoiced that "German science will give note with pleasure to new, wonderful tasks that have evolved for it everywhere. One should not deny the work of the scientist, with its emphasis on objective methods and performance, the ethos in peoplehood, national, and social regard, i.e., to look for fulfillment in the synthesis of a National Socialist interpretation of scientific questions."[59] And the respected Berlin medical historian Paul Robert Diepgen (fig. 190) wrote in 1938, "It depends how national science is defined. Certainly science, in serving all mankind, has to be cosmopolitan. But this does not contradict the fact that each people will understand and support science from its own particular vantage." Diepgen concluded: "We as Germans could not have a better ideological basis for our med-

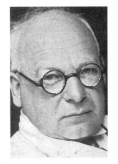

FIG 190
PAUL DIEPGEN
(1878–1966)

ical practice and course of studies than the National Socialist principles as they are embodied in the spirit of Hitler."[60]

In the face of the terrible perversion of medicine by the Nazis, German physicians acquiesced, became partisans of Nazi ideology, or did nothing. Had they been faithful to the Hippocratic Oath and to their own dignity, they could have helped prevent, in the early 1930s, the disaster that befell the German people—and so many others—in the decade that followed.

COOPERATION
WITH THE NAZIS

OW WAS IT POSSIBLE THAT AN OVERWHELMING MAJORITY OF GERMAN PHYSICIANS, MANY OF WHOM WERE CELE-brated scientists with worldwide reputations, accepted Nazi ideas about medicine without question or protest? How was it possible that the Nazis could perpetrate such cruelty without vigorous opposition from the German people in general and German doctors in particular?

There were many reasons for this phenomenon, only some of which are discussed here—namely, good feelings engendered by a sense of the resurrection of Germany as a nation; the unexpected and remarkable political success of the Nazis, especially in engineering economic recovery; massive propaganda that glorified Nazism and the new leaders of Germany; partial support for many ideas of Nazism, including euthanasia as an act to end unnecessary suffering, racial hygiene as an essential branch of preventive medicine, and the existence of a "Jewish problem"; repression psychologically by many Germans of some of the clearly stated objectives of the Nazis; rise of both oppression and violence in a gradual, hyposensitizing fashion; omnipresent control by a police state; instillation of fear; understanding that a favorable political attitude toward the state would be rewarded by the state, or, in other words, sheer opportunism; and crippling effects on the spine of a people with a centuries-long tradition of respect for authoritarianism at home and in school.

The importance of particular reasons for failure to resist the Nazis changed as the times changed. Toward the end of the twelve-year period of the Nazi regime, the cooperation of the populace had to be enforced by escalation of fear and by repressive methods; propaganda alone was no longer sufficient. Before the war, the vast majority of Germans were deeply impressed by the political and economic successes of the Nazis;

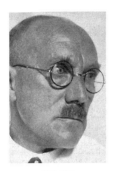

FIG 191
ERNST FERDINAND
SAUERBRUCH
(1875–1951)

they paid little or no heed to the curtailment of personal freedom and the brutal suppression of minorities. At the beginning, the most important reason for cooperation with the Nazis on the part of many Germans was the feeling that only the Nazis could restore Germany to greatness.

In the eyes of most Germans, the treatment of their fatherland by the victorious powers after the First World War had been unjust. Through the Treaty of Versailles, they believed, Germany had been reduced to a second-class nation and Germans to second-class citizens who had lost the right to be proud of themselves and their country. After the Nazis' assumption of power, the strong desire for a national resurrection enabled many Germans to overlook some harsh realities in order to protect the new government from foreign criticism. The famous surgeon Ernst Ferdinand Sauerbruch (fig. 191), for example, wrote this appeal to his foreign colleagues: "First of all, I turn to you with a confession about my native country and its people, with whom I feel fatefully united. From my love of it arises the assurance that it has an inalienable right to develop its national strength. Hence I see in our revolution the basis of a rebirth of our nation, so unworthily treated and deprived, despite initial side effects which have bothered me sincerely. Every one of you who loves his fatherland surely will understand these feelings."[1]

Sauerbruch, like millions of other Germans, considered the negative aspects of the new state to be mere "initial side effects," temporary measures that would be limited to a certain period necessary for the reorganization of public life. After the dismissal of his Jewish assistants, Walter Frieboes, chair of dermatology at the Charité Hospital in Berlin, naively asked the dean of the medical faculty when he could expect his colleagues to return to duty.[2] The actual objectives of the Nazis were repressed; their radical racial pronouncements were so far removed from fundamental principles of decency, civility, and humanity that they were not taken seriously. Even the worst anti-Semitic convulsions of leading Nazis, like Julius Streicher's diatribes in his anti-Semitic journal, *Der Stürmer*, were

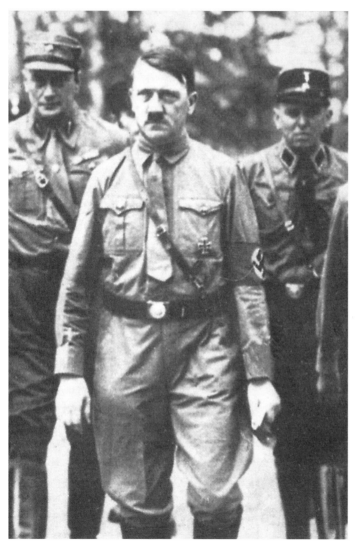

FIG 192 HITLER DRESSED AS A STORM TROOPER.

commonly excused by intellectuals as mere propaganda, aimed at winning support of "the mob." This opinion was bolstered further by Hitler himself, who changed his behavior to suit the moment and public as needed, presenting himself as a fanatical storm trooper one day (fig. 192) and as a moderate statesman the next (fig. 193). In front of conservative audiences,

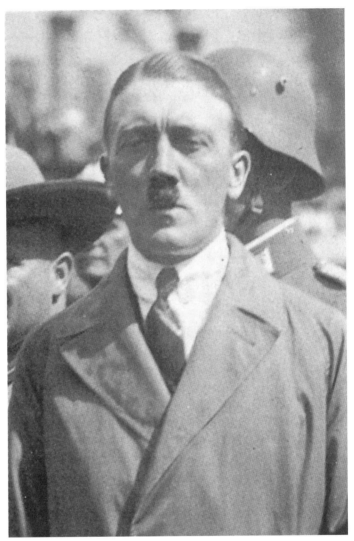

FIG 193 HITLER DRESSED AS A STATESMAN.

Hitler tended to avoid anti-Jewish remarks and to emphasize his commitment to stability and peace.[3]

The first measures against Jews, Democrats, and Socialists were conducted moderately, at least by Nazi standards. Considering the Nazis' fanaticism, it might have been expected that large-scale anti-Jewish pogroms would be conducted immediately after the assumption of power by the party.

Instead, the Nazis staged a symbolic one-day boycott of Jewish businesses on April 1, 1933, accompanied by deliberate maltreatment and illegal apprehension of Jews.

Similarly, the study of medicine at the outset of the Nazi takeover was not forbidden to Jews, but the number of them allowed to study was restricted to reflect the percentage of Jews in the general population, a policy that was perceived by many Germans as perfectly reasonable. Open violence against Jews, such as the destruction of Jewish shops, was accomplished with the blessing of the government but without its official sanction. On several occasions, Hitler even restrained bloodthirsty storm troopers, fearing that too violent encroachments might boomerang.[4] Laws that restricted Jewish rights were ostensibly enacted to protect Jews from illegal attacks by muting resentment and anger against them as a consequence of their undeserved prominence in public life.

Official regulations against Jews and political dissidents were heightened in a deliberately measured fashion, always leaving time for the public to adapt to one step before the next was taken. This gradual escalation eventually led to a degree of suppression and violence that had been unimaginable just a few years earlier. Furthermore, the worst episodes of violence were hidden from the public. After the day of the general boycott of Jews in 1933 and the pogroms that culminated in the Kristallnacht in November 1938, Hitler perceived that the response of segments of the population was not one of approval but of consternation and embarrassment.[5]

At the outset of the war in 1939, when Hitler issued a written order to kill "useless eaters"—chronically disabled patients in hospitals and nursing homes—increasing protest from some members of the clergy, some sectors of the general population, and some physicians (Ferdinand Sauerbruch among them) forced an end to the "euthanasia" killings in August 1941. Henceforth, Hitler gave only oral orders—which meant they were less likely to be publicized—and the annihilation of Jews and Gypsies (a colloquial but derogatory name given to the peoples of Sinti and Roma) was carried out in desolate abandoned regions of Poland rather than in Germany proper.

Reports about those massacres were strictly forbidden. In July 1941, the chief of staff of the German Eleventh Army, General Wöhner, informed his troops about certain codes of behavior in these words: "Considering the concept of the value of human life prevalent in Eastern Europe, German soldiers may become witnesses of events (mass executions and assassination of civil prisoners, Jews, etc.) that they cannot prevent at the moment, but that violate badly the German sense of honor. It is a matter, of course, for any human being of healthy feelings that no photographic documents are made of such abominable encroachments and that none of them be mentioned in letters home. The preparation and dissemination of pictures or reports about such events is considered an undermining of decency and manliness and will be punished severely."[6] Even Heinrich Himmler, the chief of the SS, called it a "natural matter of tact" never to speak about the killings.[7]

Although news of the gigantic mass murder occurring in Poland surely reached Germany, the crimes were not actually witnessed by most Germans and were never confirmed officially, which made it easy for the average German to ignore or deny them. Those who chose to remain ignorant about the fate of Jews were given the opportunity, and they constituted the vast majority of the population, not only in Germany but in many European countries and the United States as well.

The political successes of the Nazis led to further cooperation by the public with the party. The political vandalism and constant battles between opposing groups that had marked the last years of the Weimar Republic (fig. 194)—and to which the Nazis themselves had contributed mightily—suddenly disappeared. The streets were safe again; "law and order" seemed to have been re-established (fig. 195). In further contrast to the governments of the Weimar Republic, the Nazis refused to pay

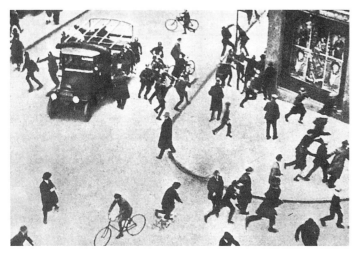

FIG 194 CHAOS IN THE WEIMAR REPUBLIC.

any more reparations for the war to the victorious Allied powers, and that refusal evoked only minor protest from the Allies.

In 1933, Germany had an army of only one hundred thousand troops, with no modern weapons and no air force. By 1938, Germany was the strongest military power in Europe. Instead of a policy of retrenchment, the Nazis expanded Germany's economy in order to overcome the economic crisis. Investments in public projects rose rapidly, especially in the armed forces, resulting in a marked increase of public debt but also an instant decrease in the unemployment rate. In 1933, more than six million people were out of work; by the end of 1937, fewer than one million were unemployed. Self-confidence and moderate prosperity had replaced misery and despair.[8]

Physicians especially benefited from the improvement in the economy. Between 1928 and 1932, the years of the Great Depression, the average annual taxable income of physicians had decreased by 34 percent. Between the summers of 1933 and 1934, a period during which Jewish colleagues were ousted from positions in universities and from insurance-fund panels, the income of Aryan physicians rose 11.3 percent, and by 1935, doctors' average taxable income had increased by 25 percent (fig. 196).

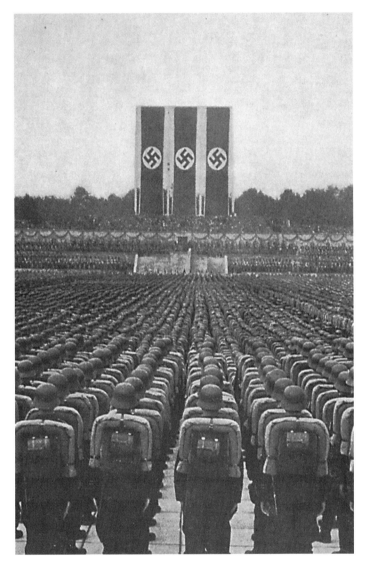

FIG 195 ORDER UNDER THE NAZIS.

Like members of no other profession, physicians placed themselves at the disposal of the new government. Karl Haedenkamp, one of the leading representatives of German physicians since the years of the Weimar Republic, stated on June 24, 1933, that "to serve this state must be the sole objective of the medical profession. We are aware of the duties that

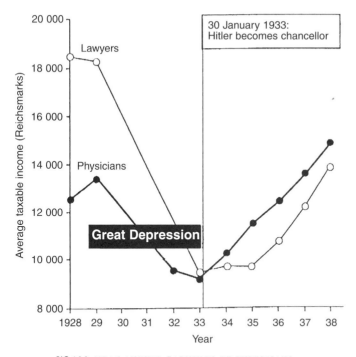

FIG 196 MEAN ANNUAL EARNINGS OF PHYSICIANS AND LAWYERS IN GERMANY DURING 1928–1939.

we have to fulfill on its behalf. Insofar as we carry them out, we shall earn the right to have our work respected."[9]

Haedenkamp's expectations were fulfilled; the cooperation of physicians was well rewarded. In the Third Reich, physicians not only were paid better than other professionals, such as lawyers and dentists, but were making more money than ever. Most physicians were able to afford and maintain well-situated and spacious offices, take vacations abroad, and buy a Mercedes at a time when even much less expensive cars were out of reach for most Germans. The favorable economic climate in the mid-1930s no doubt contributed to a marked increase in physician membership in the NSDAP, which reached its peak in 1937.[10]

The political success of the National Socialist government was evident, yet the Nazis felt compelled to trumpet it constantly through their massive propaganda machine. All

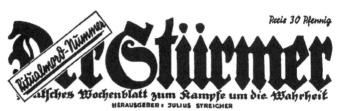

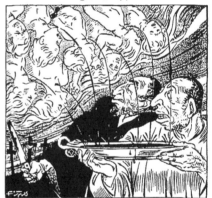

sources of information were in the hands of the party: books, newspapers, cinemas. Confronted daily by headlines praising the greatness of the new state and railing against the viciousness of Jews, many Germans were ready to believe fables like one in Julius Streicher's *Der Stürmer*: "Jewish Plan to Murder Non-Jewish Mankind Uncovered" (fig. 197).

The control of all sources of information also enabled the Nazis to change colloquial language and, through that alteration, to change the thinking of the German people. Hitler became transformed into a saint, or even more, by being referred to in the language of the Bible. Instead of "Hitler Delivers a Speech," the headlines of newspapers proclaimed "Hitler Comes to the Workers," and those workers did not simply "listen" to Hitler but "experienced" him. Phrases like "Adolf Hitler's mission" and "I believe in Hitler" became commonplace. The new standard words of welcome, "Heil Hitler," had to be used by everyone to avoid the impression of even a trace of hostility toward the state.[11] Civil servants were obliged by official decree "to carry out the German salute, while on duty and within the offices and installations, by raising the right—in case of physical disability the left— arm and by the simultaneous German saying 'Heil Hitler.'"[12] In short order, that salutation was so firmly entrenched in the German language that no one thought any longer of its literal meaning. (The German word "Heil" means health, safety, or welfare. It was used by German nationalists as a conventional salute long before Hitler appeared on the scene. Literally, "Heil Hitler" means "Well-being to Hitler.") The same was true for euphemistic expressions for the killing of mentally disabled patients and the genocide of Jews. Terms like "euthanasia" and "final solution" served the murderers well in disguising the brutal reality of their deeds and became so much a part of the language that they continued to be used long after the fall of the Third Reich.

Schoolchildren were indoctrinated early by being incorporated into the party's youth organizations. Posters proclaiming, "You also belong to the Führer," anti-Semitic cartoons in schoolbooks, and games such as "Jews out—the up-to-date and extremely funny parlor game for adults and children" were prevalent, powerful tools of propaganda (figs. 198 through 201).

The indoctrination of children was considered a key element in the Nazi goal of creating a new generation of Germans who

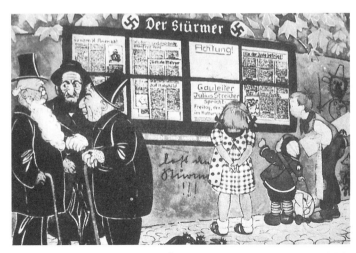

FIG 198 CARTOON FROM *DER STÜRMER* TEACHING CHILDREN NOT TO HAVE CONTACT WITH JEWS. THE GRAFFITI ON THE WALL PROCLAIMS: "READ *DER STÜRMER!*"

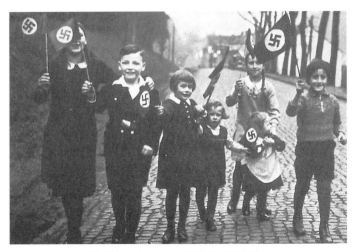

FIG 199 CHILDREN WITH NAZI FLAGS.

would be fully identified with Nazi ideology. The manner in which children were not so subtly influenced is neatly illustrated in a book titled *The Poisonous Mushroom* (fig. 202). This collection of anti-Semitic tales teaches readers how difficult it is to tell good mushrooms from poisonous ones and good people (Germans) from bad people (Jews). One of the stories in the book describes a "Jew lesson" at school, a favorite subject for the

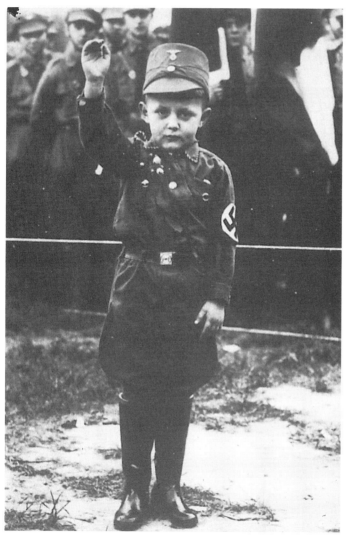

FIG 200 BOY SHOWING THE PARTY SALUTE.

pupils because the teacher is so nice and knows so much (fig. 203). When he asks them at the end of the lesson to summarize what they have learned, they show off their knowledge thus:

> *The Jew is recognized mostly by his nose. The Jewish nose is bent at its apex. It looks like a six. Therefore it is called the 'Jewish Six.' Also many non-Jews have bent*

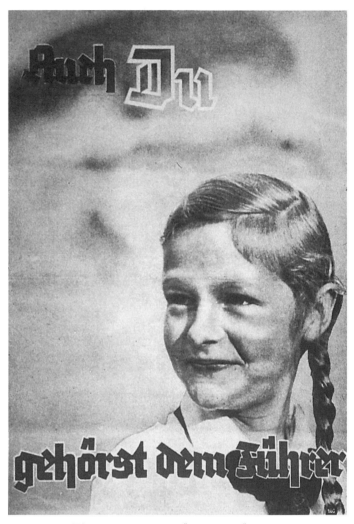

FIG 201 "AUCH DU GEHÖRST DEM FÜHRER!"
("YOU ALSO BELONG TO THE FÜHRER!")

*noses. However, their noses are not bent at the bottom but
a bit further up.... The Jew is also recognized by his lips.
His lips are mostly bulging.... And one also recognizes
the Jew by his eyes. His eyelids are usually thicker and
fleshier than ours. His look is lowering and piercing. One
already recognizes from his eyes that he is a false, mendacious man....The Jews are mostly of small or medium
size. They have short legs. Their arms are often very short*

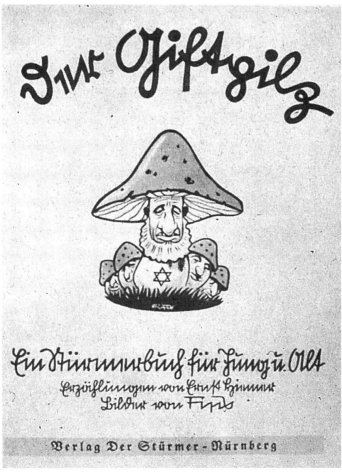

FIG 202 TITLE PAGE FROM *THE POISONOUS MUSHROOM.*

as well. Many Jews have crooked legs and flat feet. They often have a narrow, oblique forehead. One calls this is a receding forehead. Many criminals have such a forehead. The Jews are also criminals. Their hair is mostly dark and often curly as in Negroes. Their ears are often large and look like the handle of a coffee cup.... Not every Jew has these characteristic marks. Some do not have a true Jewish Six but true Jewish ears instead. Some do not have flat feet but true Jewish eyes instead. Sometimes one may not be able to recognize a Jew for what he is at first glance.

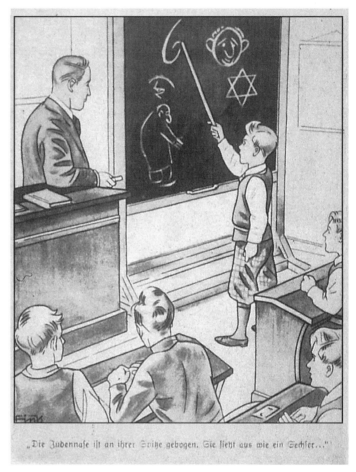

„Die Judennase ist an ihrer Spitze gebogen. Sie sieht aus wie ein Sechser..."

FIG 203 *THE POISONOUS MUSHROOM:* "JEW LESSON" AT SCHOOL.

There may even be Jews with fair hair. If we want to distinguish the Jew from non-Jews with certainty, we have to watch closely, but then one notices immediately whether one is dealing with a Jew.[13]

After his pupils' display of basic anatomic knowledge, the teacher is very pleased: "That's very good, children! You really paid attention! And if you also pay attention in daily life and keep your eyes open, then you will not be deceived by the Jew."[14]

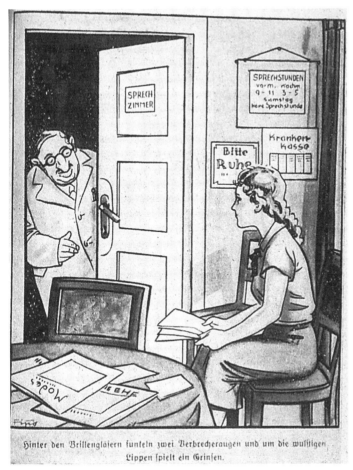

Hinter den Brillengläsern funkeln zwei Verbrecheraugen und um die wulstigen Lippen spielt ein Grinsen.

FIG 204 *THE POISONOUS MUSHROOM*: PICTURE FROM THE STORY
"HOW INGE FARED AT THE JEW DOCTOR."

Another story in the book, "How Inge Fared at the Jew Doctor" (fig. 204), tells of a little girl named Inge, who, despite her vigorous protests, is sent by her mother to a Jewish physician. Sitting in the waiting room, she recalls the admonition of the leader of the local Nazi Girls' Group that "Many a girl who sought healing from a Jewish physician found lingering illness and shame!" After a while, Inge hears a little girl cry and shout, "Doctor, doctor, leave me alone!" The story continues:

*Then the door opens. Inge looks up. The Jew appears. A
scream escapes from Inge's mouth. Scared, she drops the
newspaper. Frightened, she jumps up. Her eyes stare at
the face of the Jewish doctor. And this face is the face of
the devil. In the midst of that devil's face there is a huge,
bent nose. Behind the spectacles, two eyes are flashing,
the eyes of a criminal. And a smirk plays around the
bulging lips. A smirk that says: "Now, finally, I got you,
little German girl!" And then the Jew approaches her.
His fleshy fingers grasp at her. But now Inge has composed herself. Before the Jew can seize her, she slaps his
fat face. Then she bounds for the door. Out of breath,
Inge runs down the stairway. Out of breath, she rushes
out of the Jewish house.[15]*

Perhaps even more powerful as a tool of propaganda than
newspapers and books was the radio, at that time still a new and
highly desired item. To achieve the aim "All Germans hear the
Führer," the Nazis saw to it that radios were affordable for most
people (fig. 205). When Hitler spoke on the radio, listening not
only was obligatory but attendance at such sessions was strictly
controlled and monitored. The director of the surgical department at the Robert Koch Hospital in Berlin recorded this observation in March 1936: "I have found that all members of my
department who could be spared from duty have attended the
transmission of the Führer's speech on the seventh of this
month, and that nobody has left the assembly room before they
joined in singing the national anthem."[16]

In the Third Reich, it was impossible for a citizen to elude
such controls. Even the most private decisions, such as marriage, had to be approved by the government. The extent of
controls exceeded all expectations, and even ingrained Nazis,
such as the chair of dermatology at the University of Hamburg, Paul Mulzer, were slow in adapting to them. In 1934,
Mulzer failed to report to the authorities that he had been
elected a member of an international committee for the orga-

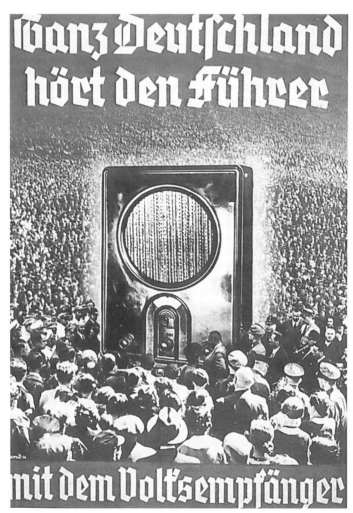

FIG 205 "ALL GERMANS HEAR THE FÜHRER."

nization of education in dermatology; he apologized for not having known that such positions were subject to approval.[17]

In 1935, the chair of dermatology in Würzburg, Karl Zieler, was made an honorary member of the Hungarian Dermatological Society and could accept that tribute only after having obtained approval from the Bavarian Ministry of Culture and Education. Eight years later, Zieler's successor, Karl Hoede, was declared a corresponding member of the

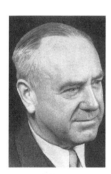

FIG 206
JOSEF HÄMEL
(1894–1969)

same society, but this time the ministry denied approval to him, arguing that "in the Hungarian Dermatological Society, there are still numerous Jewish and half-Jewish members. Therefore, until further notice, contact of German scientists with that society must be avoided."[18]

Objections to such decisions by the government were futile and could even be dangerous. The government was sacrosanct; its orders were to be carried out without delay, and execution of those orders was to be documented precisely. In 1936, for example, department chairs were forced to declare if any Jews were in their employ. A negative response was demanded. It became dangerous—if not impossible—to tolerate the presence of Jews in a department.[19]

It was equally dangerous to tolerate the presence of political opposition. Josef Hämel (fig. 206), chair of the Department of Dermatology at the University of Jena, originally a supporter of the Nazis and a party member since 1933, was imprisoned for six weeks for not having reported a "political offense." When three students smashed a bust of Hitler, Hämel failed to report them to the Gestapo. Instead, he dumped the shattered remains of the bust in the Saale River and spread the story that the bust had been damaged accidentally. After the Gestapo discovered the truth, Hämel was threatened with execution and deportation to Buchenwald. He must have considered himself lucky to get away with only a few weeks in custody. Other dermatologists were much less honorable than Hämel. For example, Walther Schultze, chair of dermatology in Giessen, did not hesitate to denounce patients to the Gestapo (fig. 207).

In the Third Reich, total control was not only practiced by the authorities but integral to everyday life. Party members were everywhere and ever willing to report "deviations" to the government. This happened to Georg Alexander Rost in Freiburg and to Erich Hoffmann in Bonn. Hoffmann enjoyed worldwide fame for his discovery of the spirochete of syphilis and for describing and naming diseases such as perifolliculitis capitis abscedens et suffodiens, lupus erythematosus tumidus,

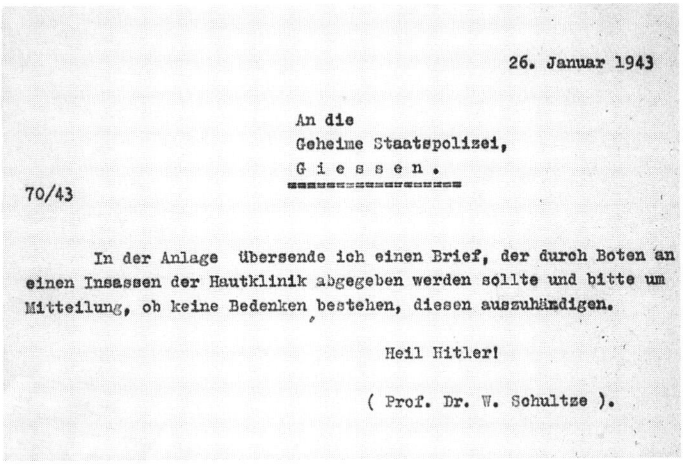

26. Januar 1943

An die
Geheime Staatspolizei,
G i e s s e n .

70/43

In der Anlage übersende ich einen Brief, der durch Boten an einen Insassen der Hautklinik abgegeben werden sollte und bitte um Mitteilung, ob keine Bedenken bestehen, diesen auszuhändigen.

Heil Hitler!

(Prof. Dr. W. Schultze).

FIG 207 LETTER BY WALTHER SCHULTZE DENOUNCING A PATIENT TO THE GESTAPO.

and dermatofibrosarcoma protuberans. As a very conservative man and member of the Stahlhelm, Hoffmann initially welcomed the appointment of Hitler as chancellor of the German Reich. Like many Germans, Hoffmann thought that representatives of the large democratic parties in Hitler's newly formed coalition cabinet would be able to act as a stabilizing force on the Nazis. In fact, on February 22, 1933, he signed a declaration in support of the new government written by some of his colleagues at the University of Bonn. He regretted this signature on the very same day and for the rest of his life. In his autobiography, this is how Hoffmann explained his action:

> *In this time of political unrest, when a return to reason still seemed to be possible, an appeal appeared in the newspaper on February 22 that also carried my signature which was said, by interested supporters of the party, to be absolutely and immediately necessary, while I, already delayed, was rushing to a lecture. I ought not to have believed the assertion that I could affix my name with a safe conscience to those of other professors who were known by me to be reliable,*

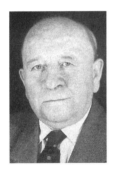

because the demonstrations of the unsatisfied with the provoking bloody-red swastika flag should have called for caution. As a consequence of this careless step, which was recognized as such immediately by my wife, those who misjudged my nature identified me with aims, such as the dismissal of capable civil servants and physicians, which I condemned rigorously and attacked vigorously from the outset.[20]

Within a few weeks, Hoffmann recognized his error and the true nature of National Socialist rule, and he changed his attitude abruptly and without compromise. He was outraged by the events on the day of the general boycott of Jews and condemned the dismissal of Jewish colleagues. He did everything possible to prevent the university from being seized by the Nazis and steadfastly refused to approve inept colleagues who had been appointed by the Nazis to direct German dermatology. Hoffmann never said "Heil Hitler" and never raised his arm in the party salute. Because of their brown party uniforms, he called the Nazis "brown shit" in public, and his saying, "I prefer a white vest to a brown shirt," was oft repeated.

Before long, Hoffmann's attitude and deportment were reported to party officials, and three of his assistants were induced by the Nazis to provide them with ammunition against him. The ignominious three were lecturers Carl Ludwig Karrenberg and Gregor Heinrich Klövekorn, and Professor Rudolf Strempel, who, after the war, was made chair of dermatology at Saar University in Homburg (fig. 208). Those three men, all members of the Nazi party, were interrogated on December 18, 1933, by the district leader of the National Socialist Lecturers' League, Professor Blumenberg, and gave a precise account of all of Hoffmann's misdemeanors:

Question: What was the precise wording of H.'s often discussed statement that addressed the Führer and what was the context of that statement?

Answer: Hoffmann praised the productivity and abilities of Jews and especially emphasized their sporting prowess. Then he said that "one cannot find a Jew who blows Hitler away; there still must be gutsy Jews." (Witnesses: Strempel, Klövekorn)

Question: What about the saying of the white vest and the brown shirt?
Answer: H. said exactly: "White vest and brown shirt are contrary to one another." (Witness: Karrenberg)

Question: Could this saying be interpreted in another way than as a disparagement of the brown shirt?
Answer: No. (Karrenberg)

Question: How did Hoffmann respond to the request for his car for the transport of war-disabled persons?
Answer: He was ready to place his car at their disposal, but only under the condition that it would not fly the Nazi flag. (Witnesses: Klövekorn, N.S.K.O.V.)

Question: Did Hoffmann make statements that criticized the measures of the government concerning the Jews?
Answer: Yes, many times, for example wild insults on the day of the boycott of Jews. H. often emphasized how able Jews were in comparison to his co-workers. (Witnesses: Strempel, Klövekorn, Karrenberg)

Question: How did Hoffmann respond to the order of the German salute?
Answer: Hoffmann initially prohibited the German salute, but following the decree he acted very reserved. He stated that it was enough to use the German salute once a day and that one did not have to say "Heil Hitler," but only "Heil" or nothing at all. He himself,

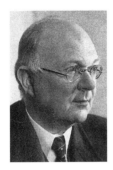

FIG 209
OTTO GRÜTZ
(1886–1963)

as a member of the Stahlhelm, would say nothing. (Witnesses: Strempel, Klövekorn, Karrenberg)[21]

In addition to the political accusations, Strempel, Klövekorn, and Karrenberg declared that Hoffmann engaged in unethical studies, performed unnecessary biopsies, and often attacked his assistants in the presence of nurses and patients. They concluded that Hoffmann was disturbed psychologically and that collaboration with him was impossible. As a consequence, Hoffmann was removed as chair of dermatology in Bonn.

The case of Erich Hoffmann was not the only example of denunciation at the University of Bonn's Department of Dermatology. Carl Ludwig Karrenberg himself had been denounced by a technical assistant for allegedly having said that Hitler had paresis. (General paresis is a late manifestation of syphilis in which a person is no longer able to cerebrate.) Although Karrenberg denied the accusation categorically and instituted legal proceedings against the assistant, he remained under suspicion. Karrenberg's cooperation with the Nazis in the case of Erich Hoffmann presumably helped to re-establish his political reliability and to resuscitate his career.[22]

A few years later, after the professionally unheralded Otto Grütz (fig. 209) had succeeded Erich Hoffmann as chair of dermatology, a member of his staff informed the headquarters of the NSDAP in Munich that portraits of the Jewish professors Neisser, Unna, and Ehrlich were still on display in the skin clinic of Bonn. After a brief inquiry by the rector of the university, Grütz removed the portraits immediately. Grütz despised the Nazis and discreetly maintained contact with "politically unreliable" colleagues who had become outcasts of the society. Nevertheless, his fear of denunciation and degradation induced him even to display a bust of Adolf Hitler at the entrance of his clinic.

Walter Frieboes (fig. 210), chair of the Department of Dermatology at the Charité Hospital in Berlin since 1932 and author of several well-known textbooks, including *Outline of the Histopathology of the Skin*, was also denounced by members of

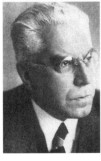

FIG 210
WALTER FRIEBOES
(1880–1945)

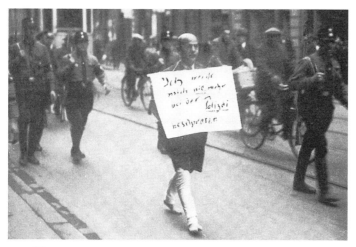

FIG 211 "I SHALL NEVER AGAIN COMPLAIN TO THE POLICE."

his staff. Frieboes was reputed to have said, in a private conversation with two nurses, that one had "to be careful of the Nazis," and that "if a Jew and members of the party share a room in a hospital and a conflict develops between them, one should not remove the Jew but rather the members of the party."[23] When confronted by party officials about these statements, Frieboes struggled to explain, to recant halfheartedly, and to justify himself without completely losing face. After lengthy clarifications by Frieboes, the issue was resolved, and Frieboes was allowed to stay at the Charité Hospital as director of dermatology.

The omnipresent sense of complete control by the Nazis generated fear—fear of degradation, of losing one's position, of finding oneself in trouble with the police. Of all the factors contributing to cooperation with the Nazis, fear was among the most compelling. There were no legal ways to prevent arbitrary acts by party members, and denouncement of such acts could result in severe punishment. In this regard, no one could feel safe, and it was made abundantly clear that there would be no tolerance of nonconformity. When it came to settling conflicts with the party, the police could no longer be counted on to uphold the law. In fact, those who did look to

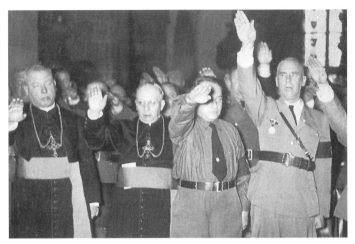

FIG 212 HIGH DIGNITARIES OF THE CATHOLIC CHURCH RAISING THEIR ARMS FOR THE PARTY SALUTE. INSTEAD OF "GRÜSS GOTT" ("BE WITH GOD"), THE WORDS OF WELCOME WERE NOW "HEIL HITLER!"

the police for protection were forced to carry signs that read, "I shall never again complain to the police" (fig. 211).

Fear kept German resistance in check until the collapse of the Third Reich near the end of the war. The churches chose to cooperate with the Nazis (fig. 212). Large socially conscious groups, such as some political parties and trade unions, faded away without even a single demonstration or a strike. Jewish organizations also tried to appease the Nazis, at first by defending the new state against protest from abroad, then by collecting vast sums of money for contribution to the government, and, finally, by aiding in the organization of transportation of fellow Jews to concentration camps and their forced labor there.

With few exceptions—such as the assassination attempt on Hitler's life late in a losing war on July 20, 1944—active resistance was carried out on a very small scale. Those activities included acts of sabotage in factories, printing and distributing leaflets, and providing false passports and secret hideaways for those who were persecuted. Most resistance groups were organized by former members of the Communist and Socialist parties. Among them was the dermatologist Otto Schlein (fig. 213), who had worked at Alfred Blaschko's clinic in Berlin and later as

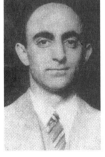

FIG 213
OTTO SCHLEIN
(1895–1944)

an associate of Carl Lennhoff in Magdeburg. In 1923, Schlein had opened a private practice in dermatology in Magdeburg. He soon became known as a "physician to the poor" who not only treated indigent patients without a fee but also shared lunch with them. Schlein was an observant Jew, being engaged in Jewish religious and cultural activities and in the Zionist movement. He also was a member of the Communist party and continued to work illegally for that party after it was banned in 1933. By 1936, Schlein had been arrested four times and accused of high treason, but each time he had to be released because of lack of evidence. In 1936, he emigrated to the Netherlands, where he was captured by the Gestapo in 1942. On October 3, 1944, Schlein, his wife, and his daughter were gassed in Auschwitz. After the war, the city of Magdeburg honored Schlein by naming one of the main streets along the Elbe River "Schleinufer" after him.[24]

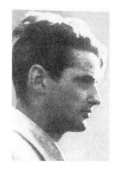

FIG 214
HANS SCHOLL
(1918–1943)

Hans Scholl (fig. 214) was one of several non-Jewish medical students who belonged to the White Rose, a group that produced pamphlets calling for an uprising against the Nazis. With his sister, Sophie, and other conspirators, Scholl was executed in February 1943.[25]

Other resistance groups were known by names such as the Red Chapel or the European Union. The latter was formed by Georg Groscurth (fig. 215), lecturer in internal medicine at the Moabit Hospital in Berlin. Among Groscurth's private patients were leading Nazis, including Rudolf Hess, from whom Groscurth secured information about forthcoming raids on the home front and, even more important, about preparations for the campaign against Russia (fig. 216). Groscurth secretly aided Jews, providing hideouts for them in his apartment, his private practice, or the hospital; supplying them with false passports; and organizing their flight from Germany. He was also involved in acts of sabotage against the armaments industry and helped soldiers to fake diseases that prevented them from being sent back to the front. Groscurth was arrested by the Gestapo in September 1943, sentenced to death, and executed eight months later. This was his farewell letter to his wife:

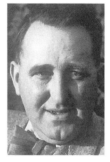

FIG 215
GEORG GROSCURTH
(1904–1944)

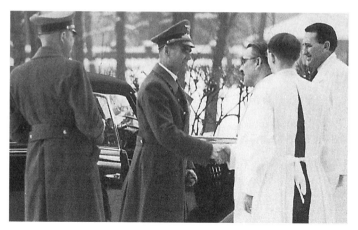

FIG 216 THE DEPUTY OF THE FÜHRER, RUDOLF HESS,
WITH PHYSICIANS FROM THE MOABIT HOSPITAL.
GEORG GROSCURTH IS ON THE FAR RIGHT.

My dear, good, true Anneliese, now the time has come. In half an hour, the sentence will be executed. I am completely calm because I anticipated it all the time. (Please excuse my poor handwriting, I write with handcuffs.) Could I only thank you, could I only express the love I always felt for you. Even in the hard days of my detention you gave me so much goodness and an infinity of love. I felt so much human greatness in you. Remain as strong as you have always been. You know it is not a mere accident but my fate. I have nothing to regret, only the great pain, the only matter for which I felt sorrow all the time, that you have to live so alone now. . . . Five more minutes! Now I cannot write to the others of the family. Your dear, good father, and Mummy, I hope they will always be well. My dear, good, true mother, do not feel sorrow, I die proud and unbroken. You had a good son. . . . I wish you a life full of happiness with the children. You will tell them that they do not have to be ashamed of their father. In a moment it is over. My love, with your noble, dear heart, you will take it well, never despair. Just think of how I

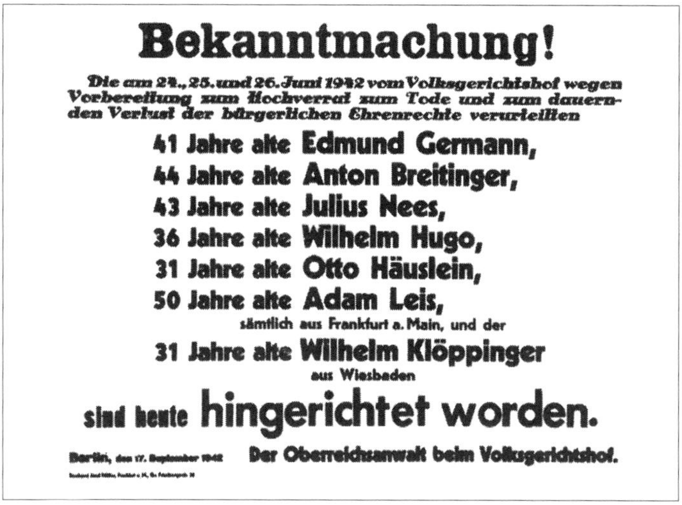

Bekanntmachung!

Die am 24., 25. und 26. Juni 1942 vom Volksgerichtshof wegen Vorbereitung zum Hochverrat zum Tode und zum dauernden Verlust der bürgerlichen Ehrenrechte verurteilten

41 Jahre alte Edmund Germann,

44 Jahre alte Anton Breitinger,

43 Jahre alte Julius Nees,

36 Jahre alte Wilhelm Hugo,

31 Jahre alte Otto Häuslein,

50 Jahre alte Adam Leis,

sämtlich aus Frankfurt a. Main, und der

31 Jahre alte Wilhelm Klöppinger

aus Wiesbaden

sind heute hingerichtet worden.

Berlin, den 17. September 1942   Der Oberreichsanwalt beim Volksgerichtshof.

FIG 217 LIST OF PEOPLE SENTENCED TO DEATH.

would have done everything. I embrace you and all the beloved. Yours, Georg [26]

For their resistance to the government, eight hundred thousand Germans—other than Jews—lost their jobs, were forced to emigrate, or were arrested and interned in prisons or concentration camps. About eighty thousand non-Jewish German citizens were killed (fig. 217).

The reality of such pervasive danger meant that most of those who disapproved of the changes taking place in Germany were forced into a kind of emigration to their inner selves. They remained as quiet and unobtrusive as possible, stayed out of political discussions, and simply tried to do their jobs without becoming affiliated with the Nazis. For someone with career ambitions, this mode of behavior was not so easy. In 1935, when Walter Frieboes, director of dermatology at the Charité Hospital in Berlin, was forced to declare in a questionnaire whether or not he was a party member, he first crossed out the statement that he did not belong to the Nazi party, thereby indicating that he did belong, when, in fact, he did not (fig. 218). That indecision likely reflected his fear of

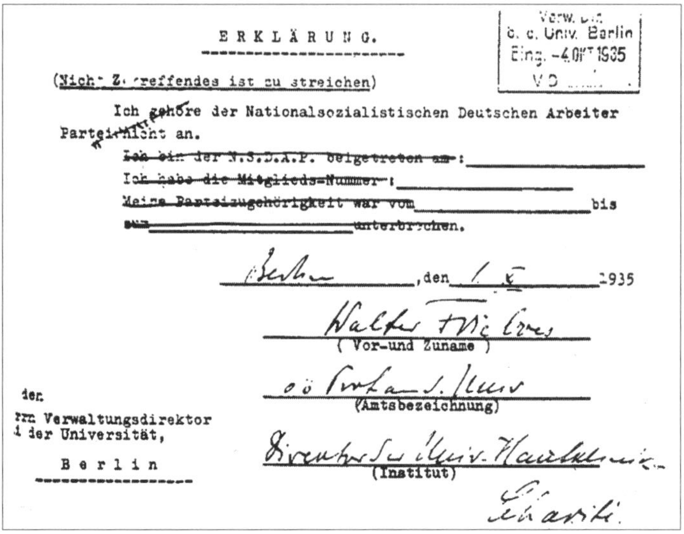

ERKLÄRUNG.

Verw. d. d. Univ. Berlin Eing. -4. OKT 1935 VD

(Nicht Zutreffendes ist zu streichen)

Ich ~~gehöre~~ der Nationalsozialistischen Deutschen Arbeiter Partei nicht an.

~~Ich bin der N.S.D.A.P. beigetreten am~~: ______

~~Ich habe die Mitglieds=Nummer~~: ______

~~Meine Parteizugehörigkeit war vom~~ ______ bis

~~zum~~ ______ ~~unterbrochen~~.

Berlin, den 1. X. 1935

Walter Frieboes
(Vor-und Zuname)

ö. Professor
(Amtsbezeichnung)

Direktor der Univ.-Hautklinik
(Institut)
Charité.

An den
Herrn Verwaltungsdirektor
der Universität,
Berlin

FIG 218 FRIEBOES'S REPLY TO THE QUESTION OF WHETHER HE BELONGED TO THE NAZI PARTY.

losing his chair if he did not appease the Nazis. To hold on to his position, Frieboes, originally a liberal and even an idealistic man, had to continually abandon his ideals and fight a losing battle with his conscience.[27]

In this regard, Frieboes was not alone. Making concessions to the "spirit of the time" was considered inevitable for anyone in a position of responsibility. Opponents of the Nazis were forced to address the question of how far they were able to compromise. In a speech on the occasion of Hitler's assumption of power, even Leopold von Zumbusch, at that time rector of the University of Munich, chose to acknowledge Hitler's work and to thank "the venerable field marshal and the leader and chancellor of the German Reich." That he did so in only a few words and without having mentioned Hitler by name contributed to his being removed from office.[28]

The chair of dermatology in Freiburg, Alfred Stühmer, also was opposed to the totalitarian state. He tried to lessen the Nazi influence in his clinic and was able to avoid joining the party for several years. However, in November 1936, when he was appointed dean of the medical faculty, Stühmer thought it might be easier to carry out his university duties as a member of the party. Six months later, he joined the NSDAP, and in a speech in 1937 to newly enrolled students, he stated that the Nazis alone had been able to solve the German crisis, to reinstitute a patriotic and military spirit, and "to cleanse the teaching staff and the student body of alien elements."[29]

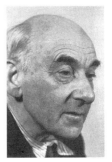

Such notions by highly regarded professors helped the Nazis consolidate their control over intellectual life in Germany. The opportunism of academics served as a model and excuse for cowardly behavior by persons of lower status and contributed to the resignation and despair of opponents of the government. In his diaries, the Jewish philologist Viktor Klemperer (fig. 219)—a brother of the renowned internist, Georg Klemperer—bemoaned the flagrant opportunism of former colleagues at the University of Dresden: "If it once came the other way round, and the fate of the vanquished persons was in my hands, I would spare all people and even some of the leaders who possibly were honest and did not know what they were doing. But I would hang all intellectuals, and the professors one meter higher than everybody else."[30] Of course, these were thoughts confided to a diary and not meant to be published, but they express the disgust aroused by learned men and former democrats who, suddenly and against their better judgment, became mouthpieces of Nazism.

As persons schooled in rational thinking, the professors were able to rationalize their opportunistic behavior. Some argued that should Hitler fail, the Communists would take over and that was thought to be even worse. Others excused opportunism by virtue of devotion to their work, which they deemed to be valuable: Work gives a sense of security and self-assurance; devotion to one's work may, in actuality, be devotion to one's own security.

Opportunistic behavior was rewarded by a certain degree of influence that could be used in salutary ways. Instead of ineffectively opposing the party—and losing their jobs in the process—Frieboes and Stühmer were able to keep their titles

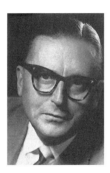

FIG 220
THEODOR
GRÜNEBERG
(1901–1979)

and discreetly support patients or colleagues who were in trouble. On one occasion, the academic promotion of Theodor Grüneberg (fig. 220) had been blocked at the University of Halle because one of his great-grandparents was Jewish. In Berlin, Grüneberg's appointment as associate professor was approved because of Frieboes's request. After the war, Grüneberg became director of the skin clinic in Halle. He died in Saarbrücken in 1979.[31]

When Alfred Stühmer was dean of the medical faculty of the University of Freiburg, he was asked by the director of the Polyclinic for dentistry, Friedrich Faber, "whether and to what degree Jewish patients may be treated or have to be treated in public hospitals." Stühmer answered, "The sick Jewish patient needs medical treatment. Therefore, if he wants to make use of our help, we have not only the right but the duty to treat him." Stühmer discouraged Faber from approaching the authorities with such questions. Had the dean of the medical faculty been an ardent Nazi, the answer to Faber's question would have been very different. In this instance, Stühmer's opportunism enabled him to serve the needs of victims of the system.[32]

The same is true of Heinrich Löhe (fig. 221), a disciple of Abraham Buschke and his successor as director of dermatology at the Rudolf Virchow Hospital in Berlin. Like Walter Frieboes, Löhe did not join the NSDAP. Nevertheless, he cooperated with the Nazis, and during the war he rose to the rank of the highest "general physician" at the Russian front and the highest consulting dermatologist and venereologist in the German army. In those positions, Löhe was well informed about the cruelties inflicted in Russia and Poland, including the annihilation of Jews and medical experiments on internees of concentration camps. In fact, in April 1945, he was scheduled to give a lecture about simulation of diseases based on data from medical experiments carried out at Auschwitz.[33] Nonetheless, he seemed to use his influence to help Buschke and his wife while they languished in the concentration camp of Theresienstadt. After the war, Löhe became chairman of

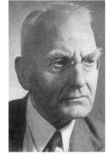

FIG 221
HEINRICH LÖHE
(1877–1961)

dermatology at the Charité Hospital in Berlin. At that time, he was already sixty-eight years of age. He retired in 1951 and died ten years later at the age of eighty-three.[34]

In contrast to Frieboes and Löhe, Hans-Theodor Schreus (fig. 222), chair of the Department of Dermatology at the University of Düsseldorf, had joined the Nazi party in May 1933, mainly at the urging of his wife, who feared for his career. Like Löhe, Schreus acquired high rank in the medical corps of the German military. As the consulting dermatologist of the air force, he knew about the cruelties carried out under German rule but saw no reason to retreat from his position. Despite this cooperation, Schreus despised Nazism and anti-Semitism. During the entire period of the Third Reich, he displayed a portrait and autograph of the Jewish dermatologist Karl Herxheimer in front of his private office. After the promulgation of the Law for the Restoration of Professional Civil Service, he kept his Jewish assistant, Fritz Bernstein, in his employ, and when Bernstein's dismissal could no longer be avoided, he tried to secure him a position in England. After the war, Schreus was dismissed by the British military government but was restored to his previous position in 1948. He retired in 1962 and died in 1970 at age seventy-eight.[35]

Heinrich Adolf Gottron (fig. 223) was also a member of the Nazi party and thus fulfilled the political preconditions for receiving a major university position. In 1935, he was called to Breslau to succeed Max Jessner as chair of the Department of Dermatology. Like many other new department chairs, Gottron was an opportunist who paid obeisance to Nazi precepts, but he was different because of his scientific achievements, including delineation of the acral papules in dermatomyositis that are credited to him eponymically. Although Gottron did not show great interest in politics, he ingratiated himself with the Nazis, integrated racist notions into his scientific papers, and acted as a representative of science in the National Socialist state. His supportive attitude was rewarded amply by the government: In 1940, Gottron was appointed dean of the

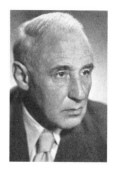

FIG 222
HANS-THEODOR
SCHREUS
(1892–1970)

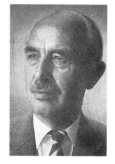

FIG 223
HEINRICH ADOLF
GOTTRON
(1890–1974)

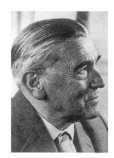

medical faculty of the University of Breslau and became the military superior of most of his colleagues. In those positions, Gottron fulfilled the expectations of the Nazis. According to the chair of surgery in Breslau, Karl-Heinrich Bauer (fig. 224), who, after the war, was rector of the University of Heidelberg and founder of the German Cancer Research Center in Heidelberg, Gottron discouraged members of the medical faculty of the University of Breslau from having social contact with Bauer solely because Bauer had a Jewish wife. Gottron also prevented Bauer from treating wounded German soldiers, even if such treatment had been sanctioned by the army.[36] On the other hand, Gottron occasionally used his influence in constructive ways. In his first years in Breslau, he defended Stephen Epstein against assaults by the party and later presumably managed the release of Franciszek Walter (fig. 225), head of the Department of Dermatology of the University of Kraków, from the concentration camp at Oranienburg.[37] How much Gottron really did for the release of Walter and whether the release was prompted by his intervention is not known. In fact, at the same time, many other Polish internees were released from the camp without having influential advocates.[38] But even if Gottron's intervention on behalf of Walter was decisive, such concessions by the government were rare and were granted arbitrarily. Any attempt to influence the government in a more consistent fashion was doomed to fail. Walter Frieboes, for instance, sent numerous complaints and petitions to the government until the Reich's Ministry of Education ordered that all his letters were to be ignored and remain unanswered.[39]

The only dermatologist who retained a certain degree of influence without embracing the party was Erich Hoffmann. When Hoffmann was attacked at the University of Bonn for his open criticism of the Nazis, his students intervened on his behalf, and after Hoffmann's dismissal had been made known, they wanted to accompany him in a triumphal march out of the lecture hall. The significance of the courage of a single

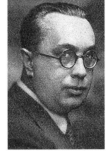

man cannot be overestimated. In Nazi Germany, cowardice and opportunism were infectious because anyone who was bothered by his conscience could easily draw a favorable comparison between himself and at least some of his neighbors and acquaintances whose behavior was even worse. In contrast, Hoffmann's behavior made opportunists and cowards feel uncomfortable and encouraged others, especially students, to emulate that courage and conviction. In a letter, one of Hoffmann's students thanked him in these words: "Out of an ocean of cringing backs, you stand out as a proud, inexorable prophet of truth. Please accept my gratitude, for your strong personality has restored in me, as well as in some other comrades, the belief in German culture and its true representatives."[40]

But Hoffmann's attitude had more than psychological effects. On many occasions, he became engaged on behalf of colleagues who were persecuted by the Nazis. Alois Memmesheimer, one of Hoffmann's former assistants, had been accused of having slandered a party member and was put in jail. Due to the intervention of Hoffmann and some of his influential friends, Memmesheimer was released after a few weeks and was even able to retain his position as chair of dermatology in Essen. Hoffmann also used his international connections to help Jewish emigrants find new positions abroad.

Why was it that Hoffmann could achieve this moderate success without provoking drastic measures against himself? Both his outstanding international reputation and his vital connections to high-ranking members of the government and the army offered him a degree of protection. Furthermore, he was said by friends and opponents to suffer from "cyclically occurring states of excitation," during which his statements could not be taken seriously. That "manic-depressive insanity" was regarded by the Nazis as an extenuating circumstance.[41] After his removal from the chair of dermatology in Bonn, Hoffmann was not harassed further and even was given the opportunity to continue his scientific studies in a private institution. For others, similar behavior had much more serious consequences.

In sum, for persons of integrity and sensitivity, life in Germany was oppressive and intolerable during the Nazi years. But for those who found the Nazis distasteful, which was only a small percentage of the German people until it became obvious that the war was lost, there were a limited number of options available. A person could feign adaptation to the mentality of the new rulers, neglect his or her conscience, comply precisely with government directives, and attempt to enhance his or her possibilities and prospects. This latter path was the easiest, and it was taken by all too many Germans who bowed to the authorities while at the same time trampling on their subordinates. In German, that behavior is likened to that of a cyclist, a *Radfahrer* who, while treading the pedals (as if kicking underlings) keeps his head bowed (as if in submission to superiors). The attitude of the *Radfahrer*, which resulted from a long history of equilibration with authoritarianism, was highly prevalent in Germany. That ingrained attitude was enhanced by the leadership principle advocated by the Nazis, a principle that permitted the disclaimer, with ease, that a person bore no responsibility for his actions because he was "only following orders."

A person who was not prepared to sacrifice conscience for the sake of success, and perhaps survival, could still try to ignore what was going on in Nazi Germany, retreat into himself, and remain silent. A person could acknowledge to himself what was going on, not like it, and resist passively. A person could speak up, but this resulted, at the very least, in immediate dismissal from a position. A person could work actively against the regime, thereby risking the constant threat of arrest, or even death. Or, a person could attempt to leave the country.

These options can be pictured schematically, based on the activities of dermatologists and the support they lent the Nazis on one extreme and the resistance to the Nazis on the other. Some dermatologists—like Wirz, Brill, and Spiethoff—were very active in the National Socialist movement. Those who rejected the Nazi party and were active in the resistance—like

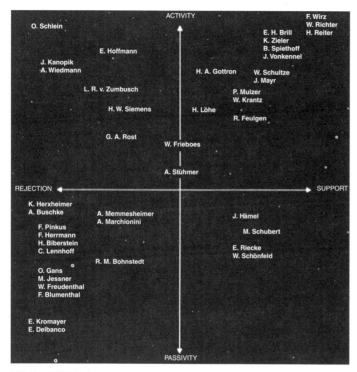

FIG 226 SPECTRUM OF RESPONSES BY DERMATOLOGISTS TO THE NAZIS.

Otto Schlein—were killed. Others did not work actively against the Nazis. Some—Ernst Delbanco among them—committed suicide. Still others—Jessner, Freudenthal, Blumenthal, Pinkus, and Gans—chose emigration as a way out. A few who despised the Nazis—such as von Zumbusch, Rost, and Hoffmann—positioned themselves on middle ground. Eventually, attitudes toward the Nazis changed over the years, usually from support at first to utter rejection when the war was lost (fig. 226).

This was the case even with such ardent Nazis as Schultze and Spiethoff, who finally came to realize that they had followed Adolf Hitler not into German greatness but into the most devastating catastrophe in German history.

THE ESCALATION
OF SUPPRESSION

THE FIRST MAJOR ASSAULT ON JEWS CAME IN 1933. A CLI-
MATE OF TERROR CREATED BY STORM TROOPERS AND
a multitude of new anti-Jewish regulations led to a first wave
of Jewish emigration. Of about six hundred thousand Jews who
lived in Germany, some thirty-seven thousand left the country
in 1933, the highest figure for any year in the five years of Jewish emigration that followed. Most Jews, however, responded to
National Socialism by reaffirming their German roots and
German identity. Immediately after Hitler's appointment as
chancellor, the largest secular organization of German Jewry,
the Central Association of German Citizens of Jewish Faith,
stated in its publication, *CV-Zeitung*, "We are convinced that
no one will dare to violate our constitutional rights." Five
weeks later, the paper reassured its readers that "Germany will
remain Germany and no one can rob us of our homeland and
of our fatherland."[1] Before the plebiscite on Hitler's policy in
November 1933, the Federal Representation of German Jews
issued this statement: "Along with the entire German people,
we Jews, as citizens also, are summoned to cast our votes on the
foreign policy of the Reich government. They are necessary to
ensure Germany's equality among the nations, the conciliation
of the nations, and the peace of the world. Despite all that we
have endured, the vote of the German Jews can only be 'Yes.'"[2]

The statement was issued under the watchful eye of the government—a recommendation to vote otherwise would not have
been permitted. Nevertheless, it illustrates the dilemma felt by
German Jews at the time. In the early 1930s, most German Jews
were liberal in religious practices, conservative in politics, and
more passionately identified with Germany than with being
Jewish. More than 80 percent had been born in Germany and
had a great sense of pride in their fatherland. They had fought

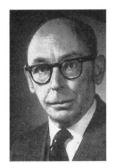

FIG 227
WALTER LEVER
(1909–1993)

for Germany in World War I, and many had belonged to right-wing antidemocratic organizations during the Weimar Republic. The Federal Union of Jewish War Veterans had thirty thousand members and was fervently patriotic. Early in 1933, Oscar Gans, the chair of the Department of Dermatology in Frankfurt, interrupted a lecture on dermatology to praise eulogistically Ernst Leo Schlageter, a highly revered hero of the Nazis who had been a nationalistically motivated terrorist sentenced to death for attacks against French facilities during the French and Belgian occupation of the Rhineland in 1923.[3]

A desire to see the strength and honor of Germany restored prompted some Jews to actually welcome the National Socialist government. Among them was Otto Lubarsch, the former chair of pathology at the Charité Hospital in Berlin and co-author of the classic text known internationally as "Henke and Lubarsch." Lubarsch died of natural causes on April 1, 1933, before the new regulations of the Nazi government he supported could affect him, as they disastrously affected so many others.[4]

Many of those regarded by the Nazis as Jews did not consider themselves to be Jews at all because their parents or grandparents had converted to Christianity. One example is Walter Lever (fig. 227), a pioneer dermatopathologist of the modern era who established bullous pemphigoid and cicatricial pemphigoid as distinct clinicopathological entities and wrote the most widely distributed dermatopathology textbook of the century. Lever was Christian, and during his medical studies in Heidelberg he belonged to a Christian dueling fraternity whose members were forbidden to socialize with Jews. One of Lever's partners in the anatomy lab was Rudolf Baer, who was Jewish and belonged to a Jewish fraternity whose members wore orange hats, while the members of Lever's fraternity wore blue ones. As they worked together on a cadaver, Baer and Lever engaged in the usual conversation expected of medical students in that endeavor, but when Lever met Baer outside the anatomy lab, he was forbidden to speak to him and he did not.

After graduation, Baer, followed by Lever, emigrated to the United States, and both had superb academic careers. Baer became chair of dermatology at the New York University School of Medicine, while Lever assumed the same position at Tufts University in Boston, after a decade of having been in the Department of Dermatology at Boston's famed Massachusetts General Hospital. When Lever arrived in New York City from Germany, he sought out his old anatomy partner, who was then a very junior physician in the Skin and Cancer Unit of New York University, working under the direction of Marion Sulzberger. Lever asked Baer to intervene on his behalf for a position in that department, but no position was available, in part because so many slots had already been taken by refugees from Europe, especially Germany.[5]

Throughout his life, Lever denied Jewish descent. When asked by A. Bernard Ackerman, then editor of the fledgling *American Journal of Dermatopathology*, whether he wished to be mentioned in a forthcoming article by Alfred Hollander about the plight of Jewish dermatologists under the Nazis, Lever responded, "Of course not. I am not Jewish."[6] When asked whether Lever had left Germany because of his Jewish heritage, his widow, Gundula Schaumburg-Lever, responded, "There was no Jewish origin."[7] In truth, Lever's father, Alexander Lever, was half Jewish. Until 1938, he had operated a private practice of dermatology in Erfurt, and his name can be found in the city archives under the heading "Jewish firms, physicians, dentists, and lawyers"[8] (fig. 228). Despite Walter Lever's denial of any Jewish origin and his own identification as Christian, the sole fact that his father was half Jewish would have made an academic career in National Socialist Germany impossible. Such was the case with Kurt Lever, Walter's twin brother, who stayed in Germany during the war and was a target of constant discrimination because of his non-Aryan descent. Kurt Lever was finally licensed as a physician as late as 1942, at which time Walter Lever had already worked productively for years in the pathology laboratory of the Massachusetts General Hospital.[9]

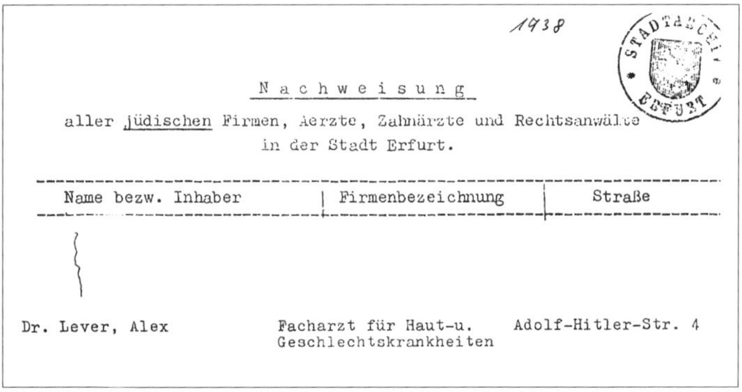

```
                                              1938      [STADTARCHIV
                                                         ERFURT stamp]

                        N a c h w e i s u n g
        aller jüdischen Firmen, Aerzte, Zahnärzte und Rechtsanwälte
                         in der Stadt Erfurt.

        -----------------------------------------------------------
          Name bezw. Inhaber    |  Firmenbezeichnung   |   Straße
        ------  --------------------------------------- -----------
                {
                {
                {

        Dr. Lever, Alex             Facharzt für Haut-u.   Adolf-Hitler-Str. 4
                                    Geschlechtskrankheiten
```

FIG 228 RECORD OF ALL JEWISH FIRMS, PHYSICIANS, DENTISTS, AND LAWYERS IN THE CITY OF ERFURT. ALEXANDER LEVER HAD HIS OFFICE ON ADOLF-HITLER-STRASSE 4.

Rudolf Baer, although acknowledging that he was Jewish, also thought of himself foremost as a German, and so did his family. Baer was born in Strasbourg when the Alsace was part of the German Reich. After the defeat of Germany in the First World War, Baer remembered vividly and painfully his elementary school class being conducted by a French military officer, with the flag and map of France prominently displayed. Suddenly, the language was French. A few years later, the Baers moved from Strasbourg to Frankfurt to be in Germany once again. In 1934, the country that Baer had embraced rejected him, and he left for the United States.[10] Within about twenty-five years, Baer became chair of the Skin and Cancer unit of the New York University School of Medicine, and in the next twenty years, he was president of virtually every major dermatological society in the United States. In 1972, Baer was president of the World Congress of Dermatology in Mexico and, in 1992, honorary president of the World Congress of Dermatology in New York City.[11] In 1977, Baer became president of the International Committee of Dermatology and the International League of Dermatological Societies. In 1987, the Rudolph L. Baer Chair was created in his honor at New York University.

Scientifically, Baer is best known for work during the 1960s pertaining to the Langerhans' cell. In fact, the seminal observation of the function of Langerhans' cells as antigen-present-ing cells in the epidermis was made by his Jewish co-worker and junior faculty member Inga Silberberg-Sinakin (fig. 229), who was born in Germany in 1934. She and her family lived in a small village in the vicinity of Kassel, whose inhabitants had known one another for years. Nevertheless, the Aryan neigh-bors did not speak to the Silberbergs. Inga Silberberg-Sinakin never had playmates and remembers vividly how other chil-dren threw stones at her and through the windows of her home. Nevertheless, her father, a German veteran of World War I, wanted to stay in Germany. Her mother, however, had the fore-sight to request an affidavit from relatives in New York City, and the Silberbergs emigrated in 1938, leaving their possessions and many relatives behind. In New York City, they lived together in a single room in Harlem, her father working as a dishwasher and saving every nickel for his daughter's educa-tion. From Harlem, the family moved to Washington Heights, where many German Jews had settled. The synagogue of Washington Heights was the major information center for news from Germany, and it was there that the Silberbergs first learned of the death of their relatives in German concentration camps. Some of Inga Silberberg-Sinakin's cousins survived and described their fate in a book titled *Muted Voices*.[12]

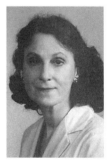

FIG 229

INGA SILBERBERG-SINAKIN
(BORN 1934)

In 1995, Rudolf Baer was invited to Berlin to present the story of the Langerhans' cell at the 38th Congress of the German Dermatological Society. He informed Silberberg-Sinakin that she would also receive an invitation that, in actuality, never arrived. Nevertheless, Silberberg-Sinakin, who had never returned to Germany, volunteered to help Baer with the prepa-ration of his lecture, noting that Baer looked forward to the event with unbridled anticipation. Baer had close friends in Ger-many, was an honorary member of the German Dermatological Society, and had used virtually every opportunity for visiting his fatherland. Even as mini-strokes progressively impaired his abil-ity to function, he struggled to complete the lecture and make it to Berlin. After a severe stroke in 1996, Baer lost control of his mental capability and died in New York City in 1997. Despite having been rejected by Nazi Germany and having been forced to emigrate, Baer never lost his German identity.[13]

Another example of the striking discrepancy between assessment of self and assessment by the Nazis is Fritz Juliusberg. For many years, Juliusberg had been director of dermatology at the Municipal Hospital of Posnan. In 1899, he had described pityriasis lichenoides chronica. At the end of the First World War, Posnan fell to Poland, and Juliusberg, who did not wish to live under a Polish government, moved to Braunschweig, where he opened a private practice. Juliusberg was a baptized Jew of Lutheran faith and had been married to a Lutheran since 1920. He felt no affiliation with Judaism or with Jews. Juliusberg was deeply devoted to his fatherland and considered himself German. When the Nazis gained power, Juliusberg suddenly found himself excluded from his own German people, a punishment undeserved, unexpected, and beyond endurance for him. Juliusberg lived in Braunschweig until 1936, at which time his name no longer appeared in the archives of the city's registration office. His ultimate fate is not known with certainty, but it is rumored that Juliusberg committed suicide in Berlin in 1936.[14]

The sudden outbreak of anti-Semitism was hard to bear, even for observant Jews who received strength and reaffirmation from their religious beliefs and from their place in the tightly knit Jewish community. But for most German Jews who had distanced themselves from Judaism or had converted to Christianity, the new situation was even more intolerable because they were suddenly deprived of an essential part of their own identity—their Germanness—and were treated just like orthodox Jews for whom they had contempt. They were forced, unexpectedly, to tolerate humiliation at the hands of fellow Germans with whom they had always shared the same hopes and ideals. It is no surprise that Jews who had based their entire existence on identification with Germany were so susceptible to suicide. Among the Jewish population of Berlin, there was a 50 percent rise in the rate of suicide from 1924 to 1926 and again from 1932 to 1934, suicide becoming the fourth most common cause of death following heart and circulatory disorders, diseases that affected the central nervous system, and malignant neoplasms.[15] In the Rhineland, the "epidemic" of suicide was so alarming that the rabbinate of Cologne, in mid-1933, issued this public appeal: "Under the shattering impact of the events of recent weeks, during which suicide claimed victim upon victim within our community, we turn to you, men and women of the Jewish community, with this appeal: Maintain your courage and will to live, preserve your confidence in God and in yourself!"[16]

In similar appeals, representatives of Jewish communities encouraged their members to remain in Germany. The upholding of a Jewish presence in Germany was considered a moral necessity and a religious imperative, essential if Jews were to achieve their universal mission in the world—the establishment of a society of human beings in which social justice obtained for each and every one of them according to the principles set forth in the divinely inspired Hebrew scriptures. German Jews in particular conceived of their mission as the establishment of liberalism and rationalism, attributes that were thought to be treasured by Jews and Germans especially. Joseph Lehmann, the rabbi of the Reform congregation in Berlin, denied that the political changes in the spring of 1933 affected "our position as Germans of the Jewish faith." Emigration might be a solution for some, but most German Jews would stay to affirm the "heritage of their German homeland."[17] Heinrich Stern, head of the Liberal Jews, argued that to flee Germany just "because five painful months lie behind us" was cowardly. "We, as Jews, reaffirm life in Germany and for Germany."[18]

Viewed in the larger context of Jewish history, the anti-Semitism of National Socialism appeared to be nothing more than a contemporary manifestation of the same persecution that had afflicted Jews throughout the ages. In the narrower context of German-Jewish history, it was seen as merely the latest phase of negative reaction in a time of otherwise dramatic progress, a temporary setback in the long process of complete emancipation. Most Jews, therefore, were willing to hold out, to endure present hardships, and to wait for things to improve, as they were confident they would.

After almost seventeen months of National Socialist reign, the time of improvement seemed to have arrived. Until then, most acts of arbitrary violence against Jews had been carried out by the SA—the storm troopers—an organization of about four million members that was led by Ernst Röhm, one of Hitler's oldest companions from the earliest days of the Nazi movement (fig. 230). By virtue of the size and the military structure of the SA, Röhm had become very powerful—too powerful for Hitler's taste. On June 30, 1934, Hitler's command for the assassination of Röhm and two hundred other SA leaders was carried out. This massacre was part of Hitler's method for consolidating power, yet it was misinterpreted—both in Germany and elsewhere—as a desire on Hitler's part to stop the arbitrary terror that had been inflicted by the Brownshirts.

After von Hindenburg's death, Hitler also assumed the presidency of Germany, and Jews continued to hope that things would now settle down. There was even a substantial return of Jews who had fled the country in 1933.[19] A hopeful sign was that no significant anti-Jewish legislation was enacted in 1934, a fact that reinforced the illusion that Jews might remain safe in Germany, albeit with decreased rights.

Those rights, however, were eroded further, and on September 15, 1935, on the occasion of the annual NSDAP Congress in Nuremberg, the Nuremberg Laws went into effect. Hitler requested that those laws be ready by the time of the festive closing of the party congress (fig. 231), and in order to accomplish that goal, the new regulations had to be feverishly worked out in only two days. Among the most significant regulations was the Law for the Protection of German Blood and German Honor, which made marriage and extramarital relations

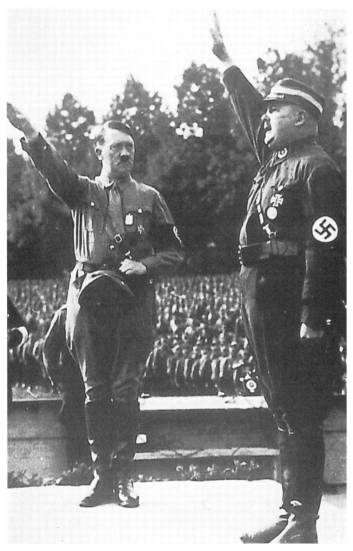

FIG 230 ERNST RÖHM (1887–1934) WITH ADOLF HITLER.

between Germans and Jews a crime. Jews were also forbidden
to employ any German woman under the age of forty-five as
domestic help or to fly the German national colors.

The announcement of the institution of the Nuremberg
Laws occurred at the same time that the International Congress
of Dermatology was convening in Budapest. Upon learning of

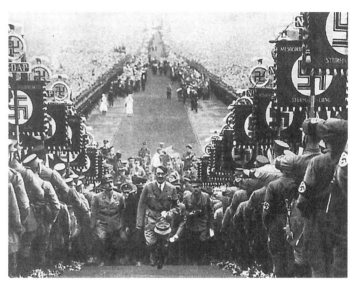

FIG 231 MASS MEETING OF THE NAZIS.

the new legislation, Alfred Hollander (fig. 232), who was one of the last students of Paul Gerson Unna in Hamburg and who would later become a clinical professor of dermatology at Boston University School of Medicine, asked the organizing committee, on behalf of himself and other Jewish colleagues who attended the congress, to be seated apart from the rest of the German delegation. Karl Zieler, who tried to avoid calling attention in any way to the new realities in Germany, was dismayed by this request, and only the intervention of Alfred Stühmer avoided severe consequences for Hollander.[20]

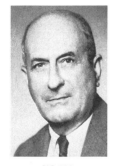

FIG 232
ALFRED
HOLLANDER
(1899–1986)

The Nuremberg Laws were soon supplemented by a decree that defined who was a Jew, a definition that was to attain unimagined importance. A Jew was defined as having at least three Jewish grandparents. Also to be regarded as a Jew was someone who had two Jewish grandparents and belonged to the Jewish religious community or was married to a Jew. Those with two Jewish grandparents but no affiliation with the Jewish community were designated "half-breed, first degree," and those with only one Jewish grandparent were "half-breed, second degree." Those with one Jewish great-grandparent or

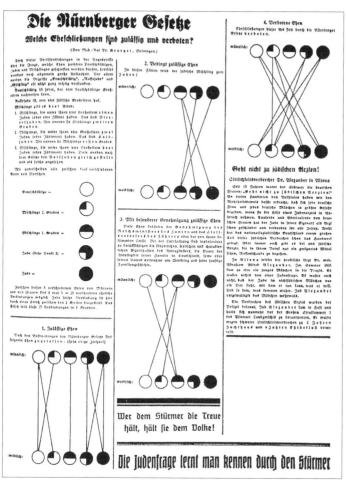

FIG 233 DEFINITION OF A JEW ACCORDING TO THE
NUREMBERG LAWS (FROM *DER STÜRMER*).

great-great-grandparent—one-eighth or one-sixteenth Jew—
were considered German, although they, too, were subject to
certain measures of discrimination (fig. 233).

The Nuremberg Laws provided the means for technocratic
classification of human beings. All full Jews were deprived of
their citizenship and were classified derogatorily as "residents"
of Germany. Because noncitizens could not hold public office,
Jewish civil servants who had been exempt because of the
"Hindenburg clauses" in the Law for the Restoration of Pro-

Hain ╪, Ursula 30, AssA a. d.
Unv▮▮Klin,~S10, Eschen-
bachstr. 14
Hain, Alfons 24, ▮▮, ~Fechen-
heim, Ueberlinger Weg 23
: Hainebach, Julius 94, SR, ~1,
Scheffelstr. 11
Hallerbach, Georg 27, ~Rödel-
heim, Alexanderstr. 5
Hammacher, Paul 10, ▮▮, ~1,
Kaiserstr. 16
Hanacek, Zdenko 12, ~1, Im
Sachsenlager 24
: Hanau, Alfred 12, ▮▮, ~1,
Steinweg 9
Hanf-Dreßler, Kurt 28, ▮▮,
▮▮, ~17, Blittersdorffplatz
43
Hanslmeier, Andreas 27, ~Nied,
Oeserstr. 31
Happel, Günther 20, ▮▮, ~
17, Rheinstr. 25

▮▮ d. Städt. Kh, ~Höchst,
Gerlachstr. 14
Hergenhähn, Eugen 91, SR, ▮▮,
~1, Gärtnerweg 16
: Hermann, Franz 23, ▮▮, ~1,
Bockenheimer Anlage 38
Herrlen, Hartmuth 34, ▮▮, OA i.
Heer
: Herxheimer, Hans 10, ▮▮, ~1,
Eschersheimer Landstr. 132
: Herxheimer, Karl 85, ▮▮,
GMR, Prof, ~17, Westend-
str. 92
: Herz, Ernst 24, ▮▮, ~1,
Bockenheimer Anlage 33
Herzog, Heinrich 31, Dr med et
med dent, ~1, Roßmarkt 12
: Hesdörffer, Julius 83, SR, ▮▮,
~1, Reuterweg 57
: Heß, Leo 25, ▮▮, ~1,
Fellnerstr. 6

FIG 234 SECTION OF THE REICH'S MEDICINAL CALENDAR OF 1937.
THE NAMES OF JEWISH PHYSICIANS ARE MARKED BY COLONS.

fessional Civil Service were to be dismissed by the end of the year. The Reich's Physicians' Ordinance of 1935 stated unequivocally that henceforth no new Jewish candidates would be licensed for medical practice. "Mixlings"—those who were as little as one-fourth Jewish but still were allowed to be citizens—and non-Jewish physicians married to Jews were to be excluded from the profession.[21] In the Reich's Medicinal Calendar of 1937, the names of all Jewish physicians—for example, the name of Karl Herxheimer, the former chair of dermatology in Frankfurt—were marked by colons (fig. 234).[22]

Other dermatologists of Jewish descent chose to give up their practices, Fritz Juliusberg of Braunschweig and Kurt Wiener (fig. 235) of Breslau among them. For many years, Wiener had organized the medical care of patients with venereal diseases and had lectured at the academy for public health. In 1936, he emigrated to the United States and, in 1937, began a new professional life in Milwaukee. Wiener wrote several textbooks, among them *Skin Manifestations of Internal Disorders* (1947) and *Systemic Associations and Treatment of Skin Diseases* (1955). He died in Milwaukee of chronic leukemia in 1960.[23]

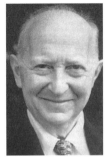

FIG 235
KURT WIENER
(1891–1960)

The Nuremberg Laws affected not only Jews but all Germans; everyone had to provide evidence of Aryan lineage. To maintain full civil rights, every person was forced to prove by certificates of birth, baptism, and marriage that none of their parents and grandparents had "fully alien, especially Jewish, blood." There were many, among them even ardent Nazis, who experienced an unpleasant surprise when examining their own family tree. The dermatologist Theodor Grüneberg, for example, a member of the Nazi party and the SA since 1933, declared in a question- naire in 1936 that he had no Jewish forebears. Subsequently, a more thorough examination revealed that Grüneberg had one Jewish great-grandparent, which was sufficient to prevent his further academic advancement at the University of Halle.[24]

For the evaluation of genealogy, the birth registers of the Catholic and Lutheran churches were invaluable resources, and the churches did not hesitate from placing them at the Nazis' disposal. Without the cooperation of the churches, the Nurem- berg Laws could not have been enforced.[25] In general, the reg- isters of the churches were remarkably well kept, but some had been destroyed by dampness or fire. If certificates of parents or grandparents were not available, a professional "tribe investi- gator" could be hired to search for missing documents, but such professional help could be costly and was not always successful.

Among those who had great difficulties in compiling docu- ments about their heritage was Rudolf Maximilian Bohn- stedt, who later became chair of dermatology in Giessen. Bohnstedt's forebears were spread throughout Europe; some were born in Germany, his mother's grandfather was born in Manchester, and Bohnstedt himself was born in St. Peters- burg, where most his family still resided. In the Russian revo- lution, Bohnstedt had volunteered to fight for the White Army, and at the end of World War I, he had emigrated to Germany to study medicine. When Bohnstedt applied for habilitation at the University of Munich in 1934, the Nazis noted that his Russian certificate of graduation from high school did not contain information about his religious affilia-

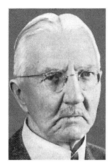

FIG 236
HJALMAR SCHACHT
(1877–1970)

tion. Further inquiries into Bohnstedt's descent revealed that one of his great-grandmothers was Jewish. As a "one-eighth Jew," Bohnstedt would still have been eligible for promotion, but he was unable to provide the birth certificate of his English-born great-grandfather, who had emigrated from Manchester to St. Petersburg; his great-grandfather's certificate of birth had been lost in the Soviet Union. The German consulate in Liverpool attested that all attempts to find that certificate had been unsuccessful. To maintain his chances for habilitation, Bohnstedt asked his brother, Edward, to search for documents that could prove that their great-grandfather was Aryan. Indeed, Edward Bohnstedt, who was still living in Leningrad (formerly St. Petersburg), produced an affidavit by the former elder of the Lutheran German Church that his great-grandfather had belonged to the Lutheran community, and the German consulate in Leningrad confirmed that he had been buried at the Lutheran cemetery. Those documents, however, were not deemed to be sufficient by the Nazis, and Rudolf Maximilian Bohnstedt was denied academic promotion. Tragically, his brother's inquiries caught the attention of the Communist authorities, who presumably found out about Rudolf Bohnstedt's counter-revolutionary activities in the White Army. As a consequence, Edward Bohnstedt was sent to Siberia and was never heard of again.[26]

Throughout the years of the National Socialist regime, enactment of anti-Jewish regulations was associated with escalation of unofficial anti-Jewish violence. The promulgation of the Nuremberg Laws was preceded in the summer of 1935 by a marked increase in arbitrary ordinances directed against Jews. Jews were prevented from going to cinemas, theaters, swimming pools, and resorts. Small Jewish businesses were effectively shut down through boycott or open violence.

Toward the end of the year, however, these assaults were suddenly interrupted on the initiative of Hjalmar Schacht (fig. 236), the president of the Reichsbank and minister of economy. Schacht condemned what he called "irresponsible

Jew-baitings" because they adversely affected foreign trade, which was desperately needed to stabilize the economy and finance the rearmament of Germany.[27] Furthermore, the party hoped to create the appearance of moderation in anticipation of the Olympic Games that were to be convened in Berlin in 1936 and were to be a celebration of the new German state for the whole world to see (see figs. 238, 239).[28]

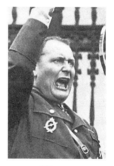

In 1938, after two years of relative moderation, the situation again changed dramatically when Nazi policy—internal and external—shifted into high gear. When Hjalmar Schacht was dismissed as minister of economy in 1937 for his opposition to the continual stockpiling of massive German armaments, Hermann Göring (fig. 237), the plenipotentiary for the Four Year Plan, succeeded Schacht and took control of the economy in its entirety. Although many Jews were without work and depended on charity at the time, about forty thousand Jewish firms were still doing business in Germany, many of them crucial to the armament industry and to import-export trade.

Göring now turned his attention to the expropriation of Jewish property. The owners of Jewish firms were threatened by rabid members of the party and even were taken into "protective custody" until they agreed to "voluntarily" transfer their

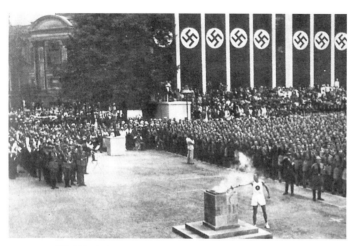

FIG 238 USE OF SPORTS FOR POLITICAL PURPOSES:
THE 1936 OLYMPIC GAMES.

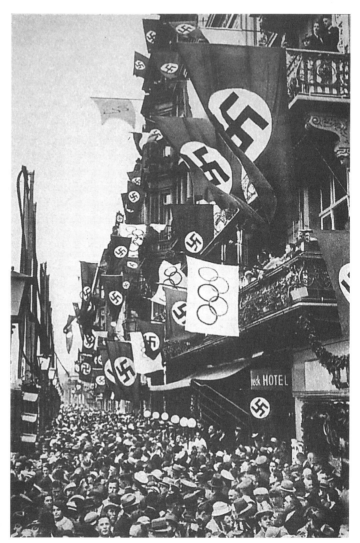

FIG 239 THE OLYMPIC GAMES IN 1936: THE OLYMPIC FLAGS
AND SWASTIKAS SIDE BY SIDE.

businesses to non-Jews, at values far below true worth. On
April 26, 1938, a decree was issued stating that every Jew had
to assess his entire domestic and foreign property and report it
to the authorities. The objective of this decree was phrased in
language that could not be misconstrued: "The plenipotentiary for the Four Year Plan may take measures to ensure that

the use of property subject to reporting will be in keeping with the interest of the German economy."[29]

The new wave of anti-Jewish regulations also affected Jewish physicians. Some three thousand—out of a count of eight thousand in 1933—had emigrated during the first year of National Socialist rule. About five hundred physicians who had lost their jobs stayed in Germany and made their living in other ways, such as in the pharmaceutical industry or as masseurs, midwives, or nurses.[30]

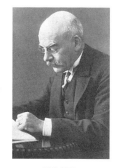

Until then, most Jewish physicians had been able to maintain their practices. Despite massive propaganda and inordinate pressure by employers and party groups, their patients continued to visit them. The reason was not only because patients deemed Jewish physicians to be more knowledgeable than the Aryan doctors—who often had been newly appointed to insurance-fund panels only because they could boast Old Fighter laurels—but also because of differences they perceived and felt in the attitude of the Aryan physicians. The Jewish internist Georg Klemperer (fig. 240) characterized that difference in these words: "The Jewish physician understands his duty as a service, he is the servant of his patient, and the Aryan physician is the commander, he gives orders."[31] The competence and gentle manner of Jewish physicians attracted patients who were unhappy with Nazi doctors. Ironically, for a brief period, some insurance-fund panel Jewish physicians had more patients and made more money than ever before, much to the dismay of their National Socialist colleagues, who responded by both systematic and capricious oppression of them.

By 1935, the radical party press demanded the death penalty for all Jewish doctors who still dared treat Gentile patients. In the same year, the Jewish general practitioner Hans Serelmann was delivered by Aryan colleagues to the Gestapo for having performed a transfusion of Jewish blood into an Aryan patient. In growing numbers, Jewish physicians were charged by young women patients with "race defilement," reporting to the authorities that the doctors had tried to kiss them or had exhibited prurient behavior. Often, these patients had been "planted" by the Nazis to lure physicians into compromising situations, at which moments Nazis would mysteriously appear in the examining room and catch the unsuspecting doctor *flagrante delicto*. By August 1936, Jewish insurance-fund panel physicians who performed surgery on Aryans were no longer paid, and in January 1938, all Jewish physicians were removed from membership in the often lucrative supplementary (private) insurance funds, which largely served upper-income business employees.[32] Furthermore, Jewish physicians were deprived of their titles. Karl Altmann, the former director of dermatology at the Frankfurt Sachsenhausen Municipal Hospital, was forbidden by the district leader of the Reich's Chamber of Physicians to maintain the word "professor" on a sign placed at the entrance of his office.[33]

As a consequence of these measures, the income of Jewish physicians, despite their dedication to patients, dropped rapidly. Their financial situation may have been bearable until the end of 1935, but in the next three years it deteriorated to a disastrous level; Jewish physicians earned next to nothing. According to data of the German Panel Fund Physicians' Union, Jewish generalists in Upper Silesia had an average yearly income of approximately 300 Reichsmarks, whereas their Aryan counterparts grossed over 13,000 Reichsmarks a year.[34]

Nevertheless, Jewish doctors did not give up. According to a 1937 survey, there were still 4,121 practicing Jewish physicians left, accounting for 7 percent of all physicians in Germany (down from 13 percent in 1933) (fig. 241).[35]

These numbers finally prompted the Reich's leader of physicians, Gerhard Wagner, to suggest to Hitler the immediate dissolution of the practices of Jewish physicians, whether or not they were attached to insurance-fund panels (fig. 242). Because of the high esteem physicians enjoyed, Hitler considered the exclusion of Jews from the profession to be an essential and crucial blow. On July 25, 1938, the decree was issued

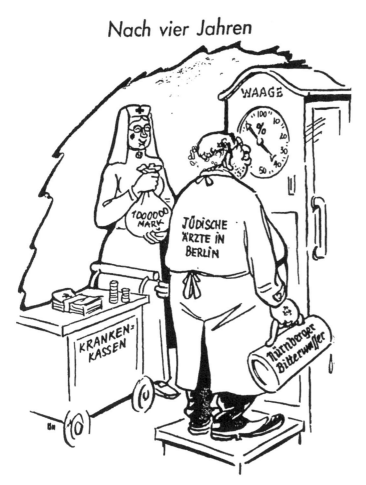

Nach vier Jahren

FIG 241 "AFTER FOUR YEARS, STILL NO LOSS CAN BE DETERMINED."
SS CARTOON COMPLAINING THAT AFTER FOUR YEARS OF NATIONAL
SOCIALISM AND DESPITE THE NUREMBURG LAWS ("BITTER WATER OF
NUREMBURG"), THERE APPEARED TO BE NO REDUCTION IN THE
NUMBER OF JEWISH DOCTORS IN BERLIN WHO WERE
GENEROUSLY NOURISHED BY INSURANCE FUNDS.

that withdrew the licenses of Jewish physicians and forbade
them to practice medicine.

Paul Richter, who wrote a lengthy chapter on the history of
dermatology for Jadassohn's *Handbuch*, was among a group of
renowned practitioners affected by the decree. Richter had
lost his wife in 1936, his son had committed suicide a year

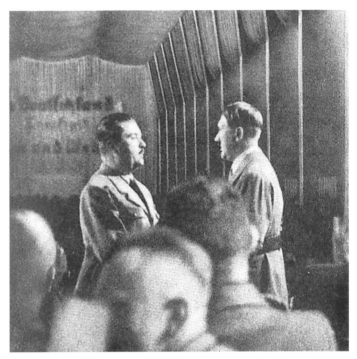

FIG 242 GERHARD WAGNER IN A DISCUSSION WITH ADOLF HITLER.

later, and his professional life—a private practice in Berlin—
was all he had left. Only a few weeks after he was denied the
right to practice medicine and care for his patients as he had
done for so many years, Richter's health deteriorated rapidly,
and he soon died of a heart attack.[36]

Because Aryan physicians were not supposed to treat Jewish
patients, 709 of the almost four thousand Jewish physicians
still practicing in Germany were given special permission by
the Ministry of the Interior to treat Jews exclusively (fig. 243).
These Jewish physicians were tolerated only in cities with
large numbers of Jews, such as Berlin and Breslau, and because
they were no longer regarded as full-fledged members of the
German medical community, they were excluded from professional organizations and denied the respected designation of
"physician." Henceforth, they were referred to as mere
"treaters of the sick."[37]

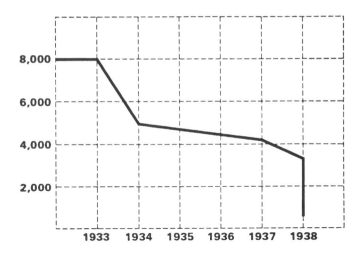

FIG 243 DECLINE IN NUMBER OF JEWISH
PHYSICIANS PRACTICING IN GERMANY.

One of those "treaters of the sick" was Felix Pinkus (fig. 244), the former secretary of the German Society for the Fight Against Venereal Diseases and of the Berlin Dermatological Society. Pinkus was one of the leading dermatopathologists of his time. Among his outstanding contributions were the first descriptions of lichen nitidus, the hair disc, and the mantle of the follicle. Pinkus also is known for his comprehensive article on the anatomy of the skin in Jadassohn's *Handbuch*. Pinkus had fought for Germany in World War I, during which he received the Iron Cross. Until 1933, he operated a large private practice in Berlin and was director of the Municipal Hospital for Women in Berlin-Reinickendorf. Shortly after the Nazis' assumption of power, he was forced out of his position at the hospital and, in 1935, had to "evacuate" his apartment and office. For some time, he resided and practiced with a Hungarian colleague, Ladislaus Bolog. After July 1938, all orders and prescriptions by Pinkus and appointment cards for visits to him had to be stamped with the Star of David and accompanied by a statement that Pinkus was allowed to practice medicine only on Jews (fig. 245).[38]

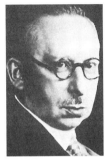

FIG 244
FELIX PINKUS
(1868–1947)

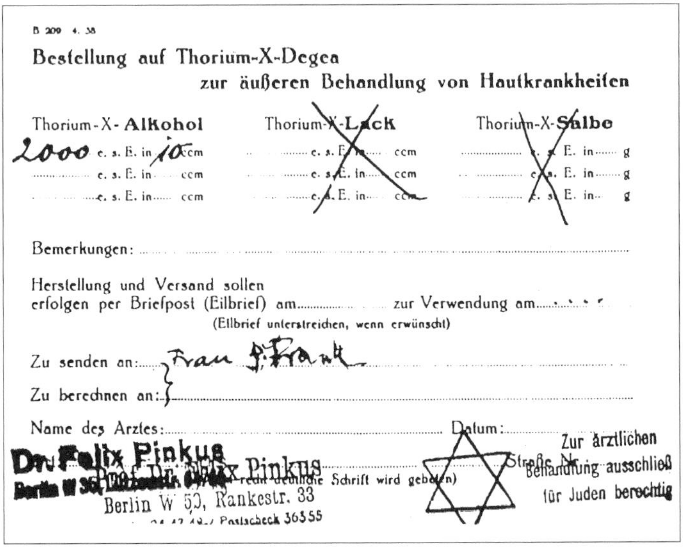

B 209 4. 38

Bestellung auf Thorium-X-Degea
zur äußeren Behandlung von Hautkrankheiten

Thorium-X- **Alkohol**   Thorium-X-**Lack**   Thorium-X-**Salbe**

2000 c. s. E. in _10_ ccm   .... c. s. E ...... ccm   .... c. s E. in .... g
.... c. s. E. in ...... ccm   .... c. s. E. in ...... ccm   .... c. s. E. in ...... g
.... c. s. E. in ...... ccm   .... c. s. E. in ...... ccm   .... c. s. E. in .... g

Bemerkungen: ....

Herstellung und Versand sollen
erfolgen per Briefpost (Eilbrief) am................... zur Verwendung am........ ...
                    (Eilbrief unterstreichen, wenn erwünscht)

Zu senden an:..... Frau J. Frank......

Zu berechnen an:.....

Name des Arztes:... Datum :......

Dr. Felix Pinkus   Zur ärztlichen
Berlin W 50, Rankestr. 33   Behandlung ausschließ
        Postscheck 36355   für Juden berechtig

FIG 245 PRESCRIPTION FORM OF FELIX PINKUS.

At that time, the last Jewish names disappeared from the frontispiece of journals; the names of Abraham Buschke and Karl Herxheimer, for example, were eliminated from the editorial board of the *Dermatologische Zeitschrift* (figs. 246, 247). For thirty-one years, the journal had been edited by Erich Hoffmann and published by Samuel Karger in Berlin. When the Nazis began to turn their attention to the Karger publishing house, a "Jewish enterprise," Karger moved his offices to Basel. For six months, Hoffmann continued to edit the journal, but he faced so many difficulties that he soon withdrew as editor. The journal continued to be published by Wilhelm Lutz in Switzerland under the name *Dermatologica*, but it was not permitted to be sold in the German Reich, and German physicians were cautioned against buying books or journals published by Karger.[39]

There was more to come. On August 17, 1938, the Law Regarding Changes of Family Names and Given Names was enacted. It provided that all male Jews must assume the first name of Israel and all female Jews the name of Sarah. The Law on Passports of Jews, announced on October 5, required all Jews to hand in their passports for foreign travel within

Dermatologische Zeitschrift

Begründet von O. LASSAR (1893)

Unter Mitwirkung von

E. A. Sainz de Aja-Burgos; J. Almkvist-Stockholm; A. Bessemans-Gent; F. Bering-Köln; H. Boas-Kopenhagen; J. S. Covisa-Madrid; C. Cronquist-Malmö; J. Darier-Paris; J. Dörffel-Halle; H. Fox-New York; R. Frühwald-Chemnitz; H. Fuhs-Graz; W. Gennerich-Kiel; H. Gottron-Breslau; O. Grütz-Bonn; R. Habermann-Hamburg; J. Hämel-Jena; L. Hauck-Erlangen; E. Hofmann-Kassel; F. Jahnel-München; P. Keller-Aachen; W. Kerl-Wien; L. Kumer-Innsbruck; v. Leeuven-Utrecht; P. Linser-Tübingen; E. G. Graham Little-London; H. Löhe-Berlin; S. Matsumoto-Kyoto; J. Mayr-München; A. Memmesheimer-Essen; H. Meyer-Bremen; G. Miescher-Zürich; C. Moncorps-Münster; P. Mulzer-Hamburg; O. Naegeli-Bern; L. Nékám-Budapest; E. Neuber-Debrecen; G. Nobl-Wien; A. Pasini-Mailand; G. Th. Photinos-Athen; R. Polland-Graz; W. A. Pusey-Chicago; C. Rasch-Kopenhagen; H. Ritter-Hamburg; G. Rost-Berlin; A. Ruete-Marburg; G. Scherber-Wien; W. I. Schmidt-Gießen; W. Scholtz-Königsberg; W. Schönfeld-Heidelberg; W. Schultze-Gießen; H. W. Siemens-Leiden; A. Stühmer-Freiburg; O. Stümpke-Hannover; L. Török-Budapest; M. Truffi-Padua; P. Uhlenhuth-Freiburg; E. Urbach-Wien; J. Vonkennel-Kiel; Ch. J. White-Boston; L. v. Zumbusch-München

herausgegeben in Gemeinschaft mit

L. Arzt
Wien

A. Buschke
Berlin

K. Herxheimer
Frankfurt a. M.

V. Klingmüller
Kiel

H. Th. Schreus
Düsseldorf

E. Zurhelle
Groningen

von Erich Hoffmann Bonn und W. Lutz Basel .

Band 77

Mit zahlreichen Abbildungen im Text

FIG 246 THE *DERMATOLOGISCHE ZEITSCHRIFT* WAS THE LAST GERMAN DERMATOLOGY JOURNAL TO HAVE JEWS ON ITS EDITORIAL BOARD.

two weeks. In return, Jews were given identity cards stamped with a large "J" (see fig. 249).

An unexpected opportunity to increase drastic measures against Jews occurred on November 7, when Ernst von Rath, a member of the German embassy in Paris, was assassinated by a seventeen-year-old Polish Jew, Herschl Grynszpan, whose parents had been among fifteen thousand Jews deported from Germany to Poland a few months earlier. Joseph Goebbels, the Reich's power-hungry minister for propaganda, used the event to initiate a nationwide pogrom and called for "spontaneous" demonstrations everywhere while at the same time ensuring that the police would not interfere. On November 9, the SA let loose its gangs throughout the entire country. They beat up Jews wherever they were found; almost one hundred Jews were killed and thirty thousand were placed in concentration camps. Jewish

Dermatologische Zeitschrift

Begründet von O. LASSAR (1893)

Unter Mitwirkung von

E. A. Sainz de Aja-Burgos; J. Almkvist-Stockholm; K. von Berde-Pécs; A. Bessemans-Gent;
H. Boas-Kopenhagen; A. Buschke-Berlin; M. Comel-Mailand; J. S. Covisa-Madrid; C. Cronquist-
Malmö; A. Feßler-Wien; H. Fox-New York; W. Gennerich-Kiel; R. Habermann-Hamburg;
F. Jahnel-München; W. Kerl-Wien; L. Kumer-Innsbruck; v. Leeuwen-Utrecht; E. G. Gra-
ham Little-London; S. Matsumoto-Kyoto; N. Melczer-Szeged; H. Meyer-Bremen; G. Miescher-
Zürich; O. Naegeli-Bern; L. Nékám-Budapest; E. Neuber-Budapest; F. S. Nohara-Bonn;
A. Pasini-Mailand; G. Th. Photinos-Athen; R. Polland-Graz; W. A. Pusey-Chicago; W. I.
Schmidt-Gießen; H. W. Siemens-Leiden; L. Török-Budapest; M. Truffi-Padua; P. Uhlenhuth-
Freiburg; E. Urbach-Philadelphia; R. Volk-Wien; Ch. J. White-Boston;
L. v. Zumbusch-München

herausgegeben von

Erich Hoffmann Bonn und **W. Lutz** Basel

Band 78

Mit zahlreichen Abbildungen im Text

FIG 247 IN 1938, NAMES OF JEWISH EDITORS OF THE
DERMATOLOGISCHE ZEITSCHRIFT WERE DROPPED, AND
HOFFMANN'S NAME DISAPPEARED SIX MONTHS LATER.

businesses and houses were destroyed, and synagogues were set on fire (see figs. 251, 252). Shattered plate glass littered the streets of all German towns and cities, accounting for the name later given by the Nazis to that night: Kristallnacht (see fig. 253).

The Kristallnacht pogroms had several major consequences, including a vehement quarrel among high-ranking party officials. Much of the property that had been destroyed belonged to Aryans and not to Jews, and therefore the damage had to be covered by German insurance companies. Hermann Göring criticized the pogroms saying, "They do not harm the Jews but me, who is the final authority for coordinating the German economy."

The repercussions as a consequence of responses from abroad were troubling. Indeed, Kristallnacht was followed by a worldwide boycott of German goods, which caused many firms to lose a large share of their export market. Goebbels (fig. 248) tried to lessen the damage by suggesting that Jews alone should be held responsible for what had happened, and after a

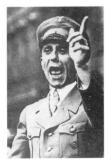

FIG 248
JOSEPH GOEBBELS
(1897–1945)

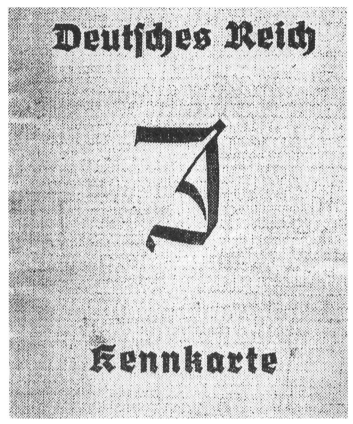

FIG 249 JEWISH IDENTITY CARD.

brief discussion with Hitler, the issue was settled: A penalty of one billion Reichsmarks—approximately $400 million—was imposed on the Jewish community in Germany.[40]

Despite this seeming triumph, and although his anti-Semitic propaganda continued unabated, Goebbels was denied his quest for greater power and for an executive role in anti-Jewish violence. That role was given to Heinrich Himmler (fig. 250), the Reichsführer of the SS that eventually was to become the instrument of the "Final Solution of the Jewish problem." Initially, Himmler concentrated his efforts on acceleration of Jewish emigration. During the Kristallnacht pogroms, he had ordered the arrest of as many Jews as could be accommodated in the space available for "protective custody" (see fig. 255). Those

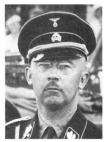

FIG 250
HEINRICH
HIMMLER
(1900–1945)

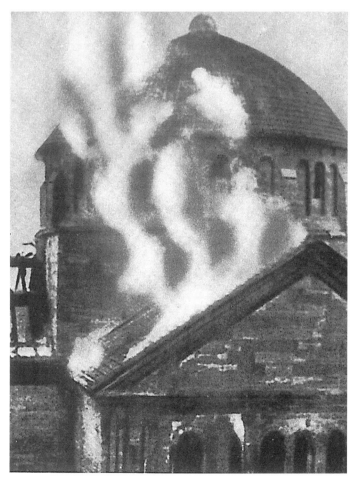

FIG 251 SYNAGOGUE BURNING DURING THE KRISTALLNACHT.

now interned in concentration camps had to buy their freedom by agreeing to leave Germany immediately upon their release. Other measures designed to speed up Jewish emigration included closing Jewish shops, barring Jewish children from schools, revoking Jews' driver's licenses, and banning Jews from public places, including resorts, theaters, and libraries. Signs that read "Access for Jews Prohibited" were posted on the entrances of public buildings, and even park benches and sidewalks were reserved "For Aryans Only" (see figs. 256, 257).

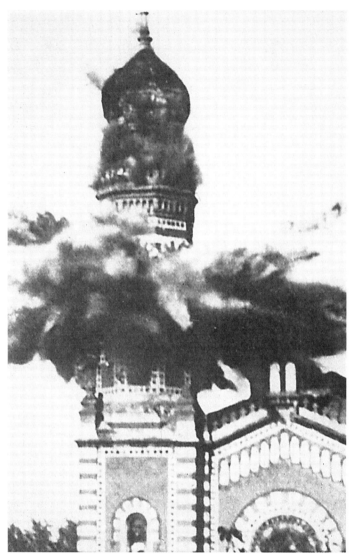

FIG 252 SYNAGOGUE BURNING DURING THE KRISTALLNACHT.

These measures destroyed any illusion that there might be a future for Jews in Germany. Many who had borne their fate stoically and patiently hoping that things would change for the better were now willing to emigrate and leave their friends and belongings behind. In the time between Hitler's assumption of power in January 1933 and the pogroms of

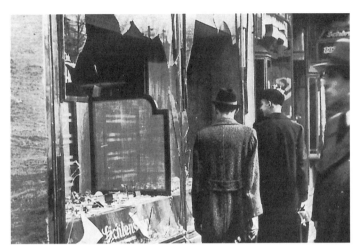

FIG 253 DESTROYED JEWISH SHOPS, NOVEMBER 10, 1938.

November 1938, some 150,000 Jews—almost 30 percent of the original population—had left Germany. After the pogroms, and under increasing pressure from the Gestapo, nearly 150,000 more Jews left, among them prominent dermatologists such as Franz Herrmann, Alfred Hollander, Erich Kuznitzky, Emil Meirowsky, and Felix Pinkus.

After emigration, Franz Herrmann worked at the Skin and Cancer Unit of the New York University School of Medicine.[41] Alfred Hollander opened a private practice of dermatology in Springfield, Massachusetts, in 1939. For forty years, he was on the faculty of the Department of Dermatology at Boston University. At eighty-seven, Hollander died in San Diego, in July 1986, only a few weeks before he was to give a major lecture about the history of dermatology to the German Dermatological Society, which had planned to honor him at the same time.[42]

Erich Kuznitzky (fig. 254), once an assistant medical director of the Department of Dermatology of the University of Breslau, was director of the Department of Dermatology at the Allerheiligen Hospital in Breslau from 1919 to 1933. In 1938, Kuznitzky left Germany following an invitation by Wilhelm Lutz to lecture in Basel. From Basel, he went to London

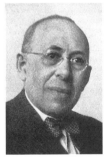

FIG 254

ERICH KUZNITZKY

(1883–1960)

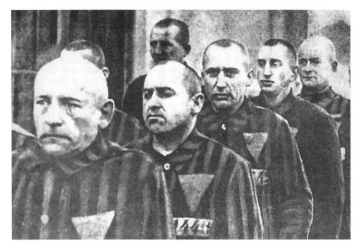

FIG 255 JEWS IN "PROTECTIVE CUSTODY"
AFTER THE KRISTALLNACHT.

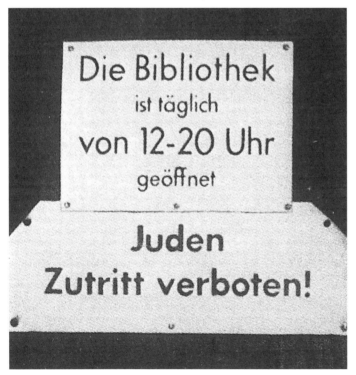

FIG 256 SIGN FORBIDDING JEWS TO ENTER THE LIBRARY.

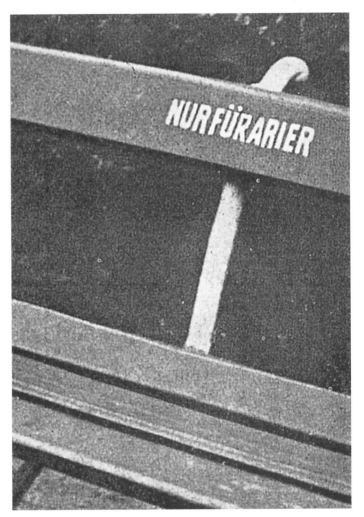

FIG 257 PARK BENCHES WERE RESERVED FOR ARYANS.

and eventually to New York City, where he worked in the department of dermatology at several hospitals but without really gaining a foothold in any of them. Like so many other physician refugees from Nazi Germany, Kuznitzky made a serious attempt to participate in professional life in the United States but never really adjusted to it. Kuznitzky, who was the first to describe involvement of internal organs in sarcoidosis, died in New York in March 1960.[43]

Emil Meirowsky (fig. 258), a pupil of Neisser and Unna, is known eponymically for his identification of postmortem pigmentation (the Meirowsky phenomenon). He also coined the term "genodermatoses." In 1933, after he had been dismissed as associate professor of the University of Cologne, Meirowsky tried to have that decision revoked by calling attention to the fact that he had worked at a military hospital during the First World War and therefore qualified for a "Hindenburg exemption" under the Law for the Restoration of Professional Civil Service. His request was denied; his work at a military hospital was said not to be comparable to duty at the front. After his dismissal as associate professor, Meirowsky continued to maintain his busy private practice in the center of Cologne. In 1939, at the age of sixty-three, he left Germany for England, where he was without employment for more than a year. From 1941 to 1947, Meirowsky worked at the Royal Surrey County Hospital in Guilford and then moved to the United States, where he performed electron microscopic studies on cancer and viruses at Indiana University Medical Center. He died in Nashville, Tennessee, in January 1960.[44]

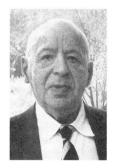

FIG 258
EMIL MEIROWSKY
(1876–1960)

Felix Pinkus left Germany for Oslo, Norway, where he remained for slightly over a year while his son, Hermann, attempted to get him an entry visa to the United States. Unfortunately, Pinkus was still in Oslo when the German army entered the city in April 1940, ending his chances of sailing for England and then the United States. In the winter of 1940, Pinkus managed to travel to Copenhagen, flew to Moscow, took the trans-Siberian railway to Vladivostok, went by boat to Tokyo, and boarded a Japanese passenger liner in Yokohama that arrived in San Francisco in January 1941. His ship was the last Japanese liner to sail to the United States before war was declared.

In the ensuing six years, Felix Pinkus resided with his son and his family in Monroe, Michigan. He saw patients in his son's office, examined histopathologic sections, started work on a dermatopathology textbook he and his son had planned to publish in Germany, resumed giving lectures, and was made an honorary

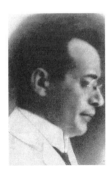

FIG 259
CARL LENNHOFF
(1883–1963)

member of the Detroit Dermatological Society and the Society for Investigative Dermatology. Pinkus died in 1947 in Monroe before the hoped-for textbook was near completion.[45]

At the same time the Nazis pressured Jewish doctors to emigrate, they also tried to extract as much profit as possible from the Jews. Carl Lennhoff (fig. 259), a student of Unna and Jadassohn, had been director of the skin clinic in Magdeburg since 1920. In 1933, because he was Jewish, Lennhoff was dismissed from his post and subsequently operated a private practice of dermatology in Magdeburg. After the riots of November 9, 1938, Lennhoff was arrested by the Gestapo and forced to turn over 35,000 Reichsmarks toward payment of the one billion–Reichsmark fine that had been imposed on the Jews. Upon receiving permission to emigrate to Norway, he had to pay an additional tax of 35,000 Reichsmarks.

In December 1940, after the German occupation of Norway, Lennhoff escaped to Sweden, where he began to work, without pay, at the skin clinic of Karoliske Sjukhuset in Stockholm. For six years he lived on the meager financial support given to him by the Committee for Intellectual Refugees. In 1946, Lennhoff was given a secure position at the clinic in Stockholm. Two years later, he was the first to propose that spirochetes were the cause of erythema chronicum migrans. In 1952, Lennhoff acquired Swedish citizenship. After all that had transpired, he returned to Germany in 1955 and died on September 9, 1963, at age eighty in Bad Reichenhall.[46]

According to a law dating from 1932, all émigrés from Germany had to pay one-fourth of their total worth as a "flight tax." Initially enacted to discourage the emigration of wealthy citizens, the law was now used to make money. In 1938, revenues to the Reich from this tax rose rapidly, reaching almost 350 million Reichsmarks. Having paid the tax, emigrants were still unable to take their fortunes with them; the Reich, in preparation for war, could not afford the loss of currency. Each emigrant was allowed to keep ten Reichsmarks; what remained was frozen and later confiscated by the state.[47]

Compounding the problem facing Jews who wanted to emigrate was the declining willingness of foreign governments to accept them. Anti-Semitism was not confined to Germany; it was common in other European countries, particularly Austria, Poland, and Lithuania. By the end of the 1930s, Nazi medical publications noted that Bulgaria, France, Hungary, Italy, Norway, Poland, and Romania had passed laws restricting the number of Jews allowed to practice medicine. In 1937, the *Deutsches Ärzteblatt* reported that "Hungarian physicians are rightly proud of the fact that they were the first among the world's medical professionals to solve the problem of the racial future of the profession."[48]

In Belgium, in 1939, as the influx of Jewish refugees increased as a result of accelerated expulsion from Germany, the Flemish Nazi leader Braun announced a campaign to exclude the "white Negro" (the Jews) from further immigration.[49] At the 1943 Casablanca Conference, even American president Franklin D. Roosevelt spoke of the "understandable complaints which the Germans bore toward the Jews."[50] Between 1933 and 1941, only 157,000 Jews were allowed to enter the United States, roughly the same number that had entered in the single year of 1906. During the entire war, only 21,000 Jewish immigrants were accepted in the United States, and opinion polls showed that 70 to 80 percent of American citizens were opposed to raising quotas to accommodate Jewish refugees.[51]

In like manner, emigration to Palestine became increasingly difficult for Jews. In political deference to the Arab nations opposed to the entry of European Jews into Palestine, the British government had imposed new restrictive regulations on those seeking entry. Some countries welcomed Jewish scientists and physicians in order to raise the standards of their universities. Oscar Gans, for example, found refuge in India. In Turkey, the government of Kemal Atatürk provided teaching positions for more than fifty Jewish and non-Jewish German and Austrian scholars, including the dermatologists Alfred Marchionini, Berta Ottenstein, and Erich Uhlmann. Although such measures might provide an answer to an indi-

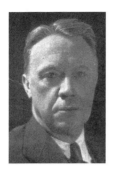

FIG 260
GEORGE MILLER
MACKEE
(1878–1955)

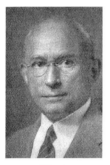

FIG 261
FRED WISE
(1881–1950)

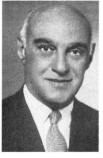

FIG 262
MARION BALDUR
SULZBERGER
(1895–1983)

vidual's problem, they were insufficient to meet the vast demand for refuge that Nazi rule had created.

Despite limitations and difficulties, the United States was still the destination most desired by German Jewish emigrants, and the prospects for building a new life seemed better there than anywhere else. Should a friend or relative in the United States provide an affidavit to cover living expenses, there was a chance of obtaining a visa for immigration. Of the physicians who emigrated from Germany, 3.5 percent went to South America, 12 percent to Great Britain, 22.4 percent to Palestine, and approximately 50 percent to the United States. Within the United States, a disproportionately high number of physicians settled in New York City, not only because it was the gateway to America for European immigrants but also because regulations on immigrants were very liberal in New York State. German physicians who had graduated before 1914 needed only to pass an English language examination to have their German doctor's degree converted into a comparable American degree.[52]

Many American dermatologists in New York City tried to help German refugees to the best of their abilities. Most notable among them was George Miller MacKee (fig. 260), the non-Jewish chairman of the Skin and Cancer Unit of the New York University School of Medicine, long-standing editor of the *Archives of Dermatology and Syphilology* and the *Journal of Investigative Dermatology*, and author of a pioneering textbook on dermatological radiotherapy.[53] Others who were exceedingly helpful in this regard were MacKee's assistant Fred Wise (fig. 261), one of the founding members of the American Academy of Dermatology,[54] and MacKee's successor Marion Sulzberger (fig. 262), who was the most active and productive dermatologic scientist in the country and whose name came to be linked eponymically to incontinentia pigmenti and to Sulzberger-Garbe's disease, a condition that today is considered to be a variant of nummular dermatitis. Wise and Sulzberger introduced the term "atopic dermatitis" in preference to "allergic eczema" and "generalized neurodermatitis." Sulzberger also was the first to apply corticosteroids topically as dermatotherapy.[55]

Through the efforts of people like MacKee, Wise, and Sulzberger, New York City became a haven for German immigrant dermatologists. Many of them, such as Hans Biberstein, Wilhelm Frei, Franz Herrmann, Max Jessner, Erich Kuznitzky, Ludwig Löwenstein, and Ernst Nathan, were given the chance to work and teach at the Skin and Cancer Unit or other New York hospitals. Infusion of them into those medical faculties greatly elevated the standards of research and practice of dermatology in the United States and was a first step toward the United States becoming preeminent in the field by the end of the Second World War. But the influx of foreign physicians soon represented a serious competitive and economic threat to their American colleagues, who called for protection.

In response, the State of New York in January 1937 adopted a regulation, already in place in other American states and in Great Britain, that made a German medical degree no longer acceptable for practice. Thereafter, newly arriving physicians were forced to take rigorous state board examinations, a task made all the more difficult by problems of language, advanced age, and financial and emotional stress. In yet another roadblock to the refugee physicians, U.S. citizenship became a requirement to take a state-sanctioned licensing examination. Despite a palpable need for doctors, many of whom were soon to be called into military service, twenty-one of the forty-eight United States categorically denied foreigners a right to practice medicine within their borders.[56]

The unhappy fate of many Jewish emigrants is poignantly expressed by the son of the Leipzig dermatologist Felix Danziger. He described the last years of his father's life in this way:

In November 1938, everything came to an end. During the "Kristallnacht" he was picked up and transported to Buchenwald. Within a short time, he fell ill . . . but

*thanks to the intervention of a colleague, he was trans-
ferred to a hospital where he was operated on and where
he recovered slowly. Now he finally realized that he
had to leave Germany, a decision that he could not face
up to before. Furthermore, he was unemployed by now!
Approximately eight weeks before the outbreak of the
next war, my brother and I succeeded in taking him to
England, where we studied at a university.*

*In the middle of 1940, one member of our family
after the other was interned as "enemy alien," and our
father was the first one. . . . After a few months he was
released and returned to our apartment in London.
Later, he was given "temporary" permission to work as
a doctor and was employed by several hospitals there.
His state of health was poor, and in the 1940s he had to
undergo several surgical procedures. . . . In 1952, he
emigrated to Canada, where my brother and I had settled. He often was very depressed and unhappy and
died the following year.[57]*

In short, the prospects for Jewish refugees were poor and emigration usually was followed by years of poverty and distress.
For these reasons, the fateful move was undertaken mostly by
younger individuals who still felt capable of building a new life
and making a fresh start. In 1933, nearly 30 percent of Jews in
Germany were under twenty-four years of age; in 1939, only 13
percent were. More than 80 percent of Jews under forty left
Germany between 1933 and 1939, whereas the emigration rate
of those forty to sixty was 50 percent, and 25 percent among
those over sixty. In 1939, 73.7 percent of the Jewish population
remaining in Germany was over forty, often unemployed, commonly disabled, and completely impoverished.[58]

WAR AND
ANNIHILATION

BY THE END OF THE 1930s, THERE WERE ABOUT 350,000 JEWS LIVING IN GERMANY, FAR LESS THAN IN MANY other European countries, such as Poland, Russia, and Lithuania. With the expansion of Nazi Germany through gains achieved by both "peaceful" takeover and war, more and more Jews came under National Socialist rule.

The first country affected by Nazi designs was Austria. In the early 1930s, the Nazi party already had a branch there, and although that party was illegal for many years, it found wide support in the population. With other right-wing organizations, Austrian Nazis created a climate of German nationalism and anti-Semitism that was particularly intense at the universities. In early 1935, the Austrian *Bulletin of the Association of Jewish Physicians* reported that for twenty-two months, young Jewish physicians were no longer being admitted to practice within government medical insurance programs or city hospitals. Since the rise of Hitler, the number of Jewish physicians employed in Austrian hospitals had fallen by more than half. In Vienna, Jews were being forced en masse out of many hospitals; by July 30, 1935, the last Jewish resident physician was supposed to leave Vienna's General Hospital. Viennese medical students were told not to attend courses conducted by Jewish instructors, which deprived the Jews of income and the medical students of knowledge.[1]

Even leading academic physicians, such as the pathologist Karl Landsteiner, who had received the Nobel Prize in Medicine in 1930 for his discovery of human blood groups, were blocked from top positions. Promotion in universities in general became increasingly difficult to obtain for Jews. The Society of German Doctors in Austria, a fast-growing pro-Nazi professional organization, published lists of non-Aryan colleagues.[2] As a consequence of this revival of a long and infa-

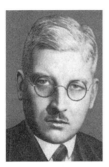

FIG 263
KURT VON
SCHUSCHNIGG
(1887–1977)

mous tradition of anti-Semitism in Austria, many Jewish physicians committed suicide or emigrated well before 1938. The number of dermatologists in Vienna fell from 160 in 1935 to 144 in 1936, and 125 by the beginning of 1938.[3]

Impressed by the remarkable political and economic successes of the Nazis in Germany, increasing numbers of Austrians called for a "return home into the Reich," an Anschluss (connection) between Austria and Germany, which was said by many Austrians and Germans to be a historical necessity. In contrast to Germany, the situation in Austria was perceived as unstable and insecure. Throughout 1937, the Austrian Nazis, financed and egged on by Berlin, stepped up a campaign of terror, with bombings occurring nearly every day in some parts of the country. In the mountain provinces—especially in Graz, the capital of Styria—huge, often violent Nazi demonstrations weakened the government's position. The Austrian police was full of Nazis, and SA brigades had formed throughout the country. On March 11, 1938, Austria's federal chancellor, Kurt von Schuschnigg (fig. 263), was forced to resign. Only a few hours later, German troops crossed the border and were welcomed enthusiastically by the vast majority of the population. While thousands of Austrian citizens were still celebrating their "return home into the Reich," drastic measures against Jews were already being instituted (figs. 264, 265, 267, 268, 270).[4]

In the days after the Anschluss, the Austrian Nazis began a campaign of sadism that far exceeded anything that had happened in Germany. Throughout the country, Jews were dragged out of their homes, beaten up by mobs, or arrested and tortured by the Gestapo. Day after day, large numbers of Jewish men and women could be seen scrubbing the sidewalks and cleaning the gutters, while jeering storm troopers stood over them and crowds gathered to taunt them. Hundreds of Jews were picked up and put to work cleaning public toilets and latrines in the SA and SS barracks. Their possessions were either confiscated or stolen. By the first night after the "marching-in," 67,000 persons, mostly Jews,

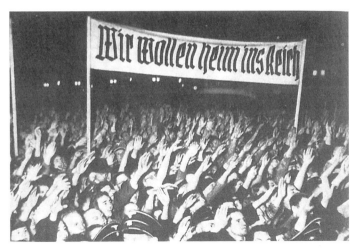

FIG 264 "WE WANT HOME IN THE REICH!"

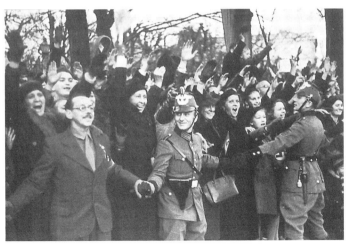

FIG 265 AUSTRIANS CHEERING GERMAN TROOPS.

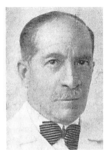

FIG 266
GABOR NOBL
(1864–1938)

had been put in jail.[5] Many others committed suicide, among them the Jewish dermatologist Gabor Nobl (fig. 266) and his wife, who killed themselves with morphine on March 14, 1938, the day that Hitler arrived in Vienna.[6] Nobl, the successor of Hans von Hebra as director of dermatology at the Vienna General Polyclinic, was greatly respected for his

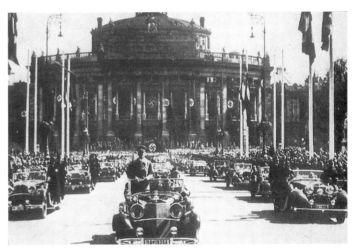

FIG 267 CELEBRATION OF THE ARRIVAL OF THE NAZIS IN VIENNA.

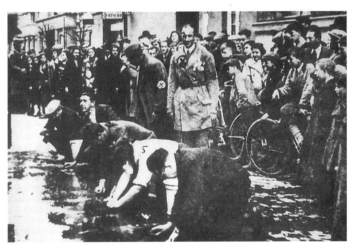

FIG 268 JEWS FORCED TO SCRUB THE SIDEWALKS OF VIENNA.

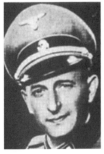

FIG 269
ADOLF EICHMANN
(1906–1962)

knowledge of syphilis and for his contributions to the under-standing of that then-common disease.

The terror that the Nazis exerted on Austrian Jews was part of a strategy to speed up the emigration of that despised minority. Upon the suggestion of Adolf Eichmann (fig. 269), a Central Office for Jewish Emigration had been founded in

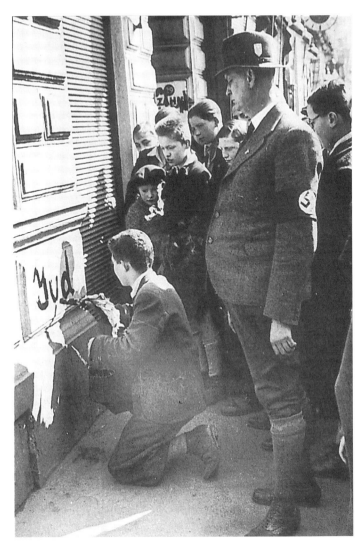

FIG 270 JEWISH BOY BEING FORCED TO PAINT
THE WORD "JEW" ON HIS FATHER'S STORE.

Germany in 1937. To enhance its successful operation, Eichmann re-established the Jewish Religious Community, then
released some of its leaders from detention and forced them
to cooperate with him in expediting emigration. The central-
ization of bureaucratic procedures, together with apposite
doses of terror, increased emigration so successfully that by six

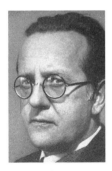

FIG 271
EDUARD PERNKOPF
(1888–1955)

months after the Anschluss, 45,000 Jews had left Austria. Over 100,000 more left before the war broke out.[7]

The de-Jewification of medicine that had taken years to bring about in Germany was accomplished in Austria within a few weeks. Of about 7,200 physicians in Austria, 3,300 were Jewish. Despite the major effect it inevitably would have on the medical care of the Austrian population, Jewish physicians from nearly the moment of the Anschluss were excluded from the practice of medicine. As of September 30, 1938, only 370 Jewish physicians remained in Austria. As in Germany, they were referred to disparagingly as "treaters of the sick" and were forbidden to treat non-Jewish patients.[8] In Vienna alone, the total number of physicians dropped from 5,700 in 1937 to 1,596 by the end of 1938.[9] The general secretary of the Reich's Association of Austrian Physicians' Organizations gratefully acknowledged that the "fervently loved" Führer had come "in the last moment to the rescue of the Aryan medical community."[10]

Three days after the Anschluss, the dean of the faculty of medicine at the University of Vienna was replaced by an outspoken Nazi, the anatomist Eduard Pernkopf (figs. 271 through 273), author of chapters on the histology of the skin in several dermatology textbooks (for example, a three-volume textbook edited by Leopold Arzt and Karl Zieler). Pernkopf was also the founding editor of a textbook of anatomy that was highly appreciated for the quality of its illustrations and that is still published by the Urban and Schwarzenberg Publishing House, a German division of Waverly, a major American medical publishing company. Some of the subjects portrayed in Pernkopf's text were probably victims of Nazi concentration camp terror, as evidenced by the fact that some illustrations were of men who were circumcised, a mark in Europe at that time of being Jewish. In the original editions of his book, Pernkopf included paintings that incorporated Nazi icons (swastikas and SS symbols) in the artists' signatures. Pernkopf had joined the Nazi party in 1933 and the SA a year later.[11] After his appointment as dean of the medical faculty, he sent a

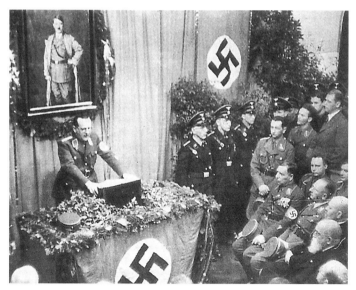

FIG 272 THE PROFESSOR OF ANATOMY, EDUARD PERNKOPF, GIVING A
LECTURE AT THE UNIVERSITY OF VIENNA IN THE FALL OF 1938.

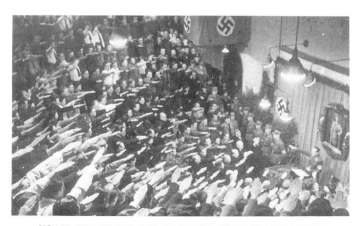

FIG 273 THE UNIVERSITY OF VIENNA BEING TRANSFORMED
INTO A POLITICAL FORUM: EDUARD PERNKOPF
AT THE ZENITH OF HIS CAREER.

letter to all university staff that advised the following: "To
clarify whether you are of Aryan or non-Aryan descent, you
are asked to bring your parents' and grandparents' birth certificates to the dean's office no later than the end of April. Married individuals must also bring the documents of their
wives."[12] In the next weeks, 153 of the 197 medical faculty
members were fired. This number (78 percent) was signifi-

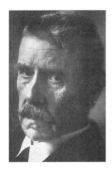

FIG 274
JULIUS WAGNER-
JAUREGG
(1857–1940)

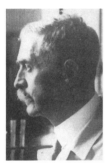

FIG 275
KARL LANDSTEINER
(1869–1943)

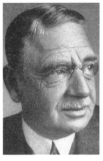

FIG 276
OTTO LOEWI
(1873–1961)

cantly larger than in any other faculty of the University of Vienna, or indeed in any university in Europe.[13]

Before the Anschluss, Vienna had the second-largest medical school in the German-speaking countries and probably the most famous one in the world. Four Nobel Prize winners originated from the faculty: Robert Barany, Julius Wagner-Jauregg (fig. 274), Karl Landsteiner (fig. 275), and Otto Loewi (fig. 276). Except for Wagner-Jauregg, all were Jewish and died in exile; Landsteiner and Barany emigrated before the Anschluss, whereas Otto Loewi left Austria shortly thereafter. To obtain permission to emigrate, Loewi had to give his Nobel Prize money, which he had won for investigations on the chemical nature of the transmission of nerve impulses, to the Nazis. In 1940, Loewi came to the United States and was appointed research professor of pharmacology at the New York University School of Medicine, a post he held until his death in 1961. Other famous non-Aryan physicians forced out of the country included otologist Heinrich von Neumann, neurologists Otto Marburg and Max Schacherl, and Sigmund Freud (fig. 277), who left with almost the entire Viennese school of psychoanalysis. Within a few months, Austrian medicine was brought from the height of excellence to consummate mediocrity and on the brink of collapse.[14]

As in Germany, punitive measures against Jews were carried out in Austria without discernible opposition, and those who remained in office often tried to minimize or ignore the removal of Jewish colleagues. In a reply to criticism from abroad, thirteen university professors—many of whom did not belong to Nazi groups—issued an official statement in the summer of 1939: "The undersigned know of not one case of prosecution of a professor for his racial or religious adherence. . . . The truth is that Jews are no longer allowed to teach non-Jews. . . . By the removal of certain influences a trend of charlatanism . . . was eliminated." Lorenz Böhler, Ernst Lauda, Wolfgang Denk (fig. 278)—who, after the war, became president of the prestigious Society of Doctors in Vienna, rector of the University of Vienna, and an unsuccessful candidate for presidency of the state of Austria in 1957—and many others who signed the infamous letter had gained worldwide professional reputations.[15]

The gaping holes left by the removal of Jewish professors were often filled by faculty of lower rank who gladly accepted the chance for advancement. Junior faculty members, in turn, were replaced by residents who were promoted without any evidence of proper scientific qualification. Between 1939 and 1944, more than 110 theses were written at the medical faculty of the University of Vienna, many of them based on specious premises.[16] In addition, professors with strong National Socialist leanings were recruited from other universities. Herbert Fuhs (fig. 279), a member of the Nazi party, the storm troops, and the National Socialist Lecturers' League, was among them. From 1936 to 1938, Fuhs had been associate professor and director of the Department of Dermatology in Graz. In 1939, he was called to Vienna as full professor and chairman of both of the Viennese departments of dermatology.[17] Because new appointments were made on the basis of political rather than academic merit, the quality of the medical school of Vienna declined precipitously. Between 1938 and 1945, not a single scientific achievement of note was attained at this once-thriving institution.[18]

The situation was worse in dermatology than in most other fields of medicine. Although many Jewish dermatologists had already emigrated before the Anschluss, Austrian dermatology was still dominated by Jewish physicians. At the beginning of 1938, there were 125 dermatologists in Vienna: 68 percent were Jewish. By 1940, only forty-eight Aryan dermatologists remained in the city; almost all Jewish dermatologists had left the country.[19]

Among the renowned Jewish dermatologists forced to emigrate was Moritz Oppenheim (fig. 280), a student of Salomon Ehrmann and Isidor Neumann. Until 1938, Oppenheim directed the Department of Dermatology at the Wilhelminenspital in Vienna, which at the time was the most modern department of

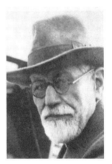

FIG 277
SIGMUND FREUD
(1856–1939)

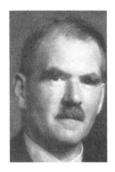

FIG 278
WOLFGANG DENK
(1882–1970)

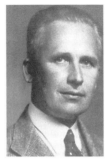

FIG 279
HERBERT FUHS
(1891–1960)

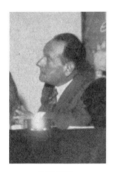

FIG 280
MORITZ
OPPENHEIM
(1876–1949)

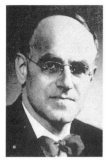

FIG 281
ERICH URBACH
(1893–1946)

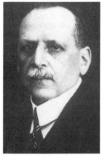

FIG 282
LEOPOLD FREUND
(1868–1943)

dermatology in the country. Upon the "return home into the Reich," Oppenheim left for the United States. From 1939 until his death in October 1949, he was chair of dermatology at the University of Chicago School of Medicine. He wrote books and monographs on occupational dermatoses and cutaneous atrophies and was responsible for the first description of dermatitis bullosa praetensis in 1927 and of necrobiosis lipoidica in 1929.[20]

Three years after Oppenheim's original report, necrobiosis lipoidica was described more precisely by Erich Urbach (figs. 281, 285), associate professor at the Department of Dermatology of the University of Vienna. In his article, Urbach clearly delineated the clinical and histopathologic features of the disease, establishing it as a distinct entity. His original description, with Camillo Wiethe, of lipoid proteinosis (known also as hyalinosis cutis et mucosae or Urbach-Wiethe disease) helped earn his renown. With his son Friedrich, Urbach emigrated to the United States in 1938 and settled in Philadelphia, where he worked unofficially at the University of Pennsylvania School of Medicine. Erich Urbach died unexpectedly in December 1946, just three days after passing the American board examinations for which he had studied fervently, and with great anxiety from fear of failing, for many months. In the same year, his son received his medical degree from Jefferson Medical College. He was trained subsequently in dermatology at the University of Pennsylvania and eventually became director of the Skin and Cancer Hospital in Philadelphia and professor and chair of the Department of Dermatology at Temple University.[21]

Leopold Freund (fig. 282), the first to use the newly discovered x-rays in the treatment of skin lesions, was arrested in 1938 but later escaped to Belgium. During the occupation of Belgium he was arrested again and in 1943 died in captivity in Brussels, allegedly of intestinal carcinoma.[22]

Stephan Robert Brünauer (fig. 283), son-in-law of the famous dermatologist Salomon Ehrmann, wrote the chapters on follicular hyperkeratoses, Darier's disease, lymphangiomas, and scleroderma for Jadassohn's *Handbuch*. In 1938, he was forced to leave the University of Vienna and emigrated to London, where he worked at the Metropolitan Hospital. In 1947, he became consultant dermatologist at Mount Sinai Hospital in Chicago, and two years later joined the staff of the Skin and Cancer Unit of New York University. Brünauer died in Palo Alto, California, in 1969.[25]

Hans Königstein (fig. 284), a pupil of Salomon Ehrmann, left Austria in 1939 and emigrated to Palestine. After several difficult years, he became a professor of dermatology at Hadassah Hospital of Hebrew University in Jerusalem. He died in Tel Aviv in March 1954. Königstein is known for a monograph on the physiology of the skin and for chapters on amyloidosis and the constitutional aspects of syphilis for Jadassohn's *Handbuch*.[24]

Robert Otto Stein, who wrote the chapter on seborrhea, acne, and rosacea for Jadassohn's *Handbuch*, was dismissed from his position as director of the Polyclinic for Cutaneous and Venereal Diseases at the Kaiser-Franz-Josef-Spital in Vienna in 1938. A year later, he became Königstein's successor

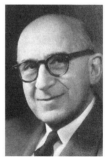

FIG 283
STEPHAN ROBERT
BRÜNAUER
(1885–1969)

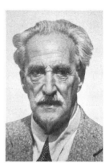

FIG 284
HANS KÖNIGSTEIN
(1878–1954)

Kartothek Nr. 6916		Geburts- Tag	Geburts- Jahr	Zuständigkeit Ort und Land
Name: U R B A C H Dr.Erich		29.VII.		Prag
Titel: Dozent		1893		
Spezialfach: Dermatologe				
Wohnort: I.Schottenring 7		wahlberechtigt		
		Eingetreten am: 1920		
Das Diplom erlangt:	an welcher Universität? Wien	Ausgetreten am: 30.VI.1938		
	in welchem Jahre? 1919			
Übt in Wien ärztliche Praxis aus:	seit?	Praxisabmeldung Z 3657/38		
	durch das ganze Jahr?			
	wenn nicht, wie lange an anderem Orte und an welchem?			
Hat eine ärztliche Anstellung als?				

FIG 285 PERSONNEL FILE OF ERICH URBACH FROM THE ARCHIVES OF
THE CHAMBER OF PHYSICIANS IN VIENNA. URBACH
LEFT THE CHAMBER IN JUNE 1938; THE REASON IS
INDICATED IN HANDWRITING: "JUDE" ("JEW").

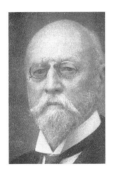

at the hospital of the Israelite Cultural Community of Vienna and remained there during the war.[25] As a professed Christian and veteran of World War I, Stein was one of the few Jews in greater Germany to survive the Third Reich. Most who survived were elderly, so their death from natural causes could be anticipated by the Nazis. Another factor that provided some degree of protection was marriage to an Aryan spouse, but if the spouse died, his or her death was nearly a death sentence for the bereaved Jew, who usually was "evacuated" to a concentration camp shortly thereafter.[26] Stein was fortunate to have a healthy Aryan wife; after seven years of humiliation, fear, and work under the most trying circumstances, he resumed his academic career and was elected president of the Austrian Dermatological Society. He died in 1951.[27]

Before 1938, the mouthpiece of German nationalism and anti-Semitism among Austrian's physicians had been the Society of German Doctors in Austria. After the Anschluss, several members of this pro-Nazi society suddenly noticed that the Nuremberg Laws also applied to them because Jews were among their own antecedents. Among the most prominent representatives of the society who experienced this unpleasant surprise were Julius Wagner-Jauregg, who was awarded the 1927 Nobel Prize for physiology and medicine for his successful treatment of syphilitic paresis by infecting patients with malaria, and Ernst Finger (fig. 286), the former chair of the second Department of Dermatology in Vienna and one of the leading syphilologists of his time.[28]

Some Aryan dermatologists, in addition to Jewish ones, were dismissed—temporarily or permanently—because they did not embrace the new policies. Among them were not only socialists but also several strictly conservative men, including Leopold Arzt (fig. 287), chair of the first Department of Dermatology in Vienna and successor of von Hebra, Kaposi, and Riehl. Arzt was dean of the medical faculty of the University of Vienna several times before 1938 and after 1945. He was highly influential politically, both inside and outside the university. In the 1920s and early 1930s, Arzt

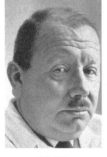

had been a close friend of Engelbert Dollfuss, who, as chancellor of Austria, aspired to a close affiliation with fascist Italy, dissolved the Austrian democratic constitution, outlawed political parties, including the Communist and National Socialist parties, and was assassinated by Austrian Nazis in 1934. Like Dollfuss, Arzt was not a democrat, and he occasionally professed anti-Semitic feelings.[29] In 1936, he complained about a decision by an American publisher in these words: "I cannot help it that there once again must be some little Jew behind it who is out for business."[30]

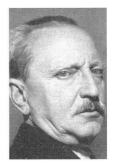

FIG 288

WILHELM KERL

(1880–1945)

This sentiment aside, Arzt was an Austrian nationalist who opposed the Anschluss and whose attitude was considered too liberal by the Nazis. After the 1934 reorganization of the German Dermatological Society, Arzt had been named president of the newly founded Austrian Dermatological Society, 80 percent of whose members were Jewish. The society was closely observed by the German Ministry of the Interior, which noted disapprovingly that the Austrian group had not adopted the racist regulations of its German counterpart.[31] Arzt's political noncompliance no doubt contributed to his removal from office in 1938. After the war, Arzt was reinstalled immediately. He died in 1955 at the age of seventy-two.[32]

The chair of the second Department of Dermatology in Vienna, Wilhelm Kerl (fig. 288), was a man of strictly conservative nationalist views, yet the fact that he had a Jewish wife was cause enough for his dismissal. Like Leopold Arzt, Kerl spent the next seven years in private practice. After the war, he was to be reinstated to his previous position, but he died of a heart attack on May 31, 1945.[33]

Leo Kumer (fig. 289), chair of the Department of Dermatology in Innsbruck, was dismissed in March 1938 because of doubts about his political reliability. One year later, however, the Nazis were less dubious about him, and he was given the chair of the dermatology section at the Wilhelminenspital in Vienna, succeeding Moritz Oppenheim. In 1941, Kumer published a textbook on dermatology in collaboration with Herbert Fuhs. He died in 1951.[34]

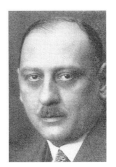

FIG 289

LEO KUMER

(1886–1951)

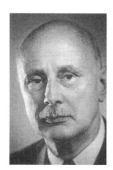

FIG 290
ANTON MUSGER
(1898–1983)

In 1941, Anton Musger (fig. 290), director of the dermatology section at the Kaiserin-Elisabeth-Spital in Vienna, had his license to teach at the University of Vienna revoked for political reasons. After the war, Musger became chair of the Department of Dermatology at the University of Graz and, later, dean and rector of that institution and president of the Austrian Dermatological Society. He died in Lienz in 1983.[35]

Albert Wiedmann (fig. 291), director of dermatology at the Rainer Hospital in Vienna, was active in the Austrian resistance. In December 1944 he was arrested by the Gestapo and three months later was sentenced to death by a People's Court; his execution was prevented by the arrival of Allied troops. In 1945, Wiedmann succeeded his mentor, Wilhelm Kerl, as chair of the second Department of Dermatology at the University of Vienna. He was elected president of the German Dermatological Society in 1965 and died in September 1970.[36]

The writer Wilhelm von Hebra, son of Hans von Hebra and grandson of the famous Ferdinand von Hebra, was not so fortunate. His crime of distributing leaflets calling for re-establishing the Austrian monarchy under the Habsburgs had aroused the attention of the Gestapo. Von Hebra was imprisoned, sentenced to death by the notorious People's Court in Berlin, and executed on October 27, 1944. Another prisoner sentenced to death along with von Hebra was not executed. The fact that von Hebra was executed shortly after the sentence had been announced may have been because his mother was half Jewish. That circumstance was underlined with a red pen in the court records.[37]

With Austria now under firm control, the Nazis turned their attention to other European countries. Their first target was Czechoslovakia. According to the Nazis, the western German-speaking region of Czechoslovakia belonged naturally to the German Reich. Shortly after the annexation of Austria, they moved with vigor to enforce this claim. They used all available means, including massive propaganda, repeated actions aimed at destabilization of Czechoslovakia, and, most important, repeated threats of a major military conflict and another

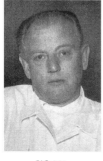

FIG 291
ALBERT WIEDMANN
(1901–1970)

world war. The Nazi position eventually came to be acceded to because of the abject submission of France and England to the bullying tactics of Hitler. Germany incorporated the western region of Czechoslovakia, the so-called Sudetenland, and, in the process, forced the dissolution of the fledgling Czechoslovakian Republic. In March 1939, as the free world stood by shamelessly, Nazi troops moved "peacefully" into Prague (see fig. 295). Once again, an annexation was followed by a series of compulsory measures against Socialists and Jews.

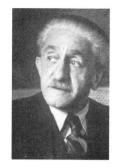

Hugo Hecht (fig. 292), one of the leading venereologists of the time, immediately emigrated to the United States, where he found a spot at Mount Sinai Hospital in Cleveland. He died in New York of a cerebrovascular accident in February 1970.[38]

Felix Sagher (fig. 293), a Jewish assistant of Kreibich's at the skin clinic in Prague, emigrated to Jerusalem, where he found a residency at the Hadassah Hospital under Arieh Dostrovsky, who later became his father-in-law. In 1956, Sagher became director of dermatology at the hospital, and two years later was appointed full professor at Hebrew University in Jerusalem. Sagher was interested in dermatopathology, but gained worldwide notice mostly because of his work as secretary of the International League of Dermatological Societies. Major publications by him concerned leishmaniasis, leprosy, and mastocytosis. He died in 1981.[39]

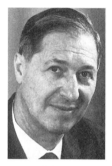

FIG 293
FELIX SAGHER
(1908–1981)

Henry Haber (fig. 294), a Jewish associate of Kreibich's at the skin clinic in Prague, left within two weeks of German troops having entered Prague and, on March 30, 1939, arrived in England with his young wife, Alice. At that time, there were about three hundred Czech refugee doctors in Britain, of whom only thirty were given an opportunity to take the basic qualifying examinations for registration in medicine. Haber was not among them, probably because he could not speak a word of English. For some time, Haber and his wife were supported by the Czech Refugee Trust Fund and by relatives who had stayed in Czechoslovakia and who thought that they were better off. After a year, letters and parcels from these relatives stopped arriving abruptly,

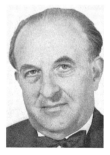

FIG 294
HENRY HABER
(1900–1962)

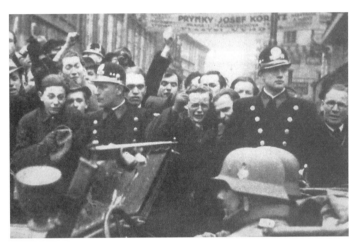

FIG 295 GERMAN TROOPS IN PRAGUE. IN CONTRAST TO THE ANNEXATION OF AUSTRIA, THERE WERE NO CHEERING CROWDS.

and neither Haber nor his wife ever heard from their families again. Until 1941, Haber worked as a photographer, but when doctors were needed during the war, he was granted a temporary medical license. Haber eventually volunteered for the British armed forces and rose to the rank of major while working at military hospitals in England and south India.

After the war, Haber returned to London and became lecturer at the Institute of Dermatology at St. John's Hospital, where he was able to establish a unit devoted to dermatopathology. Prejudice against Haber, a Jewish Czech refugee, on the part of leading figures in British dermatology prevented him from acquiring a higher academic position. Nevertheless, his vision and intellect enabled him to become one of the country's leading dermatopathologists. Several of his descriptive phrases are still in wide use today, such as "dilapidated brick wall" for the epithelial changes in Hailey-Hailey disease and "smoke from a funnel" for columns of orthokeratosis above eccrine ducts and infundibula in solar keratoses. Haber was responsible for having trained Edward Wilson Jones, who, from the 1960s to the 1990s, was one of the world's leading dermatopathologists. Haber described a familial rosacea-like eruption, a condition known today as Haber's syndrome.

In the years before his retirement, Haber found himself increasingly depressed as he recalled the fate of his relatives in concentration camps. He was also greatly disturbed by the rise of the neofascist British National Party and by his own lack of acceptance by many co-workers at St. John's. In July 1962, at the annual meeting of the British Society of Dermatology in Edinburgh, Haber committed suicide.[40]

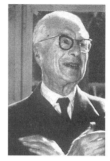

FIG 296
KAREL
GAWALOWSKI
(1890–1965)

From 1882 to 1939, the University of Prague had two separate faculties: German and Czech. The Czech University was closed by the Nazis immediately after their takeover of the country, and its professors were dismissed, among them Karel Gawalowski (fig. 296), the non-Jewish chair of the Department of Dermatology who was much respected for his work on radiotherapy of the skin. After the war, Gawalowski became chair of the First Dermato-Venereological Clinic in Prague. He died in 1965.[41]

As they had done in Austria, the Nazis tried to eliminate all political opponents from leading positions in Czech public life. Antonin Trýb (fig. 297), for example, chairman of the Department of Dermatology and Venereology at the University of Brno, was fired promptly after the annexation. Trýb was a student of Paul Gerson Unna and the most highly regarded dermatopathologist in Czechoslovakia. He was also active in politics and published several novels and collections of poems. In 1945, Trýb was reinstated in his previous position and held it until his retirement in 1956. He died in Brno in 1960.[42]

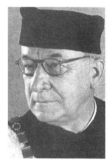

FIG 297
ANTONIN TRÝB
(1884–1960)

Jan Kanopik (fig. 298), an assistant in the Department of Dermatology of the Charles University in Prague, was arrested because of antifascist activities and was sent to the concentration camp at Theresienstadt. After his release, he rejoined the illegal organization of "revolutionary physicians" and was one of the leading figures in the uprising of Prague in May 1945. After the war, Kanopik became chair of dermatology and vice rector of Charles University in Prague. He died in December 1985 at the age of eighty.[43]

The gaps created at Czech universities were filled with loyal supporters of the Nazi party. The chair of dermatology at Charles

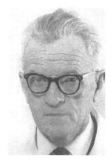

FIG 298
JAN KANOPIK
(1905–1985)

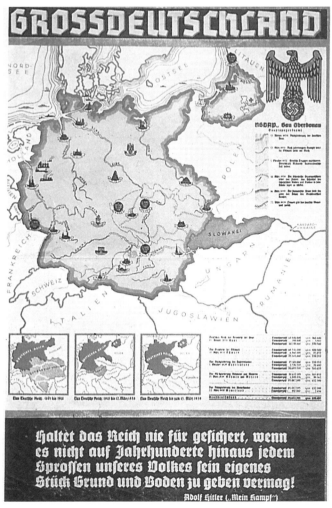

FIG 299 NAZI POSTER OF GREATER GERMANY. AT THE BOTTOM, A
QUOTATION FROM MEIN KAMPF: "NEVER CONSIDER THE REICH TO BE
SECURED AS LONG AS IT CANNOT PROVIDE FOR CENTURIES A PIECE
OF LAND AND SOIL FOR EVERY DESCENDENT OF OUR PEOPLE."

University in Prague, for instance, was given to thirty-seven-year-old Rudolf Bezecny-Greipl, a resolute Nazi who took poison when Czechoslovakia was finally liberated in May 1945.[44]

Within six years, and without any military force, Hitler had achieved what no one had thought possible—namely, retention of most of the area lost to Germany in World War I and much more (fig. 299). By the end of the 1930s, Hitler was

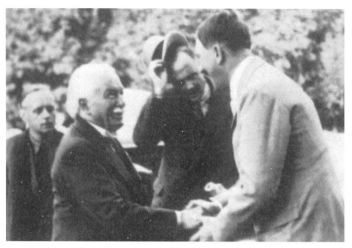

FIG 300 LLOYD GEORGE WITH ADOLF HITLER.

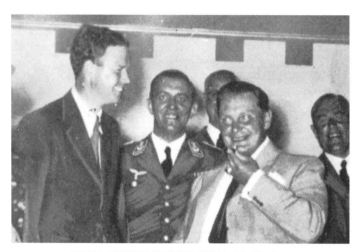

FIG 301 LINDBERGH WITH HERMANN GÖRING.

regarded by many as the greatest statesman of his time. Those who had at first jeered him now cheered him. Private audiences were sought and given to the Duke of Windsor; Lady Astor, the first female member of the British House of Commons who regarded Hitler's state as a "bulwark against communism"[45]; David Lloyd George, the former British prime minister, who compared Hitler to George Washington[46]; and Charles Lindbergh, the American flyer who called National Socialism the "wave of the future" (figs. 300, 301).[47]

Hitler's political success depended on the passivity, weakness, and opportunism of the other European nations. The Pope in Rome was no exception, having signed a concordat with Nazi Germany in July 1933, thereby increasing Hitler's prestige immeasurably. Half a year later, Poland signed a peace treaty with the German Reich that enabled the Nazi government to free itself from isolation. In 1936, when German troops moved into the Rhineland—a flagrant violation of the Treaty of Versailles, which had mandated the Rhineland as a demilitarized zone—it would have been easy for the French army, much stronger at the time, to oust them. But the French did nothing, confirming to Hitler and the entire world that any breach of contract by the Nazis would go unchallenged. Each of these successes strengthened Hitler's position and weakened what little political opposition was left within the German Reich. Representatives of foreign nations were spineless and misread completely Hitler's capability for recklessness and unscrupulousness, even though he had spelled out everything for all to see in *Mein Kampf.* Just as had been the case with most Germans—Jews and non-Jews— non-Germans did not take Hitler's statements seriously and were confident that the lunatic would disappear soon from the world's stage. Hitler's anti-Semitic ravings were seen mainly as propaganda, and his promises of a coming war to obtain new soil for Germany in Eastern Europe were dismissed as mere bombast.

In *Mein Kampf,* Hitler had indicated his willingness to sacrifice German sons for foreign soil: "We National Socialists must hold unflinchingly to our aim in foreign policy, namely, to secure for the German people the land and soil to which they are entitled on this earth. And this action is the only one which, before God and our German posterity, would make any sacrifice of blood seem justified. . . . The soil on which someday German generations of peasants can beget powerful sons will sanction the investment of the sons of today, and will someday acquit the responsible statesmen of blood-guilt and sacrifice of the people, even if they are persecuted by their contemporaries."[48]

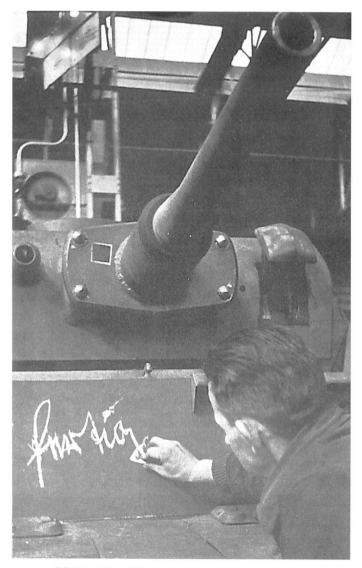

FIG 302 ARMAMENT IN THE THIRD REICH. GERMANY
WAS READY ("FERTIG") FOR WAR.

Statements such as this one were disseminated widely, and
the enormous rearmament of Germany and dramatic demonstrations of Nazi military power could not go unnoticed (fig.
302). German medicine was also affected by preparations for
a coming war. As early as September 1937, all chairs of

departments of medicine in Germany were obligated to report on work being done on war medicine, a study that from then on was to be supported chiefly by the Reich's Office of Research.[49] In the spring of 1939, the curriculum for medical students was adjusted to prepare for the inevitability of war. The subject of pathology was changed into "pathology and war pathology," the subject of surgery to "surgery and war surgery." To turn out more physicians in a hurry, the study of medicine was shortened by more than one year.[50]

Despite the obvious preparation for war on the part of Germany, some European nations still chose to believe Hitler's assertions that he only wanted peace. Like many before him, the British prime minister, Arthur Neville Chamberlain, tried to appease the Nazis by making major concessions to them. After the Munich Conference in 1938, during which Czechoslovakia had been offered up to Germany, Chamberlain proclaimed to a cheering England and the relieved Western world that as a consequence of the accommodation with Hitler, there would be "peace in our time" (figs. 303, 304). Hitler, however, was dissatisfied with the British concessions; he thought the time for war had come, and any delay would only cause Germany's modern military equipment to become outmoded and the precarious economic situation to become unmasked.

At the very time that the NSDAP celebrated the Party Congress of Peace, the invasion of Poland by German and Russian forces had already been decided on. German troops crossed the border on September 1, 1939, marking the beginning of the Second World War (see figs. 306, 307).

Once again, things went far better for Hitler than had generally been expected, even by him. Within eight months, the Netherlands, Belgium, and France were overrun, and Denmark and Norway were occupied by German forces. By mid-1941, the southeast of Europe and large areas of northern Africa were under German control (see fig. 309).

Of the many dermatologists, Jews and non-Jews, who tried to escape the rapidly advancing German troops, only a few

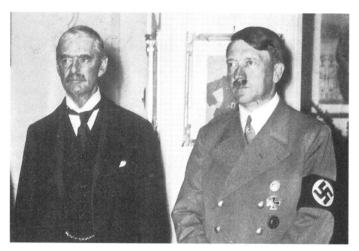

FIG 303 HITLER AND CHAMBERLAIN DURING
NEGOTIATIONS IN GERMANY, SEPTEMBER 1938.

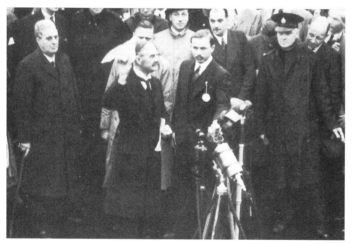

FIG 304 CHAMBERLAIN CLAIMED TO HAVE SECURED
"PEACE IN OUR TIME."

were successful. Lucien Marie Pautrier (fig. 305), the non-Jewish chair of the Department of Dermatology in Strasbourg, managed to evacuate his entire clinic to Clairvivre in southern France, where he established a new dermatological center. Subsequently, he went to the University of Lausanne and returned to his old clinic in Strasbourg after the war. He died in July 1959 at the age of eighty-three. Pautrier is known

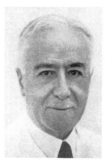

FIG 305
LUCIEN MARIE
PAUTRIER
(1876–1959)

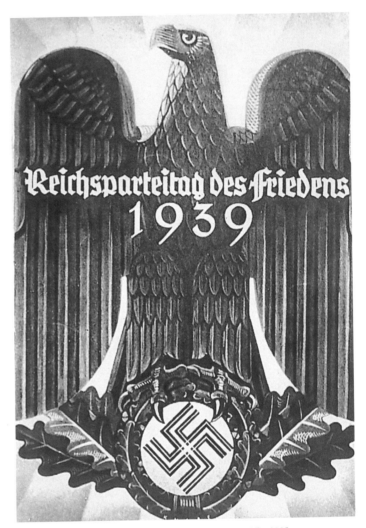

FIG 306 "PARTY CONGRESS OF PEACE 1939"
("REICHSPARTEITAG DES FRIEDENS").

for his work on mycosis fungoids, including his description of intraepithelial collections of neoplastic lymphocytes that are referred to universally as Pautrier's microabscesses.[51]

Most of Pautrier's colleagues did not fare as well. Those who were not willing to cooperate with the Nazis were either forced into silence or into hiding, or put themselves at great risk of being fired, arrested, or even killed. Franciszek Walter, the non-Jewish chair of dermatology in Kraków, attended a lecture

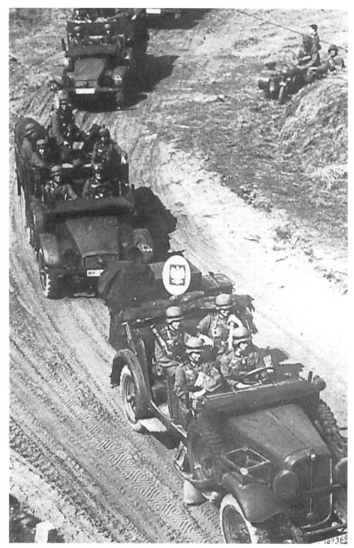

FIG 307 GERMAN TROOPS MOVE INTO POLAND.

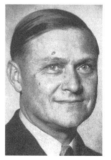

FIG 308
JOSIP FLEGER
(1896–1966)

denouncing the aims of National Socialism; this transgression alone landed him in the Oranienburg concentration camp for several months.[52]

Josip Fleger (fig. 308), an Aryan, was director of a leprosy clinic in Sarajevo. In 1942, he was arrested for contacts with the Yugoslav resistance. After his release, Fleger worked in the dermatology unit of a military hospital in Sarajevo and in 1949

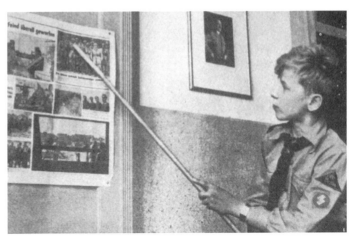

FIG 309 GERMAN SCHOOLBOY BEING TAUGHT THE VICTORIES
OF THE GERMAN ARMY AND THE RAPID CHANGES IN
THE MAP OF EUROPE.

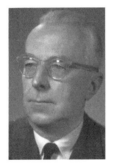

FIG 310
FRANJO KOGOJ
(1894–1983)

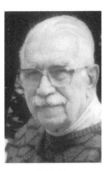

FIG 311
TIBOR SALAMON
(1914–1995)

was appointed director of the skin clinic of the University of Sarajevo; he also was elected president of the Yugoslavian Dermatological Society. Fleger died in Sarajevo in 1966.[53]

In 1941, Franjo Kogoj (fig. 310), the non-Jewish chair of the Department of Dermatology of the University of Zagreb, was dismissed by the new fascist Croatian regime and was able to resume his position only after the war. Kogoj was one of the most prominent European dermatologists of the mid–twentieth century. He identified the spongiform pustule—a collection of neutrophils in the upper part of the epidermis—a finding that is now named for him. Kogoj died in Kranjska Gora in September 1983.[54]

Kogoj's Jewish assistant, Tibor Salamon (fig. 311), was dismissed in 1941 and was interned in several concentration camps until the end of the war. In 1966, he became head of the Department of Dermatology of the University of Sarajevo. In the last years of his life, Salamon again suffered from war, this time the tribal one in Bosnia. He died in Zagreb in 1995. Salamon did important work on heritable skin diseases.[55]

Hermann Werner Siemens, chair of the Department of Dermatology of the University of Leiden, did not at first reject the Nazis, but like many other Germans, thought that they might be able to solve at last the tremendous political and economic problems facing the German people. He soon changed his mind, in part because of the influence of his father-in-law, the famous professor of internal medicine Friedrich von Müller, who had nothing but contempt for the Nazis. Siemens himself became an opponent of the Nazis, and when German troops occupied the Netherlands, he did not desist from criticizing them openly. Consequently, Siemens was removed from his position and arrested twice by the Gestapo. The first time, he was held for a few days; the second time, for three and a half months. After the war, Siemens resumed the chair of dermatology at the University of Leiden, where he stayed until his retirement in 1962. He died on November 22, 1969.[56]

Although German military aggression had severe consequences for the citizens of most European countries, no one suffered more than Jews. Beginning in September 1939, Jews living within the confines of Germany were banned from the streets after 8 P.M., were commandeered into forced labor, and saw their rations and freedoms cut. In 1941, Jews were required to wear a yellow Star of David at all times when outside their homes (fig. 312). This was intended to humiliate them and to make it easier for the authorities to identify them whenever there was the slightest violation of the countless rules and regulations. It also made it easier for the authorities to identify non-Jews who tried to help their Jewish fellow citizens by providing them with goods that Jews were no longer allowed to buy, such as onions and tomatoes, or by simply giving them a word of encouragement. With the Star of David prominently displayed, any such contact could be troublesome for non-Jews and deadly dangerous for Jews.[57] The Stars of David were distributed by the authorities on September 17 and had to be worn as of September 19, 1941. On September 18, the dermatologist Oskar Salomon, an affirming Christian who had been born Jewish, killed himself in his private medical office in Gera, along with his wife and son. Many others committed suicide in the ensuing days.[58]

After the distribution of the Stars of David, new anti-Jewish regulations were issued almost weekly. As of September 19, Jews

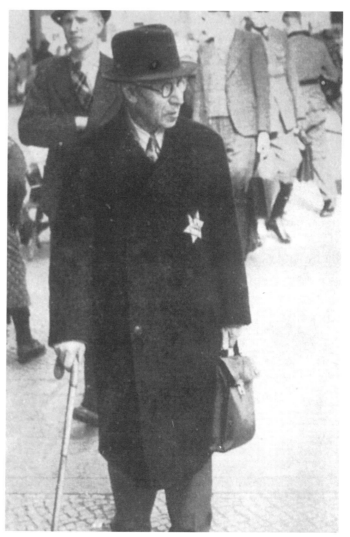

FIG 312 JEW WEARING COAT MARKED WITH A
YELLOW STAR OF DAVID.

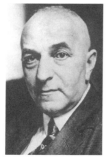

FIG 313
JULIUS MOSES
(1868–1942)

were no longer allowed to leave their city of residence. As of October, they could no longer purchase tobacco[59]; a few days later, they were ordered to deliver their typewriters. Whatever item the government needed was collected from Jews. In mid-November, the Jewish physician Julius Moses (fig. 313) received the following letter from the district mayor of Berlin-Tiergarten: "On the basis of the Reich's Contribution Law . . . I secure all

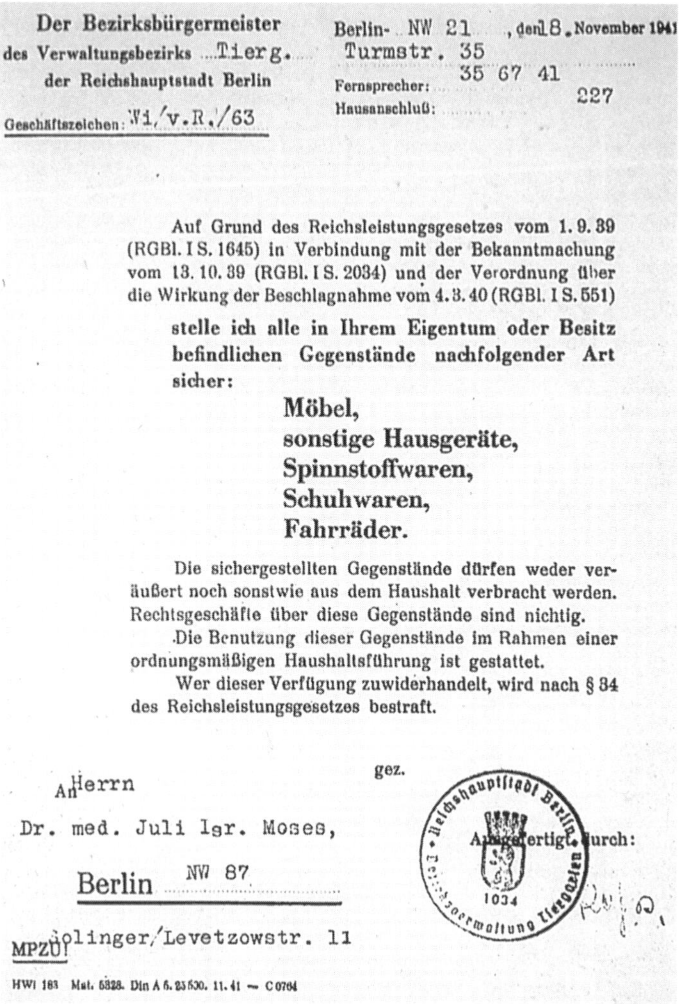

Der Bezirksbürgermeister
des Verwaltungsbezirks ....Tierg.....
der Reichshauptstadt Berlin

Geschäftszeichen: Wi./v.R./63

Berlin- NW 21 , den 18. November 1941
Turmstr. 35
Fernsprecher: 35 67 41
Hausanschluß: 227

Auf Grund des Reichsleistungsgesetzes vom 1. 9. 39
(RGBl. I S. 1645) in Verbindung mit der Bekanntmachung
vom 13. 10. 39 (RGBl. I S. 2034) und der Verordnung über
die Wirkung der Beschlagnahme vom 4. 3. 40 (RGBl. I S. 551)

stelle ich alle in Ihrem Eigentum oder Besitz
befindlichen Gegenstände nachfolgender Art
sicher:

Möbel,
sonstige Hausgeräte,
Spinnstoffwaren,
Schuhwaren,
Fahrräder.

Die sichergestellten Gegenstände dürfen weder ver-
äußert noch sonstwie aus dem Haushalt verbracht werden.
Rechtsgeschäfte über diese Gegenstände sind nichtig.
.Die Benutzung dieser Gegenstände im Rahmen einer
ordnungsmäßigen Haushaltsführung ist gestattet.
Wer dieser Verfügung zuwiderhandelt, wird nach § 34
des Reichsleistungsgesetzes bestraft.

gez.

An Herrn

Dr. med. Juli Isr. Moses,

Berlin NW 87

MPZÜ?linger/Levetzowstr. 11

Angefertigt durch:

1034

HWI 163   Mst. 6328. Din A 6. 25 600. 11. 41 — C 0764

FIG 314 LETTER TO DR. JULIUS MOSES, DATED NOVEMBER 18, 1941.

items of the following kind that are in your possession: furniture,
other household appliances, textile fabrics, shoes, bicycles. The
secured items must not be sold or otherwise removed from the
household" (fig. 314). Eleven months later, Julius Moses, a proponent of social medicine and former member of the Reichstag,
died in the concentration camp at Theresienstadt.[60]

Starting in December 1941, Jews were forbidden from using
public telephones. A month later, they were told to deliver all

their fur and woolen clothes to the authorities. In February, they were forbidden from buying newspapers or visiting Aryan hairdressers; in April, from using public transportation; in May, from owning pets; and in June, from having in their possession electrical and optical devices, bicycles, typewriters, and records. On July 1, 1942, all German Jews were placed under the law of the police, thereby officially being denied the very last remnant of their civil rights.[61]

For Jewish citizens of European countries other than Germany, the situation, unbelievably, was even worse. In Eastern Europe, where the population of Jews was greatest, there was little chance of hiding. When Poland was occupied in September 1939, more than three million Jews came under German control. The western sections of Poland were incorporated into Germany proper, and the remaining areas were used as a dumping ground for those expelled from annexed territory. On September 19, 1939, the General Government was established, in Hitler's words, as "a huge Polish labor camp" (fig. 315).[62]

Hitler's "labor camp" was not reserved for Poles; Jews were transported there from all over Europe. The extent to which Jews were deported from their native country depended on each country's wartime status within the Third Reich. Where German rule was total and supreme—in greater Germany (Germany and Austria), in the Protectorate of Bohemia and Moravia, and in occupied Poland—Jews came directly under the jurisdiction of the SS. In European countries allied to Germany, in the so-called neutral countries, and in those that retained some autonomy in spite of German occupation, the fate of Jews was determined by each country's fundamental commitment to civic equality and by its historical treatment of its Jewish citizens. In Romania, for instance, willingness to hand over Jews to the German authorities was much greater than in Bulgaria. In Denmark, anticipation of a scheduled roundup by the Germans led to an extraordinary operation in which almost all Danish Jews, who had been in hiding, were rescued by Danish citizens

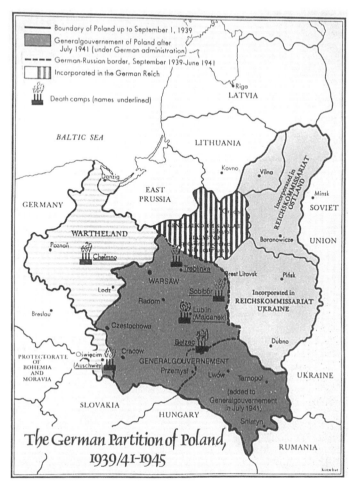

The German Partition of Poland, 1939/41-1945

Boundary of Poland up to September 1, 1939
Generalgouvernement of Poland after July 1941 (under German administration)
German-Russian border, September 1939-June 1941
Incorporated in the German Reich
Death camps (names underlined)

FIG 315 THE GERMAN PARTITION OF POLAND.

and ferried safely to Sweden. It was possible to save Jews from extermination if there was a will to do it.[63]

To avoid deportation, European Jews either had to flee or to conceal their faith and heritage. Haim A. Cohen (fig. 316), who would later become chair of dermatology at Hebrew University in Jerusalem, had been born in Greece, served as a surgeon major in the Greek army, and in the first years of the war was an assistant of Christoforos Doucas (fig. 317) at the dermatological department of the University of Athens.[64] When Greece was occupied by the Germans, Doucas—who,

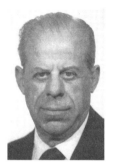

FIG 316
HAIM A. COHEN
(BORN 1914)

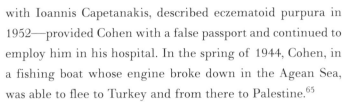

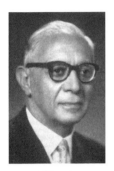

FIG 317
CHRISTOFOROS
DOUCAS
(1890–1974)

with Ioannis Capetanakis, described eczematoid purpura in 1952—provided Cohen with a false passport and continued to employ him in his hospital. In the spring of 1944, Cohen, in a fishing boat whose engine broke down in the Agean Sea, was able to flee to Turkey and from there to Palestine.[65]

As they fled, many Jews found themselves only a few steps ahead of the advancing German army. For instance, Carl Lennhoff, former director of the skin clinic of Magdeburg, initially found refuge in Norway, but, after the German occupation, was forced to move to Sweden.[66] Other physicians— such as neurologist Viktor Kafka (fig. 318), who had written several chapters on syphilis for Jadassohn's *Handbuch*—found themselves in the same position. Until 1933, Kafka had worked at the Department of Psychiatry at the University of Hamburg. By 1939, he had found a new job in Oslo, but the German occupation of Norway forced him to go into hiding again. Hounded by the Gestapo, Kafka and his wife crossed the border into Sweden in 1942, while other scientists fleeing with them were killed by German bullets. In 1943, Kafka was appointed director of the laboratory of the Lanbro Hospital in Stockholm. He died in Stockholm in May 1955.[67]

For most Jews, however, neither flight nor concealment was possible; they were detected by the Germans, taken to the General Government, and clamped into ghettos and concentration camps. Many of the camps—such as Auschwitz, Majdanek, and Treblinka—were built in remote areas that nonetheless were accessible by good railroads. They were far removed from German cities, public opinion, and too many witnesses.

Jews were treated as raw material, exploited "to the highest possible extent at the lowest conceivable degree of expenditure."[68] They were leased to German industry as cheap labor, and the SS meticulously measured profitability of Jews by subtracting from the few Reichsmarks received for each Jew per day the few Pfennigs each required for accommodation, clothing, and food. Despite the proclamation above the main gate at Auschwitz that *"Arbeit macht frei"* ("Work makes free"), hard labor com-

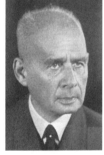

FIG 318
VIKTOR KAFKA
(1881–1955)

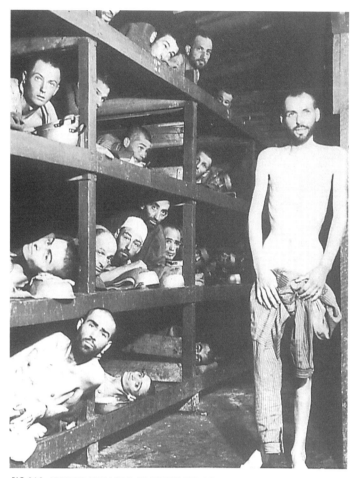

FIG 319 JEWISH INMATES AT BUCHENWALD. ON THE EXTREME RIGHT,
SECOND TIER OF THE MIDDLE COMPARTMENT, IS ELIE WIESEL,
CELEBRATED AUTHOR AND WINNER OF THE NOBEL PEACE
PRIZE IN 1986.

bined with paltry rations made life expectancy for camp inmates
somewhere between six weeks and a few months (figs. 319, 320).

Because one of the Nazi objectives in the war was the acquisition of land in the east, a German attack on the Soviet
Union was just a matter of time. In June 1941, that time
arrived. The German army, with 170 divisions, moved into
Russia. With them came "special-duty groups" that were
commissioned to eradicate the political enemy—namely, the

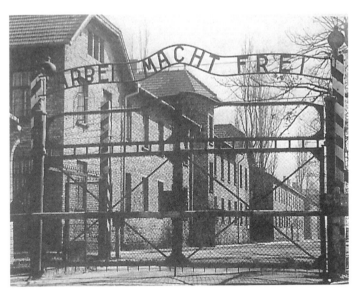

FIG 320 "ARBEIT MACHT FREI" ("WORK MAKES FREE").

Bolshevists and Jews, who were regarded as the major proponents of Bolshevism (fig. 321).

For the Nazis, the war had at last become what it was originally meant to be—a war against world Jewry, of the Aryans
against the inferior races. In an army indoctrination booklet
titled *The Jew in German History,* those objectives were set forth
clearly: "We Germans fight a twofold fight today. With regard
to the non-Jewish peoples we want only to accomplish our vital
interests. We respect them and conduct a chivalrous argument
with them. But we fight world Jewry as one has to fight a poisonous parasite; we encounter in him not only the enemy of our
people, but a plague of all peoples. The fight against Jewry is a
moral fight for the purity and health of God-created humanity
and for a new, more just order in the world."[69]

For the Nazis, "political cleansing actions" took highest priority. Special-duty groups carried out their objective with
incredible brutality and on a large scale, recruiting domestic
criminals as deputies to shoot, hang, or beat to death Communists, Gypsies, and Jews, who were often forced to dig their own
mass graves before they were killed (figs. 322 through 326).

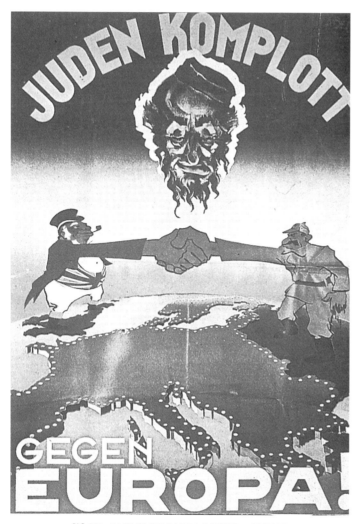

FIG 321 NAZI PROPAGANDA POSTER: "JEWISH
CONSPIRACY AGAINST EUROPE."

The regular German army and even battalions of German police contributed to these monstrosities significantly.[70]

The campaign of terror by special-duty groups resulted in the death of nearly two million people. In response to such slaughter, public opinion among non-Jewish conquered peoples in the east began to shift; many of those who initially had welcomed the Germans as liberators now preferred Stalin.

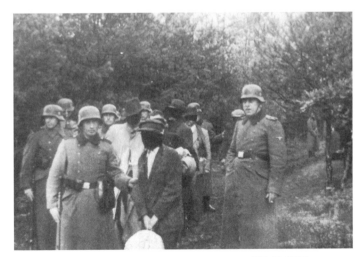

FIG 322 THE DUTIES OF THE SPECIAL-DUTY GROUPS:
BLINDFOLDED VICTIMS.

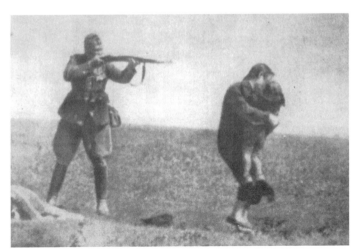

FIG 323 THE DUTIES OF THE SPECIAL-DUTY GROUPS: SOLDIER
SHOOTING A MOTHER AND HER CHILD.

A hard winter in Russia and the firm resistance of Soviet forces finally put an end to the German advance. On December 6, 1942, the Soviets began an offensive with fresh and well-armed troops called to the western front from the Asian territories, resulting in Germany's first defeat of the war. At the same time, the Sixth German Army in Stalingrad was surrounded and defeated decisively after months of struggle; 150,000 Ger-

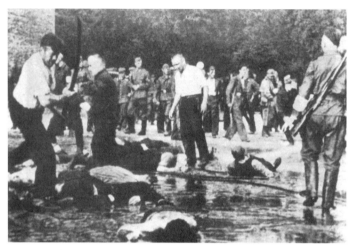

FIG 324 THE DUTIES OF THE SPECIAL-DUTY GROUPS:
SLAUGHTER OF VICTIMS.

man soldiers were killed in that battle, and almost 100,000 were
captured and sent to horrid prisoner of war camps in Siberia
(fig. 327). Although German newspapers praised the "heroes of
Stalingrad" and called for revenge, many now began to realize
that the war could not be won. According to a December 6 entry
in the daybook of the High Command of the German Army,
Hitler also was aware "that, from this culmination point on, no
further victory could be achieved."[71]

Five days later, however, Hitler surprised the world—and his
own generals—by declaring war on the United States. Judged
by standards of rationality, Hitler's decision made no sense at
all; it assured Germany's ultimate defeat. He seemed indifferent to the outcome of the war and took no action to avoid the
looming military catastrophe. Instead, Hitler concentrated his
energy on the war that could be won—the war against the Jews,
which seems to have been his real mission.

For the Nazis, the real German enemy was Jews, no matter
where they lived. In the Nazis' twisted psyche, the Allied powers were enemies because they were pawns of world Jewry
(figs. 328, 329). As early as 1939, Hitler had stated in a speech to
the Reichstag that "during my struggle for power, the Jews pri-

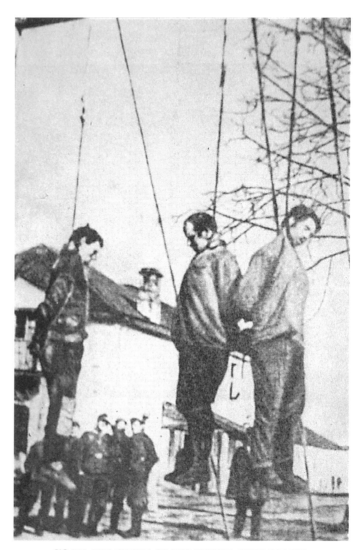

FIG 325 THE DUTIES OF THE SPECIAL-DUTY GROUPS:
HANGING OF VICTIMS.

marily received with laughter my prophecies that I would
someday assume the leadership of the state and thereby of the
entire people and then, among many other things, achieve a
solution of the Jewish problem. I suppose that meanwhile the
then-resounding laughter of Jewry in Germany is now choking
in their throats. Today, I will be a prophet again: If international finance Jewry within Europe and abroad should succeed

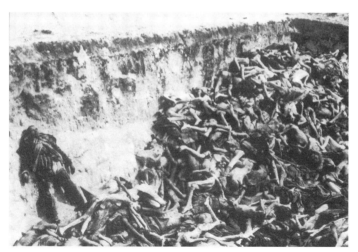

FIG 326 THE DUTIES OF THE SPECIAL-DUTY GROUPS: MASS GRAVE.

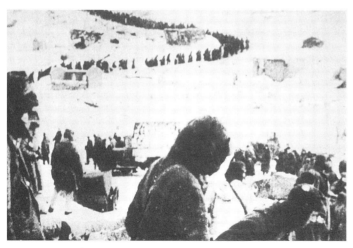

FIG 327 GERMAN PRISONERS OF WAR AFTER
THE BATTLE OF STALINGRAD.

once more in plunging the peoples into a world war, then the
consequence will not be the Bolshevization of the world and
therewith a victory of Jewry, but on the contrary, the destruction of the Jewish race in Europe."[72]

Hitler, a pathetic person with no real ego, constantly needed
the approval of others and could not accept criticism, defeat, or
mockery. In his mind, there were only two modes of action: total

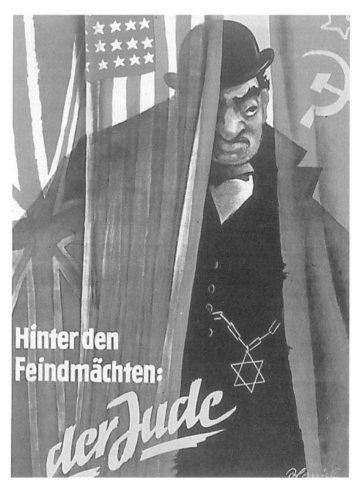

FIG 328 NAZI PROPAGANDA POSTER: THE JEW
BEHIND THE ALLIED POWERS.

victory or complete destruction. In the face of defeat, Hitler was willing to bring everything down with him, and he did. Had the means of destruction that are available today been at Hitler's disposal, he would have, with impunity, destroyed the world.

At the time, Hitler had only the means to destroy European Jewry, people who had never made war on anyone and who were utterly defenseless. This hapless people, a victim of persecution for more than a millennium, was set upon by the most mechanized military force in the history of mankind, dressed in jackboots, armed to the teeth, and joined by Ger-

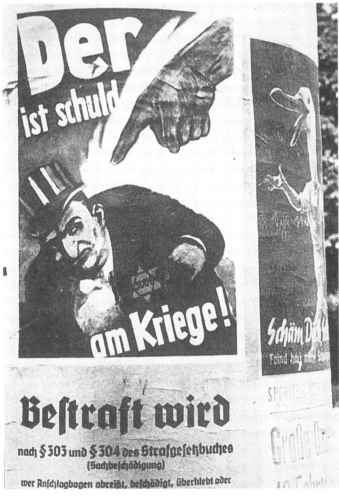

FIG 329 NAZI PROPAGANDA POSTER: "HE IS RESPONSIBLE FOR THE WAR!"

man shepherd dogs in the hunt for Jews. It was an example of unbridled, cowardly bullying unparalleled in human history.

Because shooting or beating Jews to death was found to be too time consuming and psychologically harmful, other techniques were employed, and the gassing of Jews finally proved the most efficient. The concentration camps of the General Government were transformed into annihilation camps where large gassing facilities—mobile and permanent—were

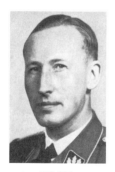

FIG 330
REINHARD
HEYDRICH
(1904–1942)

installed. Different methods of gassing were experimented with, until cyanide gas—better known under the German trade name Zyklon B—was chosen.

At a conference in the Berlin suburb of Wannsee in January 1941, Reinhard Heydrich (fig. 330), Himmler's right-hand man in the SS, elaborated on the practical realization of the annihilation of European Jewry. According to his plans, Europe had "to be combed through from west to east" for Jews, who would be evacuated "group by group into so-called transit ghettos, to be transported from there farther to the East." The official reason given for the removal of Jews was "resettlement for work in the East."[73]

In the ghettos of Poland, where hunger ravaged the population, offers of bread induced thousands of Jews to volunteer for "resettlement"(fig. 331). When rumors about the true nature of resettlement had spread and there were no more volunteers, the Nazis used force in the form of all their military might to liquidate the ghetto of Warsaw and the small band of Jewish fighters who went to their death nobly, asserting in a language of resistance the will of the Jewish people to live (figs. 332, 333).

Resistance on the part of Jews was so futile, however, that it remained an exception. In many instances, the threat of resettlement was sufficient to induce Jews to take their own lives. Franz

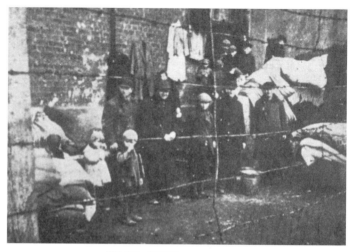

FIG 331 GHETTO IN POLAND.

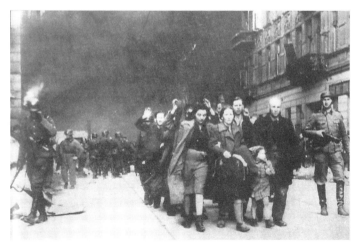

FIG 332 ROUNDUP OF JEWS DURING THE
WARSAW GHETTO UPRISING IN 1943.

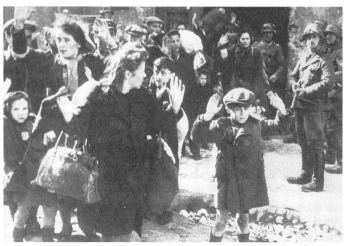

FIG 333 ROUNDUP OF JEWS DURING THE
WARSAW GHETTO UPRISING IN 1943.

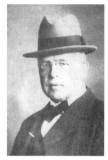

FIG 334
FRANZ SOETBEER
(1870–1943)

Soetbeer (fig. 334), professor of internal medicine at the University of Giessen and father-in-law of the dermatologist Alfred Marchionini, hanged himself in a Gestapo prison in 1943. Soetbeer, a "Jewish half-breed," had been denounced for having accepted a goose as a Christmas present from one of his former patients.[74] Rudolf Wilhelm Habermann, professor of dermatol-

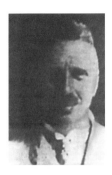

FIG 335
CARL BRUCK
(1879–1944)

ogy at the University of Hamburg, poisoned himself with potassium cyanide in 1941 just before the Gestapo was about to arrest him because of the accusation that he had issued medical certificates without having performed a physical examination. Carl Bruck (fig. 335), former director of dermatology at the Hamburg-Altona Municipal Hospital, took potassium cyanide in 1944 after having been threatened by the Gestapo. He had been denounced for having hoarded excessive amounts of butter. When Bruck categorically denied that accusation, the Gestapo declared that he had "to follow them for the purpose of further clarification." Bruck went into the kitchen in order "to drink a glass of water," came back, lay down on a sofa, and died. Bruck, a baptized Jew, was famous for having described in 1906—along with Jewish co-authors, August von Wassermann and Albert Neisser—the original non-treponemal antigen serologic test for detection of syphilis, referred to today as the Wassermann test.[75] Other dermatologists who committed suicide rather than be resettled were Martin Cohn and Dora Gerson from Dresden and Erich Oppenheimer from Görlitz. Gerson, who was in private practice from 1920 to 1935, was the first female dermatologist in Germany. Oppenheimer, also a dermatologist in private practice and, since 1938, one of 709 "treaters of the sick" who were licensed to treat Jews exclusively, killed himself in a transit camp in Rothenburg-Tormersdorf shortly before his transport was to leave for Auschwitz.[76]

The Jews selected for resettlement were herded into cattle cars with no sanitary facilities that, within hours, were filled with a pestilent smell. The cars were so crowded that one could neither sit nor fall, and a trip that lasted several days might be interrupted for biological needs for only a few minutes—if at all. Despite the transportation shortage of the German military during this critical period of the war, the SS always managed to produce enough trains to fulfill its contribution to the Final Solution of the Jewish Question: That mission always was given top priority (fig. 336).

Upon arriving at the camps, Jews were put through a series of routine procedures. At camps like Auschwitz that had labor instal-

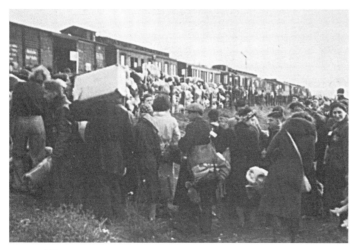

FIG 336 "DEATH TRAIN" LEAVING FOR EXTERMINATION.

lations, 10 percent of the arrivals—those who looked fittest—
were selected for work. The remainder were instructed to undress,
remove their rings, and tie their shoes together to ensure that pairs
could be identified later on (figs. 337, 338).

They then were hurried past lines of auxiliary police to the
gas chambers, which were camouflaged as shower rooms (fig.
339). Packed in, one person per square foot, they were gassed
until all were dead, a process that took between ten and thirty
minutes. Because the next trainload of new arrivals was not
far behind, bodies were burned immediately, either in the
open air or in crematoria. At night, the red sky over Auschwitz
could be seen for many miles (figs. 340, 342).

Among the countless Jews who met this fate were numerous
dermatologists and their relatives, such as the sister of Hans
Biberstein and the daughter of Emil Meirowsky, who had converted to Christianity and taken the veil but, nevertheless, was
dragged out of her nunnery in 1942 and deported to
Auschwitz.[77] Henry Haber, who had emigrated to England and
was a medical officer in the British army, lost his entire family
of parents, four brothers, and their wives and children.[78] Thousands more did not learn of the terrible fate of their relatives
until after the war and lived with that unremitting sorrow for

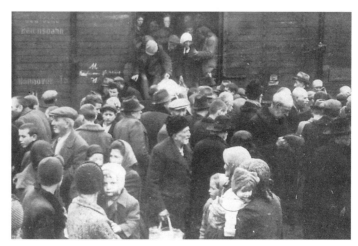

FIG 337 JEWS ARRIVING ON THE RAMP OF THE
RAILWAY STATION OF AUSCHWITZ.

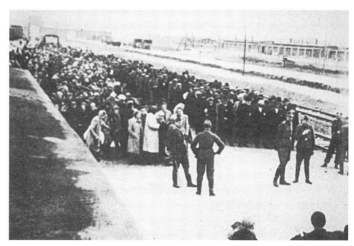

FIG 338 MEN AND WOMEN WERE SEPARATED FROM ONE ANOTHER ON
ARRIVAL. NEXT THE SS PHYSICIAN DIVIDED THOSE ABLE TO WORK
FROM THOSE CONSIDERED UNABLE TO WORK. THE LATTER WERE
SENT TO GAS CHAMBERS FORTHWITH.

the rest of their lives. Between the summer of 1941 and the end
of 1943, about two million people were gassed at Auschwitz
alone; in all, the death toll at the camps was more than five million human beings, the overwhelming majority of them Jews.[79]

In this horrible story of the deepest abyss of which human
nature is capable, physicians played a prominent role. The

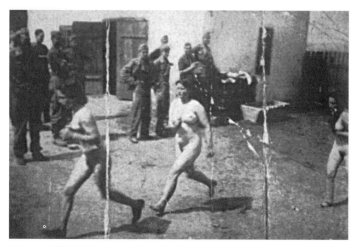

FIG 339 WOMEN BEING CHASED TO THE "SHOWERS."

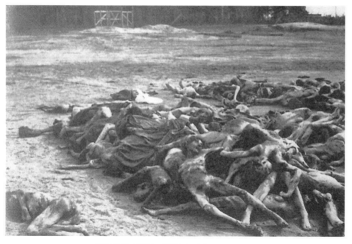

FIG 340 THE "FINAL SOLUTION."

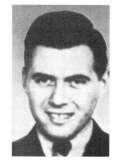

FIG 341
JOSEF MENGELE
(1911–1979)

most notorious was Josef Mengele (fig. 341), who waited at the Auschwitz railway station for arriving trains and with a wave of his hand decided who was to live and who was to die. According to Rudolf Höss (fig. 343), commander of the Auschwitz concentration camp, "Men and women are separated from one another first. Both columns are standing on the ramp. Now the SS physician begins to separate those able to work from those whom he considers unable to work. Those

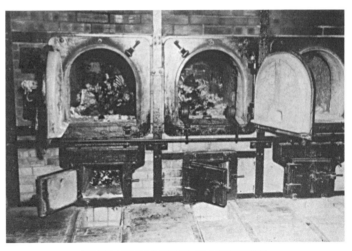

FIG 342 CREMATORIUM AT AUSCHWITZ.

good for work were sent into the camp. Others were sent to the extermination facilities immediately. Children of tender age were exterminated without exception because, on account of their youth, they were unable to work" (figs. 344, 345).[80]

In the presence of physicians, new arrivals at the camps were hit and whipped. They were disinfected with toxic solutions, such as phenol baths, which sometimes caused death (fig. 346). Hygienic conditions in the camps were deplorable. Water was scarce and unclean, lice and fleas infested the crowded barracks, and thousands of people died of typhus and other infections without receiving medical help. Medical examinations were performed only for purposes of selection for temporary life or immediate death and often were the cause of disease as columns of naked prisoners were forced to stand in the cold and rain for hours before a Nazi physician cast a glance at them (fig. 347). Prisoners were forced to undress and run in front of SS officers to demonstrate that some strength was still left in them. No matter how tired or pained they were, weakness had to be hidden if life was to be sustained.[81]

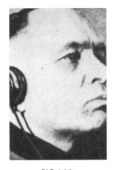

FIG 343
RUDOLF HÖSS
(1900–1947)

Many physicians in the camps practiced their surgical skills on Jews and Gypsies, performing amputations for all kinds of

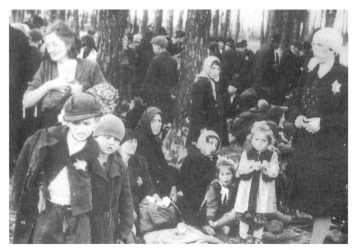

FIG 344 "USELESS" HUMAN BEINGS DESTINED FOR DEATH

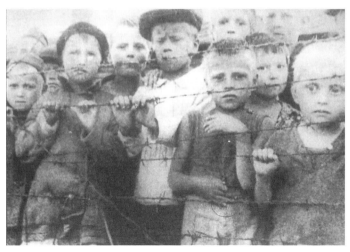

FIG 345 CHILDREN TO BE EXTERMINATED.

minor injuries and gastrectomies for stomachaches. The unfortunate "patients" were not given a chance to recover, usually being gassed to death a few days later.[82]

Prisoners were also used systematically for research purposes. It was not the first time that unethical studies on human beings had been performed. Since the 1880s when the experimental approach became *au courant* in medicine, physi-

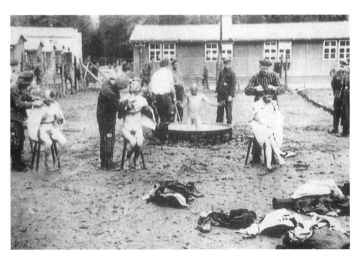

FIG 346 UPON ARRIVAL AT A CONCENTRATION CAMP, THOSE INMATES
NOT KILLED IMMEDIATELY HAD THEIR HEADS SHAVED
AND THEIR BODIES DISINFECTED.

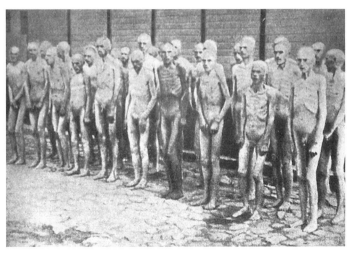

FIG 347 INSPECTION OF CAMP INMATES:
THE DECISION TO DIE OR LIVE ANOTHER DAY.

cians had become convinced of their right to undertake experiments on human beings as long as the research served a
greater good. Bacteriologists thought of themselves as "war-
riors against disease," and they averred that medical research
should be placed above the ethical code of civil life; sacrifice
of individual rights was deemed necessary if medical science

was to be advanced. That claim met fierce resistance from humanists, such as Rudolf Virchow, who condemned bacteriologists as "poisoners and murderers" for their excessive use of animal experiments. One protest against human experiments is exemplified by the row over the research conducted by the dermatologist Albert Neisser. In 1895, inspired by Emil von Behring's successes with sera against diphtheria, Neisser injected young prostitutes (the youngest was ten years old) with a cell-free syphilis serum in the hope that it would provide immunity against that spirochetal disease. The result instead was to infect some of those non-volunteers with syphilis. In 1898, a scandal erupted over the experiments and Neisser was formally censured by the state.

The animated public discussion as a consequence of the Neisser case led to the first detailed regulations in Western medicine about research that was unrelated to treatment, according to which medical intervention for other than diagnosis, healing, and immunization was forbidden when the "human subject was a minor or not competent for other reasons" or when the subject had not given his or her "unambiguous consent" after a "proper explanation of the possible negative consequences" of the procedure. In the 1920s, the socialist physician Julius Moses waged a campaign in the press and in parliament against carrying out human experiments. His efforts resulted in the Guidelines for New Therapy and Human Experimentation that were promulgated by the Reich's government in 1931. According to those guidelines, nontherapeutic research was "under no circumstances permissible without consent." Children required special protection, and experimentation on dying patients was prohibited. This legislation, which was extraordinarily advanced, was never annulled in Nazi Germany, but the Nazis ceased to enforce it, and in the concentration camps all restrictions on human research were waived.[83]

The "research" projects performed in concentration camps concerned such diverse subjects as the efficacy and side effects

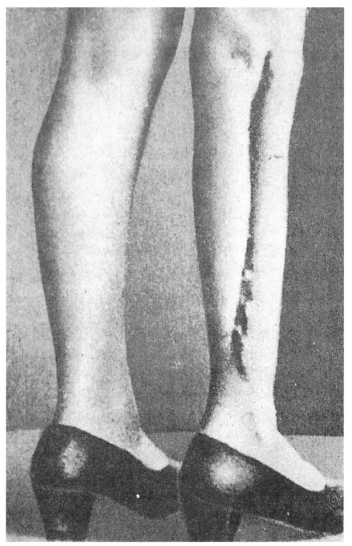

FIG 348 DISFIGURED LEG FOLLOWING A MEDICAL EXPERIMENT.

of new drugs, the effects of chemical weapons, and the efficiency of new methods of sterilization. Prisoners were subjected to extremely low atmospheric pressure and profound
hypothermia in order to discover the limits that a body could
tolerate (figs. 348, 349). The results of these experiments,
nearly all of which were pseudoscience and devoid of any
meaningful data, were published in respected medical jour-

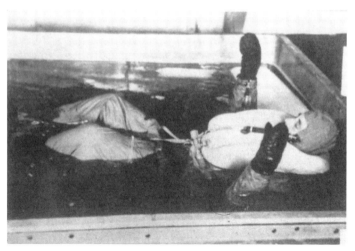

FIG 349 STUDIES ON HYPOTHERMIA IN A COLD WATER BATH.

nals such as the *Zentralblatt für Chirurgie*. Some physicians performed anthropological studies—for example, Josef Mengele, who sought academic recognition for his cruel comparative studies of Jewish twins (see fig. 351).

At that time, the only skin clinic whose research was still funded by the government was the department of Josef Vonkennel at the University of Leipzig, because Vonkennel was not only director of the skin clinic but also director of the SS Research Institute V that had been established as a separate branch of the clinic. With his assistant, Josef Kimmig, who later became chair of the Department of Dermatology in Hamburg, Vonkennel developed diaminodiphenylsulfone, a drug that has antibiotic and anti-inflammatory properties and that still is used widely for treatment of such disparate diseases as leprosy and dermatitis herpetiformis. On the initiative of Vonkennel, experiments with the new drug were carried out on internees of the concentration camp at Buchenwald, who were treated with diaminodiphenylsulfone after induction of severe burns by poison gas. Many prisoners died in the process.[84]

In the view of Nazi doctors, prisoners were merely guinea pigs, and they referred to them that way. The dermatologist Herta Oberheuser (fig. 350), the only female physician convicted by the

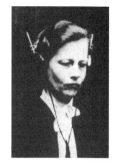

FIG 350
HERTA
OBERHEUSER
(BORN 1911)

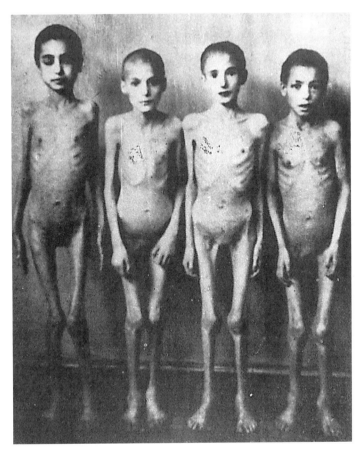

FIG 351 JEWISH CHILDREN USED FOR "RESEARCH"
(FROM THE FILES OF JOSEF MENGELE).

Nuremberg court after the war, said during her trial: "In August 1942, the so-called guinea-pig operation started in our section, I call it the experiment with living objects. I was in charge of the treatment and management of so-called guinea-pigs in section I." In the course of that operation, Oberheuser selected Polish Jewish inmates of the concentration camp at Ravensbrück for experimental bone marrow transplantation, insisted on "systematic non-care" for the persons operated on, and killed many of them by injections of gasoline. Furthermore, prisoners were infected with bacteria in order to assess the efficacy and side effects of sulfonamides; the death toll from those experiments was high.[85] Herta Oberheuser had started to work with sulfonamides during her residency in the department of dermatology of the University of Düsseldorf, whose chairman, Hans Theodor Schreus, was a pioneer in the field. During the time she was assigned to Ravensbrück, she visited Schreus repeatedly, presumably to discuss the results of her studies. She also tried to persuade assistants of the skin clinic in Düsseldorf to join her at Ravensbrück, encouraging them with the promise that any experiments on humans they desired could be performed in the concentration camp.[86] Oberheuser was sentenced to twenty years in prison, but was released after seven years because of good conduct, at which time she resumed the practice of medicine.

Many leading German physicians were involved directly in human experiments, and many more knew about them. At a meeting of the Consulting Physicians of the Academy of Military Medicine in 1943, the inhumane experiments at the concentration camp at Ravensbrück were described in detail. The audience consisted of the chief representatives of German medicine before and after the war, including dermatologists Walter Frieboes, Carl Friedrich Funk, Heinrich Adolf Gottron, Heinrich Löhe, Alois Memmesheimer, Hans-Theodor Schreus, Karl Hermann Vohwinkel, Josef Vonkennel, and Karl Zieler. None of them uttered a word of protest and none of them resigned his position.[87]

The unlimited human resources for study that the camps provided to medical schools throughout Germany prompted faculty members of university departments to ask the SS for support in creating collections of specimens for the study of anatomy and pathology. In a letter to Himmler in February 1942, August Hirt, chair of anatomy at the Reich's University of Strasbourg, asked for skulls of "Jewish Bolshevist commissaries," pointing out that

practically, the smooth acquisition and securing of those skulls is accomplished most effectively by ordering the army to henceforth turn over all living Jewish

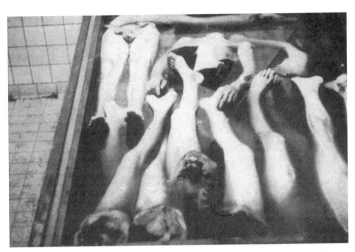

FIG 352 COLLECTION OF ANATOMIC SPECIMENS TAKEN FROM
JEWISH VICTIMS OF CONCENTRATION CAMPS ON DISPLAY
AT THE UNIVERSITY OF STRASBOURG.

*Bolshevist commissaries to the field police. The field
police, in turn, receives a special order to notify continuously the supply and whereabouts of those arrested
Jews to a certain office and to protect them until the
arrival of an especially authorized representative. The
representative (a young physician or medical student
from the army or the field police, equipped with car
and driver) has to carry out a fixed number of pho-
tographs and anthropological measurements and, if
possible, has to find out origin, date of birth, and other
personal data. After the subsequently induced death of
the Jew, whose head must not be injured, he separates
the head from the trunk and sends it, embedded in a
preservative in special, lockable sheet metal containers,
to its place of destination.*[88]

Himmler granted all requests of that kind, and the University
of Strasbourg was able to create a large collection of Jewish
skeletons (fig. 352). Shortly before the end of the war, this collection was dismantled, yet at several universities in Germany

and Austria—in Vienna, Innsbruck, and Graz, for example—
Jewish corpses acquired during the Nazi period were used for
training in anatomy until very recently.

Exceptions to the goal of extermination at the camps were
rare and were limited to German Jews over sixty-five who had
been distinguished for war service and to prominent Jews
whose disappearance would have provoked international
inquiries that could prove embarrassing to Germany. The priv-
ileged Jews were taken to Theresienstadt, a "model concentration camp" and the only one the Nazis ever allowed foreigners
to observe. Among the 65,000 inmates in Theresienstadt, about
1,000 were physicians.

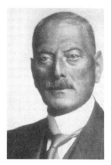

One physician at Theresienstadt was Karl Herxheimer (figs.
353, 354), the former chair of dermatology in Frankfurt and
one of the founders of Frankfurt University. Herxheimer is
identified with the Jarisch-Herxheimer reaction, a hypersensi-
tivity reaction in response to spirochetal allergens in the treatment of syphilis, and with acrodermatitis chronica atrophicans,
a disease now appreciated to be a late manifestation of an infection by *Borrelia*, that he had described in 1902. Herxheimer
had retired from his chairmanship in 1930. When the Nazis
assumed power, his friends repeatedly urged him to leave Germany, but Herxheimer insisted on staying in his hometown of
Frankfurt, like so many others who underestimated the Nazi
threat. In a discussion in 1933 about pogroms against Jews in
the Middle Ages, Herxheimer stated that while something similar might still happen, it would never be as bad as it had been
in times past. In 1936, he told his successor, Oscar Gans: "I cannot leave Frankfurt, and I do not want to leave it in my old age.
Everybody knows me. When I enter the tram, the conductor
says, 'Well, that's fine, Mr. Privy Councillor, that you stay with
us. Nothing will happen to you, every child knows you, and you
have only done good for our city. You must not leave.' Vox pop-
uli, vox Dei. And so I ask you, Mr. Gans, why should I go?"[89]

After his retirement in 1930, Herxheimer had continued to
work at the skin clinic of the University of Frankfurt in close

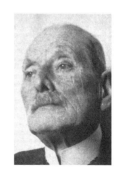

collaboration with his former assistants and his successor, Oscar Gans. After Gans had been dismissed and Martin Schubert had been appointed chair of the Department of Dermatology, Herxheimer was forbidden to enter the building. However, he lived nearby and used to take his dog to a rose garden close to the clinic. Here his former assistants used to show him patients and ask for his advice, a circumstance not approved of but tolerated by Schubert, who was far less competent than Herxheimer, and considered himself fortunate to be provided correct diagnoses for free and without losing face.[90]

At that time, Herxheimer had already been excluded from a table reserved for a group of friends to which he had belonged for many years. He still enjoyed taking his dog on a short trip to the Taunus, a mountain range northwest of Frankfurt, until he found no more benches on which a Jew was allowed to sit. In anticipation of a law that forbid Jews to possess books, he gave away his precious, priceless library to friends, including Friedrich Schmidt-La Baume, who later returned those books to the Department of Dermatology of the University of Frankfurt in memory of Herxheimer.[91]

In 1941, several of Herxheimer's friends, including a high-ranking officer of the storm troopers, made plans for Herxheimer's flight to Switzerland, where Herxheimer owned a house at Lake Thun. Again, Herxheimer rejected the offer, vowing to bear his fate until the end. By that time Herxheimer's home and cherished medical library had been seized, and he lived in humble conditions in a small apartment, existing on a modest pension he received from the University of Frankfurt.[92] On August 24, 1942, the registrar of the university wrote to the Gestapo in Frankfurt: "The former Jewish university professor, Dr. Karl Israel Herxheimer, resident here, Friedrichstrasse 26 I, identification number Q 02182, still receives public benefits from the local university cash desk. To avoid overpayment, I ask for information of my office in the case that Herxheimer should be evacuated."[93] Three days later, Herxheimer was arrested, taken to the railway station, put in a sealed wagon, and, with hundreds of other Jews, transported to Theresienstadt, where on December 6 he died of dysentery and starvation fourteen weeks after he had been "evacuated."[94]

At about the same time, another giant in dermatology, Abraham Buschke (fig. 355), arrived in Theresienstadt. Former director of the dermatological department at the Rudolf Virchow Hospital in Berlin, Buschke's name is still invoked for his description of scleredema adultorum, a rare disease of unknown cause that affects the dermis dramatically, causing it to thicken greatly, and to which his name is attached eponymically. Buschke's name also is linked to several other diseases—namely, cryptococcosis or Busse-Buschke disease, caused by the encapsulated yeast *Cryptococcus neoformans* and seen today with increasing frequency in immunosuppressed patients; dermatofibrosis lenticularis disseminata or Buschke-Ollendorff syndrome, characterized by connective tissue nevi of the skin and osteopoikilosis; verrucous carcinoma or the Buschke-Löwenstein tumor, induced by a human papillomavirus; and melanosis of Buschke, a reticulated pigmentation brought about by chronic, intense exposure to heat. As an observant Jew, Buschke was dismissed from his position at the Rudolf Virchow Hospital in 1933. In 1937, he and his wife visited the United States, where Buschke gave a lecture at the Skin and Cancer Unit of New York University. Against the wishes of their children, who lived in Chicago, the Buschkes returned to Berlin. Abraham Buschke had been working since 1933 without pay at the Hospital of the Jewish Community and did not want to give up his duties there. In 1938, he was invited to the United States again but refused to go when permission to leave Germany was granted on the condition that his wife remain behind as hostage. Four years later, both Abraham Buschke, then seventy-four years old, and his wife were taken to Theresienstadt. A few weeks after her husband's death in the camp, Erna Buschke wrote the following lines in a short, secretly kept biography: "He worked until Nov. 4, 1942, when fate caught up with us, and we were evac-

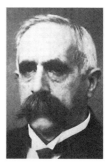

FIG 355
ABRAHAM BUSCHKE
(1868–1943)

uated to Theresienstadt. This shock was probably the beginning of the end. He could not adjust to the changed life so devoid of the possibility of working, under the dreary conditions here in Hell, and he died, totally exhausted and weakened, from severe enteritis, on Feb. 24, 1943."[95]

Of the more than 140,000 people sent to the model camp at Theresienstadt, fewer than 17,000 were alive when the camp fell to the Allies in May 1945. Among them was Erna Buschke, who spent the rest of her life with her children in the United States.[96]

THE END AND THE
YEARS AFTER

AS THE WAR NEARED AN END, IT DOMINATED LIFE IN GER-
MANY COMPLETELY. THE DAYS WERE FILLED WITH
the sound of propaganda and the nights with the wail of air-
raid warnings. Women, once glorified as the mothers of
racially pure future generations, now worked on the home
front producing bullets and bombs. Even young children were
employed in the war effort, digging shelters and collecting
metal that could be used for armaments (fig. 356).

At the universities, teaching in the usual fashion became
increasingly difficult. Congresses and scientific meetings were
canceled, not only because of a shortage of lecturers but
because there was no one left to listen to them; most students
and young physicians were at the front. Topics in medical education were devoted to problems posed by the war, however
minor in importance. For example, Walther Schultze, chair of
dermatology in Giessen, was asked to contribute to a series of
"lectures on military science" and chose to speak about "mate-
rials for washing and cleansing in the war."[1]

Medical research was restricted almost entirely to subjects of
military interest, such as aviation medicine, treatment of gun-
shot wounds, and physiological responses to heat, cold, thirst,
and pressure. In dermatology, more attention was directed
toward sexually transmitted diseases, which were occurring
more frequently. Several departments of dermatology were
commissioned to carry out projects of military interest. Carl
Moncorps in Münster, for example, received a secret order from
the highest army command to search for methods whereby
neurotoxic substances could penetrate the skin invisibly.[2]

The importance attached to various dermatological problems
is reflected in the program of the Twentieth Congress of the
German Dermatological Society, which convened in Würzburg

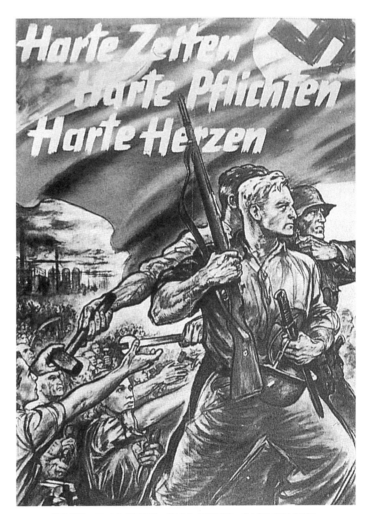

FIG 356 "HARD TIMES—HARD DUTIES—HARD HEARTS":
NAZI PROPAGANDA IN THE LAST YEARS OF THE WAR.

during October 1942. It was the first congress of any German medical society since the onset of the war. The first lecture of the congress was given by the new Reich's leader of physicians, Leonardo Conti, who spoke about the "duty of being healthy and venereal diseases." Conti exhorted his audience that the duty to seek treatment for venereal diseases, as laid down in the Law for the Fight Against Venereal Diseases in 1927, was a matter of course but insufficient. That law obligated treatment for the sole purpose of protecting others from becoming infected. In contrast, Conti argued, the "duty of being healthy meant that one and all have a moral obligation to restore and maintain health to achieve the greatest productivity" for the benefit of the people.[3]

After Conti's introduction, the program of the congress was divided into three sections. The first dealt with skin lesions produced by cold and heat, the second with metabolism of the skin and venereal diseases, and the third with infection and disinfection. Discussions ranged from skin lesions of German soldiers during the winter campaign in Russia to lesions inflicted on themselves by hard laborers from the Ukraine. The congress leader, Karl Zieler, emphasized that "also our scientific sessions are part of the total engagement in the field of health control to which we devote ourselves with all our strength and all our medical and scientific productivity, no matter if on duty in the army, at the front, or at home. Therefore, at the end, let me be mindful of a man who has devoted his entire life to the rise and the lasting safety of the German people and who, as we all hope, will also lead this hardest battle for the prosperity of our nation to a victorious end. Our leader Adolf Hitler: Sieg Heil!"[4]

As time went by, it became more and more apparent that Hitler and his minions would not be victorious. The German front shrunk mile by mile, and most major cities were under constant attack by Allied bombers, which hit civilians with the same ferocity as they did military targets.

Because Jews and people of Jewish descent were not allowed to enter public air-raid shelters, the Allied bombings claimed many victims among them. Paul Unna, Jr., for instance, was on duty in his father's private clinic in Hamburg when the entire complex of buildings, including Unna's famous Dermatologikum, was destroyed by Allied bombs in July 1943 (figs. 357, 358).[5] The Dermatologikum, founded in 1883, was a center for research in dermatology and became the cradle of dermatopathology from which emerged leading figures in that field, such as Delbanco,

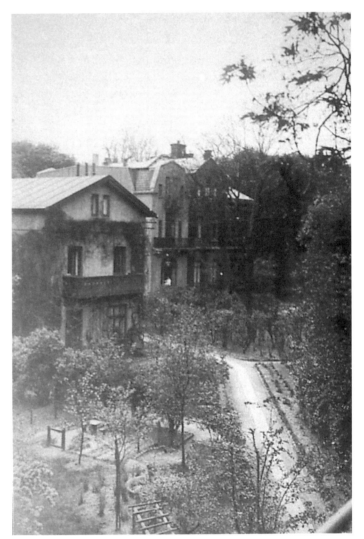

FIG 357 PAUL GERSON UNNA'S PRIVATE CLINIC BEFORE
ITS DESTRUCTION IN 1943.

Gans, Hollander, MacLeod, Meirowsky, Mibelli, Pappenheim,
Pollitzer, and Török.

Like the Dermatologikum in Hamburg, most clinics were
located in the center of large cities and often close to military
compounds, which made them particularly vulnerable to air
raids. During the firebombing of Hamburg in July and August

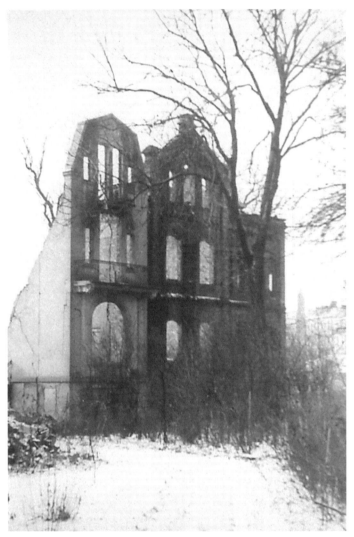

FIG 358 PAUL GERSON UNNA'S PRIVATE CLINIC
AFTER ITS DESTRUCTION IN 1943.

of 1943, 60 percent of the university clinic complex was deci-
mated (fig. 359), and among the 50,000 who perished were
many patients and physicians.[6] In Leipzig, Münster, and Düsseldorf, the university clinics were destroyed almost entirely,
and in Stuttgart, the entire municipal hospital system was
wiped out. Several hospitals under construction never came to

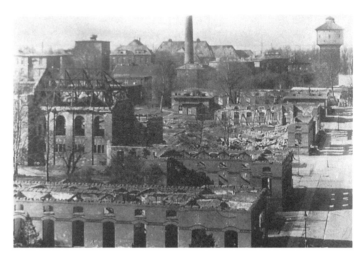

FIG 359 THE UNIVERSITY CLINIC COMPLEX OF HAMBURG-EPPENDORF AFTER ITS DESTRUCTION IN 1943.

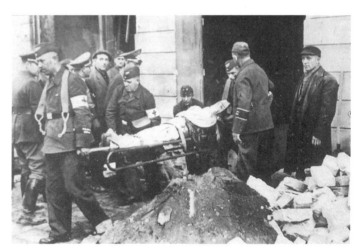

FIG 360 VICTIM OF BOMBINGS.

completion because of incessant interruptions. Toward the war's end, only a few German hospitals were intact and functioning, and these were hopelessly overcrowded. In addition to their traditional functions, hospitals now often served as military medical facilities and as emergency clinics for civilians injured during air raids (figs. 360, 361).[7]

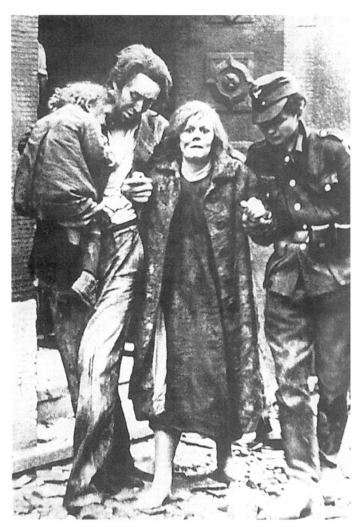

FIG 361 VICTIM OF BOMBINGS.

As the war escalated, the number of patients soared. This increase, however, was due not only to the inevitable casualties of the conflict but to the rising incidence of infectious diseases and of labor-related problems that resulted from merciless exploitation by supervisors. Industrial accidents became increasingly common because following safety regulations was considered too expensive and time-consuming. In the mines

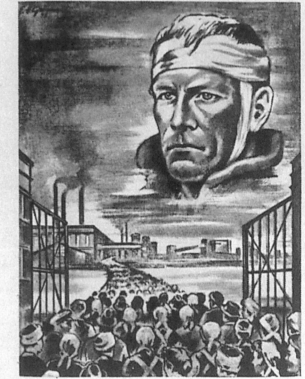

Zeichnung: E. Grunwald

*Das ich lebe, ist nicht notwendig,
wohl aber, daß ich tätig bin!*

Friedrich der Große

FIG 362 NAZI PROPAGANDA URGING WORK DESPITE ILLNESS. A
QUOTATION FROM FREDERIC THE GREAT READS: "WHAT IS ESSEN-
TIAL IS NOT THAT I LIVE, BUT THAT I AM ACTIVE!"

and on construction sites, foremen pushed laborers beyond
their limits with no consideration of the consequences. Repeatedly, workers were crushed by falling stones or burned badly
during dynamite blasting. The only official response to such
incidents were letters of condolence to the bereaved (fig. 362).[8]

Nutritional deficiencies meant that laborers also were highly
susceptible to exhaustion and disease. Soon after the start of the

war, there was an alarming increase in diphtheria and tuberculosis. Instead of warning the public and initiating preventive measures, Nazi health administrators not only hid the truth, but they propagated misinformation about the situation. Leonardo Conti, for instance, declared in 1940 that despite the false rumors "malicious Jewish emigrants" had spread abroad, the incidence of diphtheria and tuberculosis was declining. And when absenteeism from work rose and cut into efficiency of production, the Nazis responded by blaming physicians. In August 1944, Heinrich Himmler, by then Conti's superior, demanded that doctors be put on fixed salaries and made financially accountable for every day their patients were sick. The problem of absenteeism from work became so unmanageable that the Reich's mobilization minister, Albert Speer (fig. 363), contemplated using a term in a concentration camp as a proper deterrent against medically certified slackers.[9]

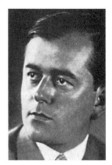

FIG 363
ALBERT SPEER
(1905–1981)

The dramatic increase in the number of patients was further aggravated by an equally dramatic drop in the number of practicing physicians available to care for them. Thousands of physicians had already emigrated, many were dead, and many others were on duty at the front. At the beginning of the Nazi regime, there were 1,351 patients for every doctor; by 1938, there were 1,380; by 1939, there were 1,432; and by 1943, there were 2,543 patients for every doctor. The ratio increased as the war drew to a close.[10]

In general, the German military paid little attention to the needs of civilians. In the last year of the war, for every male civilian doctor under the age of fifty practicing in Germany, there were three serving the needs of the armed forces. All male physicians twenty-seven years of age or younger were drafted for military service immediately upon graduation from university. Positioned just behind the front lines, these physicians were so susceptible to injury and death that their numbers could not be sufficiently replaced by those newly graduated.

In many respects, doctors on the home front were even more vulnerable. At the Charité Hospital in Berlin, surgeons oper-

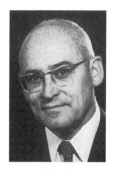

FIG 364
OTTO BRAUN-FALCO
(BORN 1922)

ated up to eighteen hours a day and suffered drastic weight loss due to food shortages. In addition, doctors were at special risk of being killed during an air raid. In the last years of the war, many physicians were assigned by the Reich's health leadership to regions where bombardment was greatest. Those who were posted in larger cities were not allowed to leave for any reason, in contrast to the option of many civilians. For instance, the dermatologist Edmund Hofmann, a student and close co-worker of Erich Hoffmann, was caught in an air raid at his residence in Kassel and perished with three of his children. By January 1943, 3,883 physicians on the home front had died, more than four times the number who died in the war zone. By 1944, physicians, after veterinarians, had become the most highly conscripted professional group in the Third Reich, and the public health administration was on the brink of collapse.[11]

Faced with this shortage, the authorities turned in desperation to medical students, who were rushed through their final examinations or pulled out of universities before completing their curriculum and obtaining their medical degrees. Among the latter was Otto Braun (fig. 364), who, as Otto Braun-Falco, was to become one of the foremost dermatologists of his time. In 1944, the twenty-two-year-old Braun was ordered to leave medical school and serve at the crumbling western front, where he was captured by the French army and sent to a prisoner-of-war camp. Shortly after his capture, he volunteered to work in the Saar Valley coal mines, believing that his chances for escape from the mines were better than his lot as a prisoner. As it turned out, many prisoners-turned-miners died working or from tuberculosis contracted in the mines. Before being sent to the mines, Braun underwent a physical examination by a young French army physician, who, on learning from Braun that he was training to be a doctor, whispered to the prisoner to begin to cough. The French doctor then declared the prisoner unfit for work in the mines and recommended he be returned to Germany for hospitalization.[12] Thus spared, Braun finished his medical studies in 1948, was appointed associate professor in 1960, became full professor and chair of the

Department of Dermatology at the University of Marburg in 1961, and assumed the chair of dermatology at the University of Munich in 1966, where he stayed for almost thirty years. Braun, in collaboration with his students, Gerd Plewig and Helmut Wolff, produced the leading textbook on dermatology in German, which now is in its fourth edition.[13]

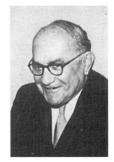

FIG 365
KARL ALTMANN
(1880–1968)

In addition to medical students, the German authorities began to conscript women doctors with young children and long-retired elderly physicians. Experienced hospital physicians were distributed as best as possible throughout the country, whereas clinics were staffed by inexperienced recent medical graduates. Even physicians of partial Jewish descent who had previously been dismissed from civil service, such as Karl Altmann (fig. 365), were suddenly given positions of responsibility. A former professor and director of dermatology at Frankfurt Sachsenhausen Municipal Hospital, Altmann was appointed leading physician in the city of Neunkirchen in August 1944.[14]

Despite the urgent need for experienced specialists, racist attitudes still prevailed. Ernst Heinrich Brill, the chair of dermatology in Rostock, wrote to the ministry about the possibility of a new assistant: "The Reich's Chamber of Physicians has offered me a Jewish half-breed of sixty-three years by the name of Dr. Lever (Levi), whom I know from my activities in Thüringen, and whom I had to refuse as a co-worker."[15] Brill surely was referring to Alexander Lever, who at the time was sixty-three and living in Erfurt, the capital of Thüringen (fig. 366). Lever was the father of Walter Lever, who would write the most widely distributed dermatopathology text of the century. Titled *Histopathology of the Skin*, the volume is dedicated thus:

In Memory of My Father
Dr. Alexander Lever
1877–1946
My First Teacher in
Dermatopathology

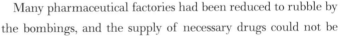

Str. 74	Lehmann, Alfred 08, ▨, Adolf-Hitler-Str. 45
Hoffmann Ernst 02, ⌀, ▨, Kartäuserring 16/17	Lehner, Eugen 31, OA a. Kath. Kh, Viktoriastr. 2
Hoffmann, Werner 35, AssA, Colmarer Str. 21 (ständ. Anschrift)	Leopolder, Karl August 19, ⌀, Anger 25
Holler, Hans 20, ▨, Salinenstr. 15	: Lever, Alex 03, ▨, Adolf-Hitler-Str. 4
Hook, Georg 09, ⌀, ▨ a. Kath. Kh, Freiligrathstr. 4	Löblich ♀, Ilse 36, VolÄ a. Städt. Kh, Kartäuserstr. 29
Horn, Gerhard 19, ▨, ▨, Schillerstr. 27	Lowes, August 06, Andreasstr.39
Huß, Enno 32, ▨, Anger 23	Marckscheffel, Ernst 92, SR, Pförtchenstr. 6
Iben, Johannes 22, Neuwerkstr. 21	Martini, Anton 22, ▨, Kasinostr. 7
: Jacobsohn, Julius 02, ▨, Schlösserstr. 2	Mechler ♀, Anne-Marie, geb. Möbuß 25 (a.ZÄ), Melchendorfer Str. 24
Jäger, Hans 26, ⌀, OA a. Städt. Kh, Nordhäuser Str. 74	Meis, Franz 22, ⌀, Johannesstr. 19
Jordan, Werner 35, AssA a. Städt. Kh, Nordhäuser Str. 74	: Moses ○, Oskar 99, Hermann-Göring-Str. 10

FIG 366 IN THE REICH'S MEDICINAL CALENDAR OF 1937, ALEXANDER LEVER WAS THE ONLY PHYSICIAN BY THE NAME OF LEVER IN THURINGEN. HIS NAME WAS MARKED BY A COLON TO INDICATE JEWISH DESCENT.

As the war hastened to an end, working conditions in German hospitals continued to deteriorate, as exemplified by the situation at the skin clinic in Münster. In 1941, the chair of dermatology there, Carl Moncorps (fig. 367), complained that "the skin clinic of the university, with 76 beds for inpatients and 135 ambulatory treatments every day, is currently equipped with only two assistants, instead of one consultant dermatologist and five assistants." After yet another induction order, however, only Moncorps, one other board-certified dermatologist, and one young resident were left in the clinic. Because Moncorps was engaged in research projects for the German armed forces and the other dermatologist had tuberculosis, the bulk of clinical work soon fell to the resident. In October 1943, the clinic was almost completely destroyed during an Allied bombing raid. Moncorps was forced to continue his work "in rooms without water and partially without windowpanes." Lectures were given in an old chapel that had neither windows nor heating. Most inpatients had to be accommodated in an old school building in the countryside.[16]

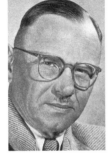

FIG 367
CARL MONCORPS
(1896–1952)

Many pharmaceutical factories had been reduced to rubble by the bombings, and the supply of necessary drugs could not be maintained. Heads of medical departments received confidential notes informing them which drugs were no longer available for prescription, including such essential items as insulin for diabetics. Some drugs and bandages were "war quality" and far inferior to the usual standards. Because glass was at a premium, by 1942 bottles for medicines, thermometers, and syringes were scarce. Furthermore, food could be purchased only with ration certificates, and physicians spent a good deal of time issuing certificates that would entitle patients with progressive diseases to receive one or two eggs or a few more grams of butter (fig. 368).[17]

Although the breakdown of the Third Reich became increasingly evident in all arenas of daily life, the Nazis continued to call for heroic resistance until the last days of the war (fig. 369, 370). Rumors abounded of "wonder weapons" currently under construction, and readers of newspapers were assured that the Führer still believed in final victory: "At the frontiers of the capital, the enemy will bleed to death." In truth, Hitler knew better than anyone that Germany's defeat was inevitable. The combination of his utter indifference to the suffering of the German people and his own overweening longing for greatness made Hitler determined to turn his own defeat into an apocalypse. In November 1942, he had declared: "As a principle, I always stop only at five minutes past twelve." The idiom "five minutes before twelve" means "just in time" or "at the very last minute." By saying "five minutes past twelve," Hitler wanted to make clear that he would not stop "at the very last minute," and this is exactly what he did.[18]

Despite the obvious hopelessness of the situation, Hitler allowed neither retreat nor capitulation, and he did not make the slightest attempt to negotiate with his enemies. To preclude the possibility of a coup d'etat, nearly 5,000 former representatives of the Weimar Republic were arrested in August 1944, among them Kurt Schumacher and Konrad Adenauer, who were to become the two leading political figures of postwar Germany. In the same month, Hitler ordered all significant buildings in Paris—including monuments and architectural

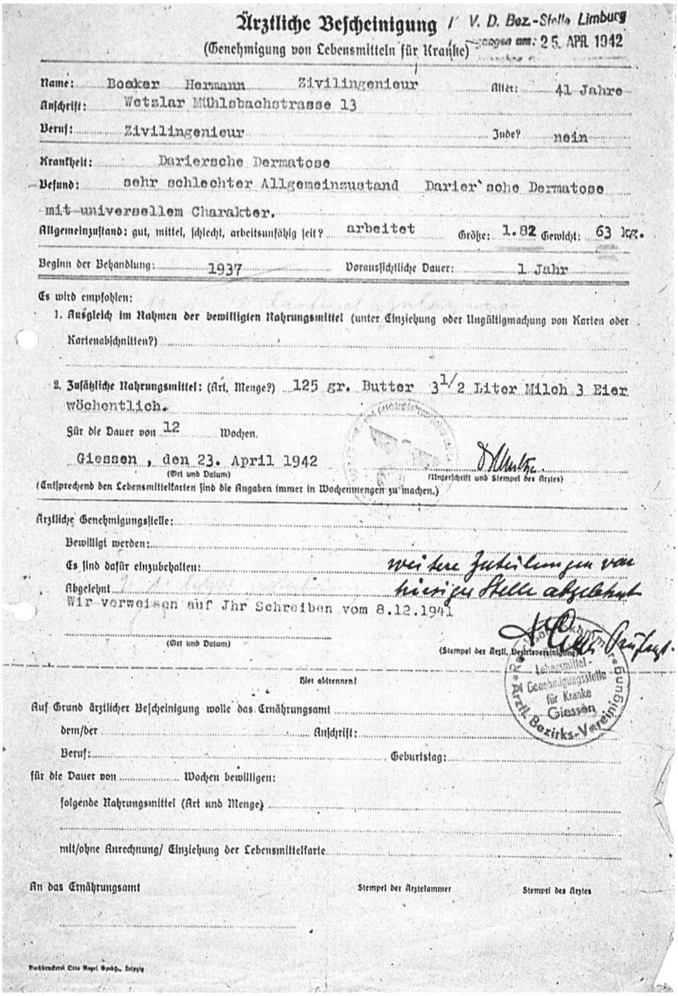
Ärztliche Bescheinigung / V. D. Bez.-Stelle Limburg
(Genehmigung von Lebensmitteln für Kranke) eingegangen am: 25. APR. 1942

Name: Booker Hermann Zivilingenieur Alter: 41 Jahre
Anschrift: Wetzlar Mühlsbachstrasse 13
Beruf: Zivilingenieur Jude? nein
Krankheit: Dariersche Dermatose
Befund: sehr schlechter Allgemeinzustand Darier'sche Dermatose mit universellem Charakter.
Allgemeinzustand: gut, mittel, schlecht, arbeitsunfähig seit? arbeitet Größe: 1.82 Gewicht: 63 kg.
Beginn der Behandlung: 1937 Voraussichtliche Dauer: 1 Jahr

Es wird empfohlen:
1. Ausgleich im Rahmen der bewilligten Nahrungsmittel (unter Einziehung oder Ungültigmachung von Karten oder Kartenabschnitten?)
2. Zusätzliche Nahrungsmittel: (Art, Menge?) 125 gr. Butter 3 1/2 Liter Milch 3 Eier wöchentlich.

Für die Dauer von 12 Wochen.

Giessen, den 23. April 1942
(Ort und Datum) (Unterschrift und Stempel des Arztes)
(Entsprechend den Lebensmittelkarten sind die Angaben immer in Wochenmengen zu machen.)

Ärztliche Genehmigungsstelle:
Bewilligt werden:
Es sind dafür einzubehalten: weitere Zuteilungen von
Abgelehnt hiesiger Stelle abgelehnt
Wir verweisen auf Jhr Schreiben vom 8.12.1941
(Ort und Datum) (Stempel der Ärztl. Bezirksvereinigung)

Lebensmittel-Genehmigungsstelle für Kranke Giessen Ärztl. Bezirks-Vereinigung

Hier abtrennen!

Auf Grund ärztlicher Bescheinigung wolle das Ernährungsamt
dem/der Anschrift:
Beruf: Geburtstag:
für die Dauer von Wochen bewilligen:
folgende Nahrungsmittel (Art und Menge)
mit/ohne Anrechnung/ Einziehung der Lebensmittelkarte
An das Ernährungsamt Stempel der Ärztekammer Stempel des Arztes

FIG 368 CERTIFICATE FOR FOOD RATION ISSUED BY WALTHER SCHULTZE, THE CHAIR OF DERMATOLOGY IN GIESSEN, FOR A PATIENT WITH DARIER'S DISEASE. ALTHOUGH THE PATIENT WAS NOT A JEW ("JUDE? - NEIN"), SCHULTZE'S REQUEST TO GRANT HIM SOME MORE BUTTER, MILK, AND EGGS WAS DENIED.

works of art—to be destroyed, and six months later issued the same order for major cities in Germany. Neither order was ever carried out by commanders of the army.

In the last days of the war, sixteen-year-old boys were sent to the front (fig. 371). In the end, Hitler did not want anybody—

Württemberger Zeitung

Das nationalsozialistische

Morgenblatt in Stuttgart

Der Führer gibt die Parole für das Jahr 1945

Dem Geist unseres Volkes gehört die Zukunft

Stuttgarter

NS-Kurier

Gauorgan der NSDAP

Der Führer: Noch in diesem Jahr tritt die große geschichtliche Wende ein

Adolf Hitlers Siegesglaube auch unser Glaube

Schlacht an der Rur nimmt an Heftigkeit zu

Wortlaut der Ansprache des Führers

Reichsminister Dr. Goebbels: Wir werden auch diese Krise meistern

Hinter dem Führer steht ein Volk, das auf ihn baut

Heimat und Front einander würdig im Leiden und Arbeiten, im Kämpfen und in der Tapferkeit

Im Februar 288 480 BRT.

Wortlaut der Rundfunkansprache von Dr. Goebbels

Württemberger Zeitung

Das nationalsozialistische

Morgenblatt in Stuttgart

Der Führer: Vor der Hauptstadt wird der Feind verbluten

Tagesbefehl an die Ostkämpfer: In diesem Augenblick wird sich die Wende des Krieges entscheiden

Ein erstaunliches Volk

Im Unglück nicht feige, sondern trotzig werden

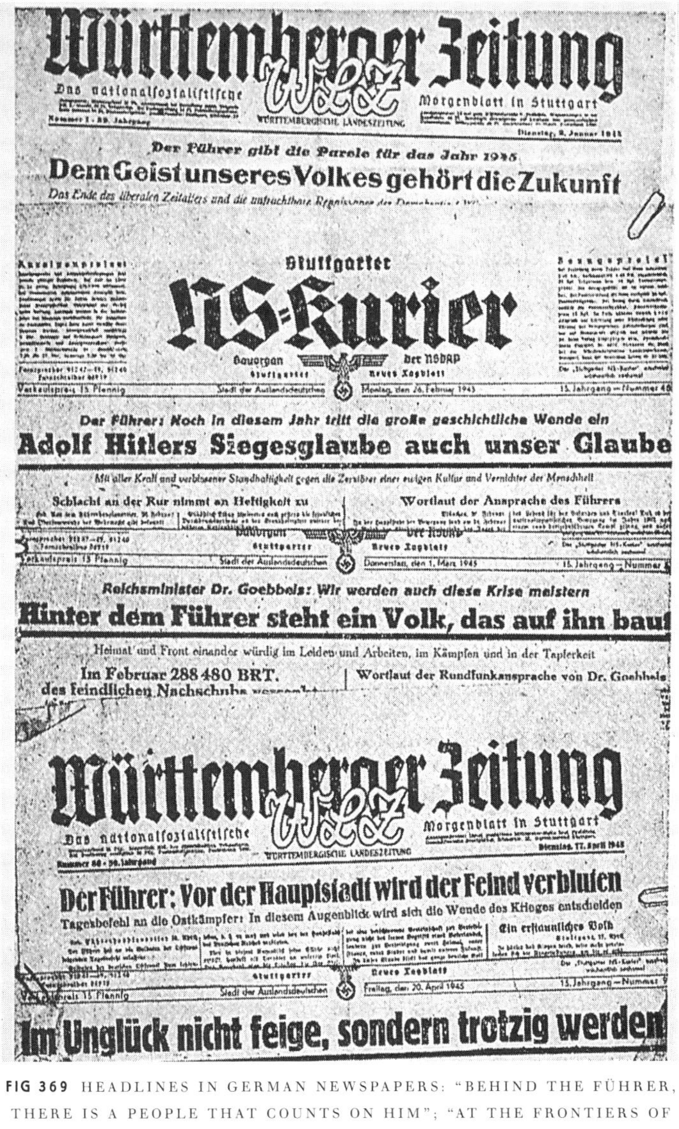

FIG 369 HEADLINES IN GERMAN NEWSPAPERS: "BEHIND THE FÜHRER, THERE IS A PEOPLE THAT COUNTS ON HIM"; "AT THE FRONTIERS OF THE CAPITAL, THE ENEMY WILL BLEED TO DEATH"; "IN MISFORTUNE, DO NOT BECOME COWARDLY, BUT DEFIANT."

Jews or Germans—or anything to survive his personal disaster. On March 18, 1945, he told Albert Speer, his minister for armament and war production: "If the war is lost, the nation will also perish. This fate is inevitable. There is no need to take into consideration the basis which the people will need to continue

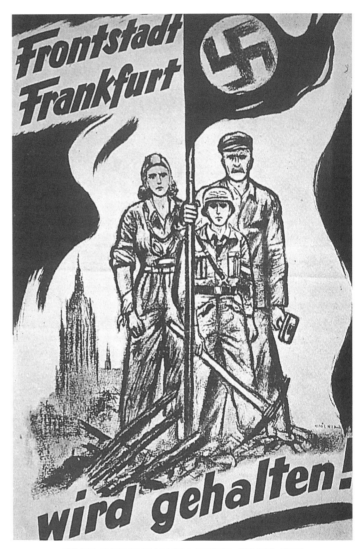

FIG 370 NAZI PROPAGANDA POSTER: "FRONT CITY
FRANKFURT WILL BE HELD."

a most primitive existence. On the contrary, it will be better to destroy these things ourselves because the nation will have proved to be the weaker one and the future will belong solely to the stronger eastern nation. Besides, those who will remain after the battle are only the inferior ones, because the good ones have been killed."[19] On April 30, 1945, Hitler committed sui-

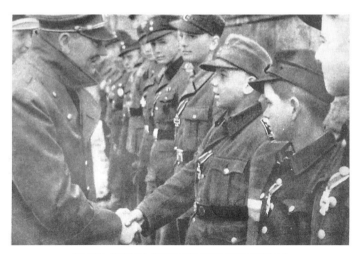

FIG 371 HITLER WITH HIS NEW "SOLDIERS."

cide, thereby exempting himself from responsibility that, from the beginning, he had never truly accepted (fig. 372).

There were many Germans who also did not wish to survive the demise of the Third Reich. Walter Frieboes was among them. As acting chair of the Department of Dermatology at the Charité Hospital in Berlin, he volunteered for the "Volkssturm," a military brigade of men between the ages of sixteen and sixty who previously had been found to be unfit for military service, as well as of girls, women, and older, infirm people. In a letter to a brigadier general on January 30, 1945 (fig. 373), Frieboes wrote: "I have volunteered, at sixty-four years of age, for the 'Volkssturm' with the serious intention to serve the fatherland with a weapon in my hands. . . . Because until now there has been no decision in this matter, I again ask respectfully—with the knowledge of my company commander—to discontinue my employment as a physician under these special circumstances and to release me to fight with a weapon as a 'Volkssturmmann.' Heil Hitler! Respectfully yours, W. Frieboes."[20] Frieboes, almost completely deaf and incapable of fighting, could not have defended his fatherland because there was not much left in Berlin to defend. His true intention was self-sacrifice. Whether

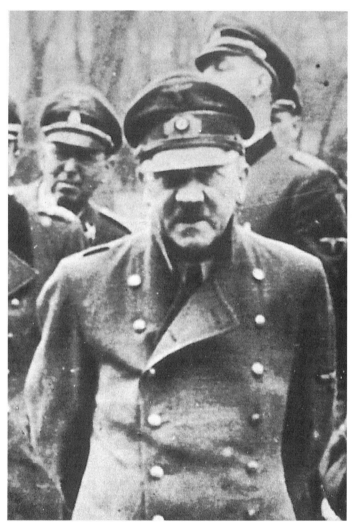

FIG 372 ONE OF THE LAST PICTURES OF ADOLF HITLER.

he was compelled by feelings of guilt for having been unable to behave in a manner consonant with his earlier humanistic ideals, or shame for not having resisted the Nazis (and thereby serving his country better), is not known. Frieboes was killed "in battle" on May 2, 1945.

Seven days after Frieboes died, the war was over. In Europe alone, it had claimed fifty-seven million victims, most of them

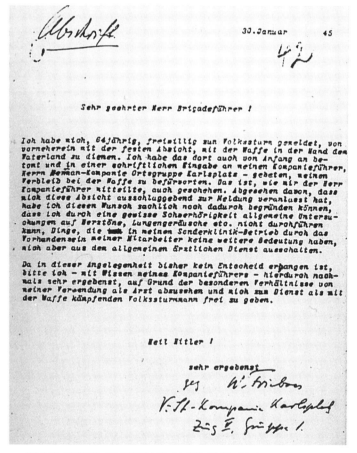

FIG 373 LETTER OF FRIEBOES TO HIS BRIGADE COMMANDER IN
BERLIN, JANUARY 30, 1945. IT WAS EXACTLY TWELVE YEARS
EARLIER, IN THE SAME PLACE, THAT HITLER HAD ASSUMED POWER.

Soviets, Germans, Poles, and Jews. As a result of more than two
years of constant bombing, German cities were mostly demol-
ished. In Cologne, only the two spires of the Gothic cathedral
stood majestically amid the devastation (figs. 374, 375).

When the Allied forces swept through Germany, they found not
only prominent Nazis, such as Joseph Goebbels and Heinrich
Himmler, dead, but also lower-ranking party members who had
committed suicide rather than face the consequences (figs. 376
through 378). Among them were the then leading dermatologists

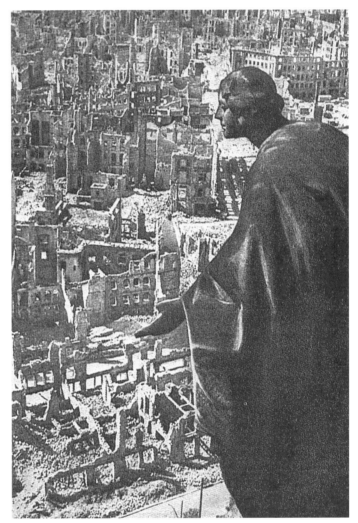

FIG 374 THE RUINS OF DRESDEN.

Ernst Heinrich Brill, chair in Rostock, and Karl Zieler, former chair in Würzburg and president of the German Dermatological Society. Brill left his clinic in the first days of May, announcing to his staff that he and his wife were going to commit suicide. Zieler spent his last days with his spouse in a villa in the countryside. On March 27, he wrote these lines to Karl Hoede, his student and successor as chair of dermatology in Würzburg: "We do not feel able

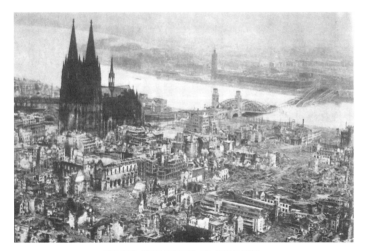

FIG 375 THE RUINS OF COLOGNE.

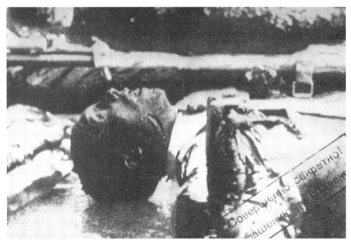

FIG 376 THE CORPSE OF GOEBBELS.

to cope with the task of surviving the fall of our German Fatherland and, therefore, will depart from life voluntarily when we
consider the moment to have arrived." One day later, Zieler and
his wife were found dead, leaning against the wall of a cemetery,
a half-empty glass of water next to them and a calling card
attached to Zieler's lapel that proclaimed: "President of the German Dermatological Society."[21]

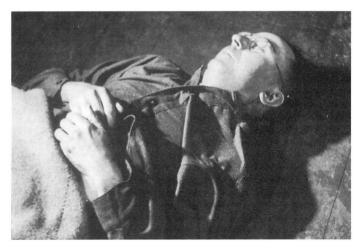

FIG 377 THE CORPSE OF HIMMLER.

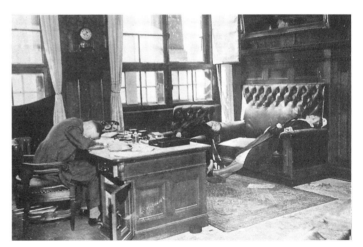

FIG 378 SUICIDE OF ACTIVE MEMBERS OF THE
NAZI PARTY AT THE END OF THE WAR.

At the Conference at Yalta in February 1945, the Allies had expressed their will to eradicate German militarism and Nazism, to guarantee that Germany would never again be able to disrupt the peace of the world, and to remove all National Socialist and militaristic influences from political, cultural, and economic life of the German people. After the defeat of Nazi Germany, all Germans older than 18 years of age were compelled to specify in a questionnaire their political engagement in the Third Reich. Those who had been involved in Nazi organizations were summoned to denazification tribunals, which judged the severity of involvement and imposed punishments ranging from fines to dismissal and prohibition to work in one's profession. In addition, lists had been prepared with the names of teachers, professors, and administrative officers who were known to be Nazi supporters and who were dismissed immediately. Among them were numerous dermatologists, such as Julius Mayr in Munich, Walther Schultze in Giessen, Julius Dörffel in Halle, and Martin Schubert in Frankfurt, who were never active in academic life again.

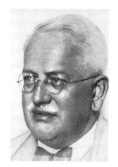

FIG 379
PAUL MULZER
(1880–1947)

Such was the case, too, with Paul Mulzer (fig. 379), chair of dermatology in Hamburg and an ardent Nazi. As early as 1923, Mulzer had belonged to the Deutscher Kampfbund, an association of three right-wing military movements—Reichsflagge, Oberland, and NSDAP—whose political leader was Adolf Hitler. The Kampfbund had three military leaders: Hermann Göring, Captain Heise, and Captain Mulzer, a brother of Paul Mulzer. At that time, Mulzer was still an associate professor at the University of Munich and was involved in Hitler's attempted putsch in Munich in 1923. One year later, Mulzer was appointed chair of the Department of Dermatology at the University of Hamburg. In 1931, he became a member of the National Socialist Physicians' League, and when Hitler assumed power on January 30, 1933, Mulzer joined the Nazi party within two weeks. At the same time, he renounced his membership in the Hamburg Rotary Club because he had been seated at a table with two Jews.[22] At the university, Mulzer closed ranks with the National Socialist Students' League in order to enforce the medical faculty's appointment of professors with Old Fighter laurels.[23]

Mulzer was also held responsible for the arrest of Rudolf Degkwitz (fig. 380) by the Gestapo. Degkwitz, known for the introduction of passive vaccination against measles, was director of the pediatric clinic of the University of Hamburg. Dur-

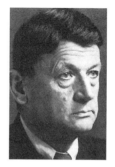

FIG 380
RUDOLF DEGKWITZ
(1889–1973)

ing the war, he repeatedly criticized the Nazis, opposed the euthanasia program in Hamburg, and tried to employ antifascist physicians in his department. For these misdemeanors, he was sentenced to "seven years in prison and seven years of loss of honor," and only the fact of his great service to the health of thousands of children saved him from death.[24]

After the war, Degkwitz accused Mulzer of having denounced him to the Gestapo, an accusation that was substantiated by other members of the faculty. After a short investigation by the advisory council of the university, Mulzer was dismissed on May 3, 1945, five days before his sixty-fifth birthday. Because his dismissal had major consequences—the loss of his pension and the right to open a private practice—Mulzer tried to have it reversed and applied for an ordinary emeritus status. This request was rejected, and in February 1947, Mulzer committed suicide.[25] His photograph, unaccompanied by any biographic information concerning his despicable career as a Nazi, still hangs prominently in a major amphitheater at the Medical School of the University of Hamburg.

In general, the dismissal of former Nazis was accomplished using a standard form to which only names and positions had to be added. Walther Schultze, for example, was informed of his dismissal in January 1946 in the following way: "According to an order by the military government, you are dismissed, with immediate effect, from your position as ordinary professor. A legal claim to a pension or a pension for surviving dependents does not exist. Without being summoned, the access to the rooms of your office as well as its branches is prohibited to you. Papers, receipts, valuables, official documents, and other properties of your office which are still in your hands have to be returned immediately" (fig. 381).[26]

For many longtime university chairs who felt they had "only done their duty" as a citizen of the Third Reich, short and impersonal notes such as the one to Schultze came as a shock. But for Schultze, the note could not have been a surprise. During the years of the National Socialist regime, he

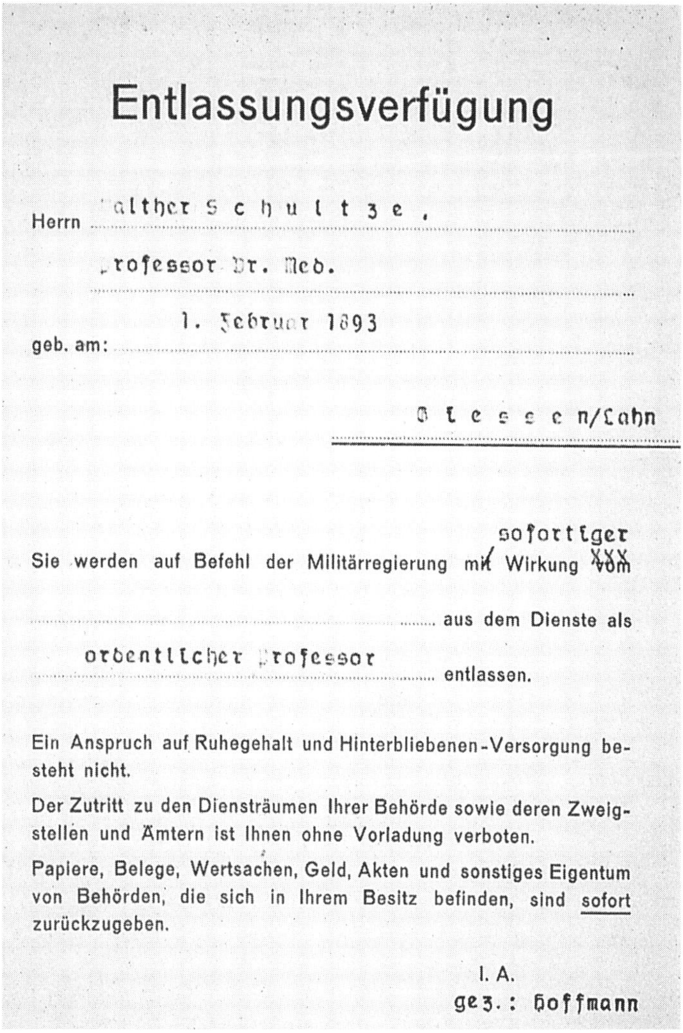

Entlassungsverfügung

Herrn ......'alther S c h u l t z e ,

......rofessor Dr. Med.

geb. am: ......1. Februar 1893

......Giessen/Lahn

Sie werden auf Befehl der Militärregierung mit Wirkung vom sofortiger XXX

...... aus dem Dienste als

ordentlicher professor

...... entlassen.

Ein Anspruch auf Ruhegehalt und Hinterbliebenen-Versorgung besteht nicht.

Der Zutritt zu den Diensträumen Ihrer Behörde sowie deren Zweigstellen und Ämtern ist Ihnen ohne Vorladung verboten.

Papiere, Belege, Wertsachen, Geld, Akten und sonstiges Eigentum von Behörden, die sich in Ihrem Besitz befinden, sind sofort zurückzugeben.

I. A.

gez.: Hoffmann

FIG 381 LETTER OF DISMISSAL TO WALTHER SCHULTZE.

had been active in several Nazi organizations, proved himself to be an ardent anti-Semite, refused to treat prisoners of war, and repeatedly had denounced patients to the authorities. A Polish hard laborer, for instance, who had not followed the instructions of male nurses, was identified by name to the Gestapo, with the added suggestion from Schultze that an eye be kept on him after his release. When two other Polish hard

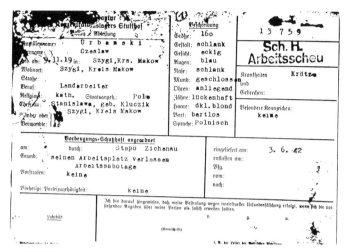

FIG 382 THE FATE OF A POLISH HARD-LABORER IN GERMANY:
THIS TWENTY-TWO-YEAR-OLD MAN LEFT WORK WITHOUT
PERMISSION AND WAS INCARCERATED IN THE
CONCENTRATION CAMP AT STUTTHOF.

laborers violated the house rules of the dermatology clinic,
Schultze asked the Gestapo to take them into "protective custody" and assured the secret police that both laborers were
physically able to tolerate detention.[27] Schultze surely knew
that "requests" such as his nearly always were synonymous
with incarceration in a concentration camp and, in many
instances, death of the prisoner within weeks (figs. 382, 383).

Schultze was never readmitted to the university, yet only
seven months after his dismissal he was awarded a pension, and
at retirement age he was given an ordinary emeritus status.
According to the judgment of the denazification trial tribunal
at Giessen, Schultze was incriminated only slightly because

> it could not be proven that the person concerned was a
> political leader (leader of the district office). It also tells
> to his credit that he contributed to the removal of party
> members from his clinic who had acted illegally. . . .
> During the persecution of Jews, the person concerned
> always treated Jewish patients. Furthermore, he contin-
> ued to employ Catholic nurses—in contrast to orders by

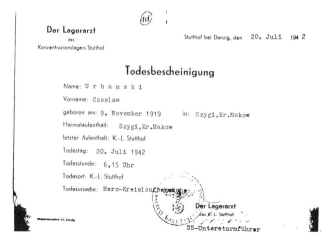

FIG 383 THE POLISH HARD-LABORER DIED SEVEN WEEKS AFTER
HAVING BEEN INTERNED AT STUTTHOF. ON THE DEATH CERTIFICATE,
THE SS PHYSICIAN'S PHONY DIAGNOSIS READS:
"WEAKNESS OF THE HEART AND CIRCULATION."

*the district leader Sprenger—and he has engaged him-
self on behalf of colleagues—Profs. Boening and
Weber—who had different political opinions. Because
of all these doings, he had sincere controversies with the
district leader Sprenger and came into danger himself.
In consideration of all these points, the court had to
deviate from the petition of the public accuser.[28]*

The dismissal of university professors by military governments was usually carried out without interrogation of the person charged, and sometimes wrong decisions were made on the
basis of incorrect information. Such was the case with Alfred
Ruete (fig. 384), chair of the Department of Dermatology at the
University of Marburg. Ruete was dismissed on September 28,
1945, and was informed that he had "to cease work immediately.
The cashier of the university has been ordered to stop paying
your salary on September 30, 1945." This decision by the military government was a consequence of the registrar of the University of Marburg having indicated erroneously that Ruete had
belonged to the SA. In reality, Ruete had never been a member

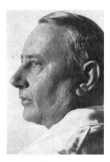

FIG 384
ALFRED RUETE
(1882–1951)

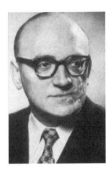

FIG 385
HORST-GÜNTHER
BODE
(BORN 1904)

of the storm troops or the Nazi party. As a result of this "new" information, he was reinstated only two weeks later as chair of dermatology. Ruete retired in 1949 and died in 1951.[29]

At the University of Göttingen, the chair of the Department of Dermatology, Walther Krantz, was dismissed on November 4, 1945. Krantz had belonged to the SA and the National Socialist Lecturers' League, but he had not been a member of the Nazi party. Like Ruete, he tried to obtain a reversal of his dismissal. In a letter to the military government, he explained: "In 1933 I became a member of the 'Stahlhelm' in Cologne in order to avoid entering the NSDAP. . . . When afterwards the Stahlhelm, gradually and compulsorily, was united with the SA, I was deceived by the promise that the Stahlhelm as such was to exist further. Thus I became a member of the SA, much against my will. By 1934, I could not resign without endangering my whole career." After this plea, the military government revoked its decision and granted Krantz the status of emeritus, but Krantz wanted more. In a series of lawsuits that lasted for more than two years, he attempted to enforce his reinstatement as chair of dermatology, arguing that his successor, Horst-Günther Bode (fig. 385), a former assistant to Riecke, Frieboes, and Gottron, had been more closely affiliated with Nazism than Krantz himself. Those efforts, however, were denied in court, and Krantz was never readmitted to the university. He died in 1970.[30]

In the confusion after the war, it was difficult to come to a balanced judgment about personal guilt of physicians. Of twenty-three chairs of dermatology at German universities, eleven were dismissed in 1945 for political reasons.[31] Some of them who had never been inordinately active in the National Socialist cause were terminated mainly because of their membership in a Nazi organization. For some, like Krantz, this was the end of their professional careers, whereas for others, like Willy Engelhardt, the former chair of dermatology in Tübingen, their professional lives continued in private practice. Still others, like Friedrich Bering in Cologne, Hans Theodor

Schreus in Düsseldorf, and Alfred Stühmer in Freiburg, resumed their positions at universities. When questioned about his personal history, Stühmer explained how he had joined the party for family reasons and for professional necessity. Because he had not gained personal advantages through that membership, he was reinstated and died in Freiburg in 1957 at the age of seventy-two.[32]

In contrast to the situation of Schreus and Stühmer, many physicians who had gained personal advantage and had assumed leading positions in the National Socialist state were not prosecuted at all. When summoned by the military government, former Nazis usually had no difficulty finding a friend who was able to recall exactly when, where, and how they had engaged themselves on behalf of victims of the system. When it came to elaborating on their own or their friends' activities within the Nazi party, their memories suddenly failed them.

One example of this selective amnesia was exhibited by Josef Vonkennel, chair of dermatology in Leipzig, a high-ranking SS commander and the consulting dermatologist of the Waffen SS. In 1945, Vonkennel was arrested and spent several months in custody. Three years later, after an inquiry, the University of Leipzig declared that there was no evidence of any NSDAP activity on the part of Vonkennel, and in 1950, he was appointed chair of dermatology in Cologne, a position he held until his death on June 13, 1963.[33] A few months before Vonkennel's death, his involvement in unconscionable medical experiments during the Nazi period had been uncovered. When legal proceedings were instituted against him by the Department of Public Prosecution of Cologne, Vonkennel presumably committed suicide.[34]

The chair of dermatology in Breslau, Heinrich Adolf Gottron, fled the city shortly before it was occupied by Soviet troops, leaving behind all his personal belongings. In search of a new position, Gottron contacted several universities in West Germany and finally was successful in the zone occupied by the French military, where the authorities were less strict about former Nazi activities than they were in the zones under American control. The University of Tübingen was particularly well known as a gathering place for academics with former Nazi affiliations.[35] It was there, in 1946, that Gottron assumed the chair of dermatology, succeeding Willy Engelhardt. The military governor called attention to the fact that "Monsieur Gottron was a member of the party and his nomination has a precarious character of which you should be aware."[36] Gottron's reputation as a scientist, however, overrode all political considerations, and he was appointed chair despite his Nazi past.

Indeed, Gottron eventually did turn the Skin Clinic of Tübingen into one of the leading centers of dermatology in Germany. Gottron described several "new" diseases, among them amyloidosis nodularis atrophicans and scleromyxedema, and, with Walther Schönfeld, published a five-volume textbook, *Dermatologie und Venerologie*, which became a standard resource.

Gottron was probably the most charismatic dermatologist in postwar Germany, a man who thought very well of himself. When a new president of the German Dermatological Society was to be elected, Gottron boasted that if he wanted the position, he could get it. He was wrong. Although he had chosen to deny his prominent role in National Socialist Germany, others had not forgotten it. American dermatologists warned their German colleagues that if Gottron were elected president of the German Dermatological Society, they would break off all contact. As a consequence, Gottron was no longer considered for the post.[37]

In subsequent years, Gottron tried to alter his image as a former proponent of the Nazi cause. At international congresses he went out of his way to assure participants that he had never really been a Nazi and elaborated on how much he had done on behalf of Jews. Among the foreign colleagues Gottron attempted to sway was Rudolf Baer, then chair of dermatology at New York University School of Medicine, who had emigrated from Germany in response to the Nazi's intimidation of

Jews. Baer was both surprised and irritated by Gottron's unso-licited assertions.[38] Gottron eventually achieved his goal: sub-mersion of his ignoble role in Nazi Germany. Celebrated as one of the most valued members of the academic world, he was elected president of the German Cancer Association, received two honorary doctoral degrees, and became an honorary mem-ber of eighteen international medical societies. After his death in 1974, numerous brief biographies were written about Got-tron and they either omitted completely his activities during the years of the Nazi regime or transformed his behavior in those days into that of a rebel, a man of the resistance.[39] In a 1983 article by Leyh and Wendt that they foisted on the editor of the *American Journal of Dermatopathology*, the Nazi period of Gottron's life is mentioned in three apologetic sentences: "The most striking examples of Gottron's high ethical stan-dards were evident during the Nazi regime. Gottron defended the Jewish dermatologist Stephan Epstein against assaults by the Nazi party until he could emigrate to Madison, Wisconsin, in the United States. After internment of the Polish dermatol-ogist Franz Walter in the concentration camp of Oranienburg, Gottron managed to effect Walter's release some months later."[40] Gottron's membership in the Nazi party and his sup-port of racial hygiene in some of his publications went com-pletely unnoted by his surviving colleagues, which is characteristic of the way the postwar German medical commu-nity came to terms with the past.

For many years, critical assessment of the inglorious role of physicians in the Third Reich was taboo, a mentality that, in part, persists.[41] Three of the four postwar presidents of Ger-many's Chamber of Physicians were early active members of the SA or SS—namely, Ernst Fromm, Hans Joachim Sewering, and Karl Haedenkamp, who had masterminded the de-Jewifi-cation of German medicine in the 1930s. Fromm was president of the World Medical Association from 1973 to 1974, and Sew-ering (fig. 386) was elected president of the World Medical Association in 1992. Only after Sewering's unquestionable com-

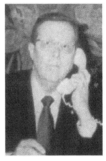

FIG 386
HANS JOACHIM
SEWERING

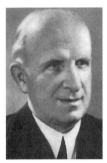

FIG 387
OTMAR FREIHERR
VON VERSCHUER
(1896–1969)

plicity during the 1930s in the killing of a fourteen-year-old patient became known was he forced to step aside.[42] Karsten Vilmar, Sewering's successor as ranking medical functionary of the Federal Republic of Germany since 1978, continued to deny the involvement of German physicians in the crimes of the Nazis. In 1986, he contended that "only a minority of German doctors—one might justifiably call them a macabre 'order'—spoiled the reputation of our profession."[43] Revisionism universally attributed to Communist Russia and China was very much en vogue in postwar democratic Germany.

The statement by Vilmar is patently false and seeks to conceal the true, disproportionate number of physicians involved in the NSDAP. It ignores the flagrant violation of medical ethics by German physicians during the Nazi period. Only a minority of physicians were actively involved in killing patients and in performing macabre experiments on internees of concentration camps, but many, many more were aware of those activities and even used results of such "research" for their own pragmatic purposes. After the war, almost all of these physicians were readmitted to medical practice, including former killers like Herta Oberheuser, who participated in cruel experiments on female internees in the concentration camp at Ravensbrück, and Werner Heyde, who played a prominent role in the euthanasia program.

Some of the worst Nazi physicians resumed academic careers. Hans Bertha, a key figure in the killing of disabled children at the Pediatric Hospital at the University of Vienna, obtained a professorship in 1954 and later became head of psychiatry at the University of Graz in Austria. Fritz Lenz, who, in 1933, was given the first full chair of racial hygiene by Hitler, was reappointed professor of human genetics at the University of Göttingen in 1946. He continued to publish the results of his work into the 1970s.[44]

Another example of restoration to acceptability is Otmar Freiherr von Verschuer (fig. 387), who gained an international reputation for his comparative research on twins. As chair during the Nazi period of the Department for Genetics and Racial Hygiene at the University of Frankfurt, von Verschuer taught that it was the duty of a people to reject "alien race elements, if it wants to preserve its own kind. Once such elements have entered, they must be forced out and destroyed. There is no denying that the Jew is of a different kind and hence is to be resisted, if and when he seeks to enter." In 1944, von Verschuer acknowledged that Germany was waging a "racial war" against "World Jewry" and demanded as a "political priority of the present, a new, total solution of the Jewish problem."[45]

At that time, von Verschuer held the prestigious chair at the Kaiser Wilhelm Institute in Berlin, and his assistant, Josef Mengele, had joined the "medical staff" of the concentration camp at Auschwitz. In return for academic promotion, Mengele carved from prisoners—often twins or dwarfs—organs such as heterochromatic eyeballs or unborn fetuses, which were then sent to von Verschuer, who used them for his anthropological studies. Despite these undeniable facts, von Verschuer claimed after the war that he had been opposed to National Socialist ideology, bemoaned the "dreadful annihilation of Jews" that "as an extralegal, politically motivated act of violence, has nothing to do with eugenics," and deplored the "misuse of science" by the Nazis. In 1947, von Verschuer was chosen as an expert consultant of the state of Hesse for a "Bill Concerning Sterilization and Refertilization" that was worked out in the zone under American administration. Because the terms "eugenics" and "racial hygiene" were no longer agreeable, von Verschuer introduced the term "human genetics" and, in 1951, became chair of the newly founded department of human genetics at the University of Münster. He praised that university "because the faculty has called back all its members, has filled not a single chair with somebody else, and has not stumbled over political trip wires. It is truly pleasant to belong to such a faculty who, despite differences in regard to personal views and contents, is of rare unanimity and has demonstrated character in a politically difficult situation." When old companions faced difficulties because of a Nazi past, von Verschuer was ready to help, arguing that "the freedom of science is in danger as long as there are still faculties at German universities who . . . give way to political influences."[46] As a protagonist of the "freedom of science," von Verschuer contributed to the reappointment of several high-ranking Nazis to university chairs. Von Verschuer's own professional reputation was not impaired by his Nazi past. He was lionized in international academic circles and, in 1961, was one of the honored guests at the Second International Conference of Human Genetics in Rome. Von Verschuer died in Münster in 1969.[47]

In addition to Bertha, Lenz, and von Verschuer, many other former Nazis reoccupied or were elevated to university chairs after the fall of the Third Reich. It was easy for them to alter former beliefs, to conceal their pasts, and to pretend that they never had anything to do with Nazism. Articles with racist content were no longer cited, and those passages in textbooks considered to be politically objectionable were rewritten or expunged. In 1952, the J. F. Lehmann Verlag, which had been a pioneer in publications about racial hygiene and physical Semitic traits, issued the thirteenth edition of *Racial Hygiene and Population Policy: Foundations of Genetics* by the dermatologist Hermann Werner Siemens, with a new introduction that denounced "racial fanaticism."[48] In 1947, the textbook *Medicine and the Medical Profession* (first published in 1938) by Paul Diepgen, a medical historian and enthusiastic supporter of the Nazis, went into its second edition. In the preface, Diepgen wrote about his purpose: "This book . . . is meant to help educate the young physician, from the outset of his studies, to that combination of medical and scientific thinking from which alone a true medical attitude can develop, and to alert him early on to doubts and controversial problems in order to make him think."[49] Although Diepgen's book was intended to enhance a medical student's capability for critical analysis, it did not induce the same process in himself. It called attention to the problem of an inadequate general education but made no reference to the delusion of physicians and other educated people in Germany during the time of Nazi rule, including his own terrible misperceptions. For the 1947 edition, all he did was change the title of one chapter, remove all references to racial hygiene, racial science, and National Socialism, and reword offending passages.

In one passage, common to both editions, Diepgen referred to the importance of a worldview (*Weltanschauung*) in regard to the development of medicine. By "worldview," he wrote, "one means the standpoint from which someone will answer questions about the meaning of Being and Becoming in the world. . . . And when one examines the history of medicine, one can clearly see that over the course of time, first one and then another of these worldviews has shaped the thinking of the physician." After this, the two editions begin to diverge. In the first edition, Diepgen wrote: "And yet never before has the question of Weltanschauung become of such immediate importance for public and private life, as in our own times. For us in Germany, more immediately than ever before, the most important decisions in recent years have been those in the sphere of Weltanschauung. And this Weltanschauung is the National Socialist Weltanschauung." In striking contrast, the 1947 edition reads as follows: "And yet one-sidedness has always taken its toll. He who truly wants to help his fellow man must see the world as a physician. His entire worldview must be determined by his character as a physician, a position that recognizes no differences in religion, nationality, or race when it comes to help. Science serves the entire world and must be cosmopolitan."[50] Expounding such a noble view, Diepgen continued his academic career in postwar Germany and built a new Institute for the History of Medicine at the University of Mainz. In obituaries, Diepgen was praised as one of the greatest medical historians ever.

The first major effort to uncover the inglorious role of physicians in the Third Reich was a study by Alexander Mitscherlich and Fred Mielke titled "The order to despise man." When this work was to be published in 1947, it included the statutory declaration of a physician who had worked at the concentration camp at Ravensbrück. According to the declaration, leading physicians such as the pharmacologist Wolfgang Heubner and the surgeon Ferdinand Sauerbruch had been informed about medical experiments on internees of the camp, had discussed them in an open forum, and had spoken not a word of disapproval. Through an injunction, Heubner and Sauerbruch were able to enforce complete deletion of that paragraph from Mitscherlich's and Mielke's book, and it never appeared again in subsequent editions.[51]

Franz Büchner, director of the Institute for Aviation Pathology at the University of Freiburg, also knew about those medical experiments without denouncing them publicly. Furthermore, his name has been found repeatedly in conjunction with unethical medical experiements on human beings—for example, studies on the consequences of deprivation from oxygen or exposure to underpressure. In 1941, Büchner published an article titled "The Oath of Hippocrates: Fundamental Laws of Medical Ethics," in which he praised the Nazis for having thwarted the Marxist attitude in regard to ethical questions in medicine. Because of this article, Büchner was lauded as a preserver of ethical principles, and he even became a member of a denazification tribunal.[52]

In short, the denazification of German medicine was little more than whitewash. It was carried out with emphasis only in the American zone, where the number of Nazis convicted as "principal offenders" was more than one hundred times higher than in the French and British zones. As a consequence, many former Nazis moved to the zones under French and British government, where their chances for reappointment to leading positions were much higher, Heinrich Adolf Gottron being but one example. Even in the American zone, the vigor to identify and convict former Nazis soon decreased, as the division of Europe into two political blocks became more and more obvious and the Germans were sought as allies. In February 1948, when the U.S. government pressed to terminate the political cleansing in Germany, about 450,000 denazification trials were still pending.[53]

Demands for stricter measures against former Nazis were ignored. Professors who criticized the inadequacy of denazification subjected themselves to attacks and accusations by colleagues. Among them was Erich Hoffmann who, like no other German dermatologist, had publicly attacked National Socialism. When he criticized the University of Bonn as being too easy in regard to former Nazis, he was informed by the dean of the medical faculty, Professor von Redwitz, that several faculty members "have uttered their amazement about your attitude regarding the denazification of the faculty and declared that they could not concede to the attitude expressed in your letter. You have signed the declaration, along with four other members of the faculty, in support of Hitler published in the press (General-Anzeiger) in 1933. In public, your name stands next to names whose bearers have at least contributed to thrusting National Socialism into power. The majority of members of the faculty would consider it to be more appropriate if you exercised more restraint in regard to the question of denazification."[54]

At the same time, the University of Erlangen employed only one physician who had been a victim of the Nazis—namely, Robert Ganse, an assistant at the Department of Gynecology, who had been interned in a concentration camp for many years. When Ganse submitted his thesis for habilitation, an examination of the causes of death among women who had been subjected to enforced sterilizations at the Department of Gynecology, the acting chair and former assistant medical director of that department, Professor Rech, not only rejected Ganse's thesis but also forced his dismissal in 1947.[55]

In regard to denazification, the universities—administrators, professors, and students—demonstrated what they had never shown under National Socialist rule: resistance. Apart from this resistance and the support former Nazis continued to grant each other, denazification was complicated by the serious lack of experienced physicians available to occupy positions. The expulsion and extermination of Jewish physicians and the deaths of countless non-Jewish doctors during the war had thinned severely the ranks of the German medical community, and capable juniors were nowhere in sight. When asked for his opinion on candidates for the chair of dermatology at the University of Greifswald, Egon Keining wrote in 1945:

> *Dermatology, which before 1933 was marvelously developed at German universities, suffered its first serious setback through dismissals that were motivated politically. Almost half of the widely known chairmen of dermatology were removed from their positions and replaced by representatives of the Third Reich. In the last 12 years, German dermatology could not recover from this grievous blow because of various shortcomings. It must, especially, be called a sin of omission that no qualified junior academic generation has been trained, a fact that has contributed staggeringly to the current misery. . . . This short summary indicates clearly that German dermatology can no longer be considered to exist.*[56]

In dermatopathology, the plummet of a specialty was even more striking than that of clinical dermatology. Before the Nazi period, Germany and Austria had been the mecca for study of dermatopathology, both countries being far ahead of any other. Of the first eight textbooks on dermatopathology published between 1848 and 1928, seven had been written by German-speaking authors. In contrast, after 1933, eight of eleven dermatopathology texts were published in the United States and only one in Germany. The leading textbooks of the postwar period—Lever's *Histopathology of the Skin* and Pinkus's *Guide to Dermatohistopathology*—were written by German emigrants of Jewish descent who had brought the fundamental knowledge they had acquired in Germany to the United States. Not a single capable dermatopathologist was left in Germany; until recently, there was no place in Germany to study dermatopathology.[57]

To fill the gaps created by war and annihilation, the universities often had no other choice but to hire staff that was compromised politically. Furthermore, some physicians who had been denied academic careers under the Nazis were now asked to return to universities and contribute to the reconstruction of German medicine.

One of them was Rudolf Maximilian Bohnstedt, who, at the end of the war, was engaged in private practice of dermatology in Berlin. After the eleven-year interruption of his academic career, Bohnstedt resumed his research in 1946 at Humboldt University in Berlin. Two years later, he became temporary director of the skin clinic in Marburg and in 1949 was called to Giessen as chair of the Department of Dermatology. In 1955 and 1956, Bohnstedt was also dean of the medical faculty of the University of Giessen. He retired in 1969 and died a year later at the age of sixty-nine.[58]

In Leipzig, Oskar Kiess (fig. 388) was appointed chair of the Department of Dermatology. Kiess had been an assistant to Johann Heinrich Rille and, in July 1934, had been appointed associate professor at the University of Leipzig's skin clinic, a position from which he was dismissed only a few months later. After eleven years in private practice, Kiess returned to the university as temporary chair and in 1947 was succeeded by Karl Linser, then director of the skin clinic at Dresden-Friedrichstadt. Kiess died in 1954 at the age of seventy-two.[59]

From 1946 to 1949, the Department of Dermatology at the University of Munich was temporarily directed by Heinrich Höcker, a physician who never received the status of professor. Until 1933, Höcker had been an assistant to Leo Hauck at the skin clinic of the University of Erlangen. He had submitted his thesis, a prerequisite for acquiring a higher academic rank, and his academic promotion was under way when the Nazis' rise to power put a sudden end to his career. Höcker was Aryan, but his wife had one Jewish grandmother, which was cause

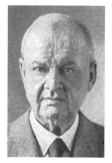

FIG 388
OSKAR KIESS
(1882–1954)

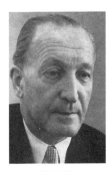

FIG 389
ERICH LANGER
(1891–1957)

enough for his dismissal. For three years Höcker was denied an opportunity to work as a physician. Eventually, he received permission to treat his patients outside the scope of health insurance, but throughout the war Höcker and his wife were under close surveillance by the Gestapo.[60]

Erich Langer (fig. 389) had been dismissed as director of dermatology of Berlin-Britz Municipal Hospital in 1933. Langer was one of fifteen Jewish dermatologists to survive within the confines of Germany. He spent the last months of the Third Reich hiding on an island in Lake Tegel in Berlin. After Germany's capitulation, he immediately resumed his former position at Berlin-Britz Municipal Hospital. In 1946, Langer founded the *Zeitschrift für Haut und Geschlechtskrankheiten*, one of the most important dermatologic journals in the German language. Five years later, he succeeded Heinrich Löhe as director of dermatology at the Rudolf Virchow Hospital. He died of a heart attack in 1957.[61]

In Frankfurt, the chair of dermatology was temporarily filled by Karl Altmann, a former pupil of Paul Ehrlich and Karl Herxheimer. At the time of his appointment, Altmann was sixty-five and handicapped by a recent cardiac infarction. To present his lectures, he had to be carried to the auditorium on the second floor; there were no elevators in the building. He died in 1968.[62]

Georg Alexander Rost, at sixty-eight years old, was asked in August 1945 to take over the Dermatological Department of Berlin-Spandau Municipal Hospital. In conjunction with Erich Langer, Rost reestablished the Berlin Dermatological Society in 1948. Two years later, he was appointed honorary professor of the Free University of Berlin. Until his ninetieth birthday, he continued to run a busy private practice. He died in Berlin at the age of ninety-three.[63]

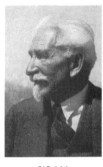

FIG 390
JOHANN HEINRICH
RILLE
(1864–1956)

Even at the age of eighty, Johann Heinrich Rille (fig. 390) was asked to resume, albeit temporarily, the chairmanship of dermatology at the University of Innsbruck, a position that he had held from 1897 to 1902, before accepting a call to the University of Leipzig, where he worked until his retirement in 1934. Rille was the author of several textbooks on dermatology and was the first to describe non-bullous ichthyosiform erythroderma. He died on December 14, 1956, four days after his ninety-second birthday.[64]

Of those who had been forced to emigrate, only a few returned to their native countries. In Austria, no attempt was ever made to invite back those physicians who had been thrown out in 1938. In fact, the new president of the Austrian Medical Association, Alexander Hartwich, actually wrote to emigrants in London and New York in an effort to discourage them from returning. He informed them that there were "no Jews left to treat," that there was a "shortage of housing and work," and that Nazi physicians were "unlikely to leave their posts."[65]

In Germany the situation was not much different from that in Austria, and only about 5 percent of the emigrant physicians returned.[66] Some of those who were invited back to Germany rejected the offer. Among them was the Jewish dermatologist Emil Meirowsky, who explained his reasons in a letter to the dean of the medical faculty of the University of Cologne:

Dear Sir,

I have received your offer to return to Cologne and to take up again my previous appointment as professor extraordinary of your faculty. I regret to be unable to accept your offer. The atrocities that were committed after Hitler had become your leader were mainly due to the lack of resistance by those who were "professors," which means "Bekenner" (passionate advocate) of truth and decency. You stood for freedom of science and research, but you did not hesitate to give up your privilege of being a team of "Bekenner" and to betray the ideals which once made Germany a fortress at the front of science. You did not protest against the removal of your colleagues of Jewish extraction who have contributed so very much to the outstanding success of German science in pre-Hitler times.

*You even silently and without opposition accepted the fact
that members of your faculties were murdered in concentration camps together with millions of innocent men,
women, and children. For all these reasons you have for-
feited your call as professors in the sense of "Bekenner"
or your call as doctors, as protagonists of humanity irrespective of race, creed, and color. I am called upon by my
conscience to ask you to delete my name from the archives
of your faculty.*

Yours truly,
Emil Meirowsky[67]

Among the emigrants who returned to Germany were Oscar
Gans, who came back from Bombay to reassume his chair of
dermatology in Frankfurt; Franz Herrmann, who left New
York University in 1959 to become Gans's successor in Frankfurt; and Alfred Marchionini, who became chair of dermatology first in Hamburg in 1948 and then in Munich in 1950.

The decision to return to Germany after many years of
exile was not an easy one. Apart from the righteous wrath felt
and expressed by Emil Meirowsky, the prospects for a fulfill-
ing professional life in what was now a poor country marked
by the disasters of war were dubious. Furthermore, some of
the emigrants had attained leading positions in their countries
of refuge and this success could not be discarded cavalierly.
Herrmann, for instance, a full professor of experimental dermatology at New York University School of Medicine, hesi-
tated for almost two years before he accepted the call to the
University of Frankfurt.[68]

Marchionini had built a sound Department of Dermatology at the University of Ankara and enjoyed a splendid reputation and great popularity there. His decision to return to
Germany emanated from his wish to accept responsibility for
his native country and for his compatriots, and from a desire
to work and help. His inaugural lecture in Hamburg was

turned into a celebratory party, and Marchionini's wife organized a tombola in which rare and highly desired items that
she had brought from Turkey were given away—the first
prize being a can of coffee. As chair of dermatology at the
University of Hamburg, Marchionini tried to restore old tra-
ditions and to establish bonds with foreign colleagues. Shortly
after his arrival in Hamburg, he reinstalled the bust of Paul
Gerson Unna, which had been removed by the Nazis, and, on
that same occasion, organized the first postwar dermatologic
international meeting in Germany, with participants coming
from many foreign countries—an important event for isolated German dermatology.[69]

As president of the German Dermatological Society, Marchionini worked diligently to alter the picture of Germany
and Germans in the eyes of foreign colleagues and to help
reestablish German dermatology's place in the international
community. In 1950, he founded the *Hautarzt*, today the most
important journal of dermatology in the German language.
In assembling the editorial board, he gathered together, in his
own words, "renowned German clinicians and many superb
foreign colleagues in order to turn the *Hautarzt* into a European platform for practical and scientific dermatology."[70] As
the editor of nearly twenty supplementary volumes to Jadassohn's *Handbuch*, Marchionini saw to it that the articles were
written not only by German dermatologists but by the best
dermatologists in the world.

Marchionini was an ambassador of the new German democracy, often far ahead of politicians in government. Using dermatology as a vehicle, he promoted international understanding,
respect of people for one another, and friendship. He traveled
extensively, visited foreign departments of dermatology, and, in
his own department, invited many students from abroad with
whom he discussed medical as well as cultural and political
issues, such as the horrors of the Auschwitz concentration camp
that he was one of the first Germans to witness firsthand after
the war. With all these efforts, Marchionini attempted to close

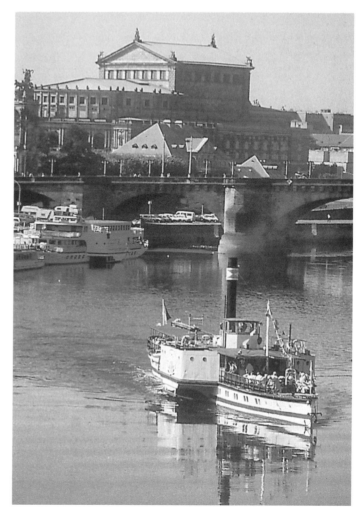

FIG 391 DRESDEN TODAY.

the wounds caused by war and genocide; he was a teacher not only of dermatology but of humanity, and as such he is still remembered in Germany and abroad. The extraordinary reputation he enjoyed is reflected by the honors bestowed on him, such as an honorary doctoral degree from the University of Strasbourg and honorary membership in forty-one dermatological societies throughout the world. Marchionini died in Munich in 1965 at the age of sixty-six.[71]

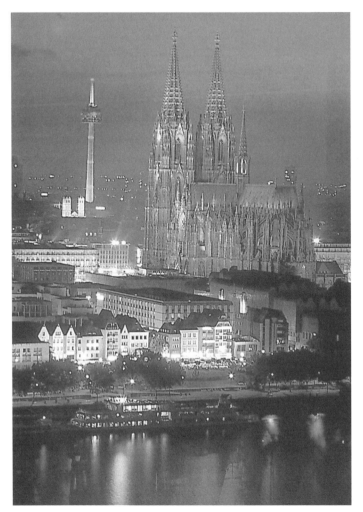

FIG 392 COLOGNE TODAY.

Many years have passed since the horrors perpetrated by the Nazi regime, and those who can testify firsthand about them are becoming fewer. Dermatology in Germany enjoys a splendid reputation again, as does democracy in Germany. Its cities, even those that had been completely destroyed, like Dresden and Cologne, are beautiful and thriving once again (figs. 391, 392).

Nevertheless, it will forever remain essential to remember, reconsider, and reflect on what happened in Germany during the Nazi regime. For societies that are now democratic, it is essential to understand the forces that led to the Nazis' rise to power. Similar mechanisms are still at play: poverty, fanaticism, intolerance, and racism. Those who would use them for their own advantage still exist and always will. For dermatologists and dermatopathologists in particular, it is interesting to learn about the fate of so many people whose names are invoked often and are found in every textbook in connection with the diseases that they described: Buschke's scleredema adultorum, Jessner's lymphocytic infiltration, Gottron's papules, the Herxheimer reaction, and the Meirowsky phenomenon, to mention but a few.

For every one of us, it is important to examine how we behave each day and to wonder how we might behave under the conditions that prevailed in National Socialist Germany. Let us return now to the schema with the four poles found in fig. 226 in Chapter 7: activity and passivity, rejection and support. Based on limited data, classification of individuals like Delbanco, Frieboes, and Gottron according to these poles alone is unjust. But the schema was not meant to be just; it was meant to force confrontation with the question of where would we stand—where would I stand—if exposed to pressure and control like that exerted by the Nazis? On the upper right-hand side of the schema, together with Wirz, Richter, Reiter, and Brill? At the lower left pole, committing suicide like Delbanco? At the upper left pole, actively engaged in resistance, like Schlein? Or somewhere in between?

If we are to be prepared for the future, these are the kinds of questions we must ask ourselves today.

NOTES

NOTES TO INTRODUCTION

1. Ferdinand Hebra was the most important dermatologist of the nineteenth century. Together with his distinguished pupils—among them Auspitz, Kaposi, Neumann, and Pick—he turned Vienna into the mecca of dermatology to which physicians from countries around the globe came for training. Early in his career, Hebra presented a new classification of skin diseases that was based on pathological anatomy and that almost immediately superseded previous classifications. Hebra demonstrated that many cutaneous diseases are caused by parasites or external irritants, removed hundreds of useless medications from the dermatologic armamentarium, and established the value of proper local therapy. In his famous textbook of skin diseases (the second edition of which was written in collaboration with Moriz Kaposi), he gave the first definitive description of several cutaneous diseases, among them erythema multiforme, a distinctive clinical and histopathological reaction usually caused by drugs or infectious agents. J.T. Crissey and L.C. Parish, *The Dermatology and Syphilology of the Nineteenth Century* (New York: Praeger, 1981), pp. 163–177.

2. Heinrich Auspitz was one of the first dermatologists to use the microscope as a tool for a more profound understanding of pathologic processes in the skin. He tried to improve the clinical classification of skin diseases proposed by his teacher, Ferdinand Hebra, and suggested a "system of skin diseases" that was based on changes seen by microscopy. This system, however, was too complex and theoretical to be of practical value. Many of Auspitz's concepts were far ahead of his time, and his uncompromising insistence on them put him in conflict with the Viennese medical establishment. As a result, Auspitz never received a university chair in dermatology. Nevertheless, his influence on dermatology was profound and was sustained by his pupils, among them Paul Gerson Unna. K. Holubar, "Remembering Heinrich Auspitz" in *American Journal of Dermatopathology* 8(1986):83–85.

3. Moriz Kaposi was born in Kaposvar, Hungary, as Moriz Kohn. He studied medicine in Vienna and became an assistant to Ferdinand Hebra who, at that time, was one of the leading figures of the Viennese Medical School. In 1869, Moriz Kohn converted to Christianity and married Hebra's daughter; two years later, he changed his name to Kaposi. In 1880, Kaposi became Hebra's successor as chair of dermatology. Apart from the disease, Kaposi's sarcoma, which is seen commonly in patients with acquired immunodeficiency syndrome, Kaposi is known for his descriptions of xeroderma pigmentosum, acne keloidalis, and Kaposi's varicelliform eruption, a widespread infection

by the virus of herpes simplex in patients with atopic dermatitis. Kaposi also was the first to describe systemic lupus erythematosus and to delineate the histopathologic findings of it. G. Gottlieb and A.B. Ackerman, *Kaposi's Sarcoma: A Text and Atlas* (Philadelphia: Lea & Febiger, 1988).

4. Isidor Neumann was one of the first dermatologists to use the microscope as an instrument for diagnosis. He was also one of the leading syphilologists of his time. In 1881, he was appointed director of the clinic for syphilis of the University of Vienna. Among his pupils were renowned scholars such as Ernst Finger, Samuel Ehrmann, and Johann Heinrich Rille. In addition to pemphigus vegetans, Neumann provided the original descriptions of seborrheic keratosis and "alopecia circumscripta orbicularis," later designated "pseudopelade of Brocq." Crissey and Parish, *The Dermatology and Syphilology of the Nineteenth Century*, pp. 253f.

5. Filip Josef Pick was chair of dermatology in Prague. Together with Heinrich Auspitz, he founded the *Archiv für Dermatologie und Syphilis*, which was the leading dermatologic journal in the world for many decades. In 1888, he and Albert Neisser began the German Dermatological Society. G. Sebastian and A. Scholz, "Zum 150. Geburtstag von Filip Josef Pick" in *Dermatologische Monatsschrift* 171(1985):123–127.

6. Heinrich Köbner was one of the pioneers of dermatology in Germany. His efforts resulted in establishment of the first separate department of dermatology at a German university, the skin clinic of the University of Breslau. Today Koebner is remembered especially for his description of Koebner's phenomenon, the tendency of lesions of a dermatitis to develop after trauma in clinically normal skin. A. Scholz, "Zum 150. Geburtstag von Heinrich Köbner" in *Dermatologische Monatsschrift* 175(1989):111–117.

7. Albert Neisser was chair of dermatology at the University of Breslau, where he created his own school of dermatology. Among Neisser's pupils were Arning, Buschke, Herxheimer, Jacobi, Jadassohn, Jessner, and Pinkus. Together with Filip Josef Pick, Neisser started the German Dermatological Society, and with Alfred Blaschko, he initiated the German Society for the Fight Against Venereal Diseases. Crissey and Parish, *The Dermatology and Syphilology of the Nineteenth Century*, pp. 179–182.

8. Edmund Lesser received his education in dermatology from Ferdinand Hebra in Vienna and Oskar Simon in Berlin. In 1892, he was appointed professor of dermatology in Bern. In 1896, Lesser received a call to the Charité Hospital in Berlin, where he took over the department for syphilis and, a few years later, the department for skin diseases as well. Among Lesser's most prominent pupils were Abraham Buschke, Erich Hoffmann, and Georg Arndt. F. Blumenthal and H. Löhe, "Edmund Lesser zum 100. Geburtstag" in *Dermatologische Wochenschrift* 125(1952):457–459.

9. Paul Gerson Unna was the most prominent dermatohistopathologist of the late nineteenth and early twentieth centuries. He directed a private clinic in Hamburg and an associated laboratory for research in dermatology, the Dermatologikum, where he

trained students from Germany and many foreign countries. His textbooks *Die Histopathologie der Hautkrankheiten* (1894) and *Histochemie der Haut* (1928) remained standard references for many decades. Unna also is known for his original description of seborrheic dermatitis in 1887, the recognition of plasma cells in 1891, and the introduction of numerous compounds into dermatologic therapy, including ichthyol, Eucerin, salicylic acid, and cignolin. A. Hollander, "Development of dermatopathology and Paul Gerson Unna" in *Journal of the American Academy of Dermatology* 15(1986):727–734.

10. C. Schmidt, "Dermato-Venerologie im Nationalsozialismus—Die Neuordnung des Fachgebietes durch personelle Veränderungen im akademischen Bereich, in den Fachgesellschaften und Herausgeberkollegien der Fachzeitschriften" (M.D. diss., Carl Gustav Carus Medical Academy, Dresden, Germany, 1990); A. Scholz and C. Schmidt, "Decline of German dermatology under the Nazi regime" in *International Journal of Dermatology* 32(1993):71–74.

11. Schmidt, "Dermato-Venerologie im Nationalsozialismus."

12. C. Schmidt, "Dermato-Venerologie im Nationalsozialismus—Die Neuordnung des Fachgebietes durch personelle Veränderungen im akademischen Bereich, in den Fachgesellschaften und Herausgeberkollegien der Fachzeitschriften" (M.D. diss., Carl Gustav Carus Medical Academy, Dresden, Germany, 1990); A. Scholz and C. Schmidt, "Decline of German dermatology under the Nazi regime" in *International Journal of Dermatology* 32(1993):71–74.

13. A. Scholz, "Eugen Galewsky (1864–1935)" in *Dermatologische Monatsschrift* 158(1972):53–68.

14. Werner Jadassohn (1897–1973), the son of Joseph Jadassohn, was chair of dermatology at the University of Geneva from 1948 to 1968. Samuel Jessner, the father of Max Jessner, was lecturer in dermatology at the University of Königsberg (now Korolev, Russia).

15. A. Scholz, "Der Suizid von Dermatologen in Abhängigkeit von politischen Veränderungen" in *Hautarzt* 48(1997):929–935.

16. A. Scholz, S. Eppinger, S. Löscher, S. Scholz, and W. Weyers, "Dermatologie im Nationalsozialismus" as part of the poster presentation at the 39th Congress of the German Dermatological Society in Karlsruhe, Germany, 1997.

NOTES TO CHAPTER 1:
THE HISTORY OF ANTI-SEMITISM

1. P.A. Johnson, *A History of the Jews* (New York: Harper/Perennial, 1987), pp. 133ff.

2. R. Hilberg, *Die Vernichtung der europäischen Juden* (Frankfurt: Fischer Taschenbuch Verlag, 1990), pp. 17f.

3. D.J. Goldhagen, *Hitler's Willing Executioners: Ordinary Germans and the Holocaust* (New York: Vintage, 1997), pp. 27–48.

4. Johnson, *A History of the Jews*, pp. 205–232.

5. Hilberg, *Die Vernichtung der europäischen Juden*, pp. 22–23.

6. J.H. Schoeps and J. Schlör, *Antisemitismus: Vorurteile und Mythen* (Munich: Piper, 1995), pp. 153ff.

7. Johnson, *A History of the Jews*, p. 343.

8. Johnson, *A History of the Jews*, p. 342.

9. Jacob Henle was one of the most prominent anatomists and microscopists of the nineteenth century. After an assistantship in Berlin under Johannes Müller, he became chair of anatomy in Zurich, Heidelberg, and Göttingen. Apart from the anatomic structures he described, his name is linked to the establishment of criteria for proving the infectious cause of disease. B. Kisch, "Forgotten leaders in modern medicine" in *Transactions of the American Philosophical Society* 44(1954):227–296.

10. Kisch, "Forgotten leaders in modern medicine," pp. 193–226.

11. Johann Lucas Schönlein was professor of pathology and therapy in Würzburg, Zurich, and Berlin. He changed medical education radically by teaching at the bedside and by using the German language instead of the traditional Latin.

12. Kisch, "Forgotten leaders in medicine," pp. 227–296.

13. E.R. Long, *A History of Pathology* (Baltimore: Williams & Wilkins, 1928), pp. 134–136.

14. Paul Ehrlich was one of the most ingenious and innovative physicians ever. At the outset of his career, he analyzed chemical reactions of various dyes with organic material, resulting in the development of new staining procedures and the identification of cells previously unrecognized—namely, basophilic and eosinophilic granulocytes. He also pursued the idea that chemical reactions of external substances with organic material could be used for therapeutic purposes, and he eventually developed Salvarsan for the treatment of syphilis, the first chemotherapeutic drug ever used.

15. M. Berenbaum, *The World Must Know: The History of the Holocaust as Told in the United States Holocaust Memorial Museum* (Boston: Little, Brown, 1993), p. 15.

16. Ibid.

17. Goldhagen, *Hitler's Willing Executioners*, pp. 27–48.

18. Technically, *Aryan* refers to those who speak any of the family of Indo-European languages that include Iranian, Sanskrit, and most European languages, as well as of the Indic or Iranian branches of the Indo-European family of languages. It is also used to refer to the hypothetical parent language of the Indo-European family of languages and to the ancient people who presumably spoke this language. Aryan was misused by the Nazis to refer to persons of non-Jewish Caucasian descent. The use of the word in connection with race arose from the idea, regarded by ethnologists as false, that peoples who speak the same or related languages had a common genetic origin. Misuse of the term *Aryan* has led to its replacement in scientific discussion by the term *Indo-*

European. Webster's New World Dictionary of the American Language, College Edition (New York: World Publishing Company, 1966).

19. J. Bleker and N. Jachertz (eds.), *Medizin im "Dritten Reich"* (Cologne: Deutscher Ärzte–Verlag, 1989), pp. 11–21.

20. Ernst Haeckel was professor of comparative anatomy and zoology at the University of Jena. As the first German biologist, he supported fully the theory of evolution proposed by Charles Darwin and formulated a "biogenetic law" according to which each organism, as it grows, repeats each stage of development experienced previously in the evolution of species. He also tried to apply the doctrine of evolution to morphology, classifying in this way various orders of animals based on their evolutionary relationships, as well as on religion and philosophy.

21. Max Schultze, professor of pathology in Bonn, was one of the pioneers of microscopy in pathologic anatomy. Apart from his studies on the structure and function of the cell, he contributed through his work on the histologic structure of the retina.

22. Rudolf Virchow was the most influential pathologist ever. Born in Schivelbein, Pomerania, and educated at the University of Berlin, he became prosector at the Charité Hospital in Berlin in 1843 and was appointed lecturer in pathology in 1847. In 1849, he was called to the University of Würzburg as chair of pathologic anatomy, having been dismissed from his posts in Berlin because of his involvement in the revolution of 1848. In 1856, he returned to Berlin as chair of pathology. Virchow was the first to attribute diseases to changes in cells. His most important works were *Cellular Pathology as Based on Histology* in 1850 and *The Pathologic Neoplasms* in 1868. Other publications by him include discussions of political and social issues. From 1880 to 1893, Virchow served as a Liberal in the German Reichstag, where he opposed the policies of the German chancellor Otto von Bismarck.

23. P. Weindling, *Health, Race and German Politics Between National Unification and Nazism, 1870–1945* (Cambridge: Cambridge University Press, 1989), pp. 38ff.

24. Bleker and Jachertz, *Medizin im "Dritten Reich,"* p. 14.

25. Ibid.

26. Paul Schiefferdecker was professor of pathology in Bonn. He described eccrine and apocrine glands and introduced celloidin as a substance in which to embed specimens before cutting sections from them.

27. B. Hamann, *Hitlers Wien. Lehrjahre eines Diktators* (Munich: Piper, 1996), pp. 467ff.

28. M. Hubenstorf, "Der Wahrheit ins Auge sehen" in *Wiener Arzt* 5(1995):14–27.

29. Hamann, *Hitlers Wien*, pp. 467ff.

30. Ibid., pp. 472–473.

31. Hubenstorf, "Der Wahrheit."

32. K. Holubar, "Hans von Hebra (1847–1902) zum 150. Geburtstag: Ein Epitaph" in *Hautarzt* 48(1997):276–277.

33. Hamann, *Hitlers Wien*, p. 474.

34. L.S. Dawidowicz, *The War Against the Jews, 1933–1945* (10th anniversary ed.) (New York: CBS Educational & Professional Publishing, 1986).

35. W. Busch, *Die schönsten Bildergeschichten in Farbe* (Cologne: Buch und Zeit Verlags-gesellschaft mbH, 1974).

36. Dawidowicz, *The War Against the Jews*, pp. 34ff.

37. A. Holitscher and A. Turek (eds.), *Internationales ärztliches Bulletin: Zentralorgan der Internationalen Vereinigung Sozialistischer Ärzte*, reprint, vol. 3, no. 1 (Berlin: Roth-buch Verlag, 1989), pp. 15f.

38. H. Freund and A. Berg (eds.), *Geschichte der Mikroskopie: Leben und Werk großer Forscher*, vol. 2 (Frankfurt: Umschau–Verlag, 1964), pp. 221–228.

39. Ernst Toller was one of the most highly regarded German writers of the early part of the twentieth century. After World War I, in 1919, he participated in the short-lived Communist uprising in Bavaria. As a consequence, he was imprisoned between 1919 and 1924. In 1933, he left Germany for the United States, where he committed suicide in 1939. The passages quoted are from his autobiography, *Eine Jugend in Deutschland*, published in 1933; Schoeps and Schlör, *Antisemitismus*, p. 211.

NOTES TO CHAPTER 2:
THE ASSUMPTION OF POWER

1. J.H. Schoeps and J. Schlör (eds.), *Antisemitismus: Vorurteile und Mythen* (Munich: Piper, 1995), pp. 212f.

2. K. Atermann, W. Remmele, and M. Smith. "Karl Touton and his 'xanthelasmatic giant cell'" in *American Journal of Dermatopathology* 10(1988):257–269.

3. W.L. Shirer, *The Rise and Fall of the Third Reich: A History of Nazi Germany* (30th anniversary ed.) (New York: Touchstone, 1990).

4. Ibid., pp. 150–288.

5. R.N. Proctor, *Racial Hygiene: Medicine Under the Nazis* (Cambridge, MA: Harvard University Press, 1988), pp. 156f.

6. M.H. Kater, *Doctors Under Hitler* (Chapel Hill, NC: University of North Carolina Press, 1989), pp. 150ff; Proctor, *Racial Hygiene*, pp. 156ff; C. Pross and R. Winau, *Nicht misshandeln: Das Krankenhaus Moabit* (Berlin: Edition Hentrich im Verlag Frölich & Kaufmann, 1984), p. 194.

7. R. Jäckle, *Schicksale jüdischer und "staatsfeindlicher" Ärztinnen und Ärzte nach 1933 in München* (Munich: Liste Demokratischer Ärztinnen und Ärzte München, 1988), p. 20.

8. C. Reiter, "Albert Jesionek: Sein Leben und wissenschaftliches Werk zur Tuberkulose der Haut unter besonderer Berücksichtigung seiner lichtbiologischen Forschung" (M.D. diss., Justus Liebig-University, Giessen, 1992). H.W. Spier, "In memoriam Stephan Rothman (1894–1963)" in *Hautarzt* 15(1964):145–146.

9. A. Scholz, F. Ehring, and H. Zaun, *Exlibris berühmter Dermatologen* (Dresden, Germany: Institute for the History of Medicine, Carl Gustav Carus Medical Academy, 1995), pp. 6f.

10. G. Stresemann, *Wie konnte es geschehen? Hitlers Aufstieg in der Erinnerung eines Zeitzeugen* (Berlin: Ullstein, 1987), p. 57.

11. Ibid., pp. 48ff.

12. Shirer, *The Rise and Fall of the Third Reich*, pp. 200ff.

NOTES TO CHAPTER 3:
THE REORGANIZATION OF MEDICINE

1. R. J. Lifton, *The Nazi Doctors: Medical Killing and the Psychology of Genocide* (New York: HarperCollins, 1986), p. 22.

2. In Germany, medical care was financed by public health insurance in which membership was compulsory for everybody earning an income. Half of the contributions for the public health insurance had to be paid by the employer, half by the employee. The KVD, the organization of physicians working under the scope of public health insurance, was mainly responsible for negotiating with the insurance companies about fees for medical procedures. Only persons with a relatively high income had the option to leave public health insurance and be insured privately. Treatment of those patients could be carried out by any doctor and was more lucrative for the doctor because the fees were independent of the negotiations between the KVD and the public health insurance companies. This system, introduced under Bismarck and modified by the Nazis, proved to be valuable for the organization of health care. It is still in effect in Germany.

3. M. Rüther, "Zucht und Ordnung in den eigenen Reihen" in *Deutsches Ärzteblatt* 94(1997):A434–439; M. Rüther, "Mit windigen Paragraphen wider die ärztliche Ethik" in *Deutsches Ärzteblatt* 94(1997):A511–515.

4. H.M. Hanauske-Abel, "Not a slippery slope or sudden subversion: German medicine and National Socialism in 1933" in *British Medical Journal* 313(1996):1453–1463.

5. Ibid.

6. Kater, *Doctors Under Hitler*, p. 183.

7. Hanauske-Abel, "Not a slippery slope."

8. S. Drexler, S. Kalinski, and H. Mausbach. *Ärztliches Schicksal unter der Verfolgung 1933–1945 in Frankfurt am Main und Offenbach: Eine Denkschrift* (Frankfurt: VAS Verlag für Akademische Schriften, 1990).

9. J. Bleker and N. Jachertz (eds.), *Medizin im "Dritten Reich,"* (Cologne: Deutscher Ärzte-Verlag, 1989), p. 72.

10. C. Schmidt, "Dermato-Venerologie im Nationalsozialismus—Die Neuordnung des Fachgebietes durch personelle Veränderungen im akademischen Bereich, in den Fachgesellschaften und Herausgeberkollegien der Fachzeitschriften" (M.D. diss., Carl Gustav Carus Medical Academy, Dresden, Germany, 1990), p. II/44.

11. A. Hollander, "Geschichtliches aus vergangener Zeit: Politische Bekämpfung der Geschlechtskrankheiten?" in *Fortschritte der Medizin* 99(1981):927–928.

12. V. Klemperer, *Ich will Zeugnis ablegen bis zum letzten: Tagebücher 1933–1941*, vol. 1 (Berlin: Aufbau Verlag, 1995), p. 98.

13. M.B. Sulzberger, "Joseph Jadassohn. A personal appreciation" in *American Journal of Dermatopathology* 7(1985):31–36; Schmidt, "Dermato-Venerologie im Nationalsozialismus," pp. 37ff.

14. Schmidt, "Dermato-Venerologie im Nationalsozialismus," pp. 82f.

15. Gustav Riehl, Sr., studied medicine in Vienna, where he also received his dermatologic education under Moriz Kaposi. In 1902, after several years as chair of dermatology at the University of Leipzig, Riehl became Kaposi's successor in Vienna and held that position for 24 years. His name is attached to Riehl's melanosis, a reticulated hyperpigmentation seen most commonly on the face of women. It probably represents the end stage of different unrelated inflammatory processes.

16. Schmidt, "Dermato-Venerologie im Nationalsozialismus," p. II/64.

17. K. Zieler, "Rede zur Eröffnung des 17. Kongresses der Deutschen Dermatologischen Gesellschaft am 8.10.1934 in Berlin" in *Archiv für Dermatologie und Syphilis* 172(1935):3–6.

18. J. Schumacher, "Bekanntmachung über die Deutsche Dermatologische Gesellschaft" in *Dermatologische Wochenschrift* 47(1934):125–126.

19. Notice about Erich Hoffmann in *Zentralblatt für Haut- und Geschlechtskrankheiten* 48(1934):752.

20. A. Holitscher and A. Turek (eds.), *Internationales ärztliches Bulletin: Zentralorgan der Internationalen Vereinigung Sozialistischer Ärzte*, reprint, vol. 3, no. 1 (Berlin: Rothbuch Verlag, 1989), p. 16.

21. H. Sarkowski, *Der Springer Verlag: Stationen seiner Geschichte, vol. 1, 1842–1945* (Berlin: Springer–Verlag, 1992), pp. 331f, 376ff.

22. A. Scholz, S. Eppinger, S. Löscher, S. Scholz, and W. Weyers, "Dermatologie im Nationalsozialismus" as part of the poster presentation at the 39th Congress of the German Dermatological Society in Karlsruhe, Germany, 1997.

23. Schmidt, "Dermato-Venerologie im Nationalsozialismus," pp. II/125f.

24. University Archives of Giessen, PrANr. 349, p. 36.

25. The mention of Emil von Behring's name was forbidden temporarily by the Nazis according to Erich Hoffmann. Hoffmann also noted that one of von Behring's sons committed suicide because of disgraceful treatment of his Jewish mother by the Nazis. E. Hoffmann, *Ringen um Vollendung: Lebenserinnerungen aus einer Wendezeit der Heilkunde, 1933–1946* (Hannover: Schmorl & von Seefeld Nachf., Verlagsbuchhandlung, 1949), p. 234.

NOTES TO CHAPTER 4:
THE REMOVAL OF JEWS FROM THE UNIVERSITIES

1. C. Pross and R. Winau, *Nicht misshandeln: Das Krankenhaus Moabit* (Berlin: Edition Hentrich im Verlag Frölich & Kaufmann, 1984), pp. 172, 186.

2. B. Bromberger, H. Mausbach, and K.D. Thomann, *Medizin, Faschismus und Widerstand* (Frankfurt: Mabuse-Verlag, 1990), pp. 160ff.

3. H.A. Strauss and W. Roeder (eds.), *International Biographical Dictionary of Central European Emigres, 1933–1945, vol. 2: The Arts, Sciences, and Literature* (Munich: Saur-Verlag, 1983).

4. J.J. Herzberg and G.W. Korting (eds.), *Zur Geschichte der deutschen Dermatologie: Zusammengestellt aus Anlass des XVII. Congressus Mundi Dermatologiae* (Berlin: Grosse Verlag, 1987), p. 150; A. Scholz, "Der Suizid von Dermatologen in Abhängigkeit von politischen Veränderungen" in *Hautarzt* 48(1997):929–935.

5. N. Goldenbogen, S. Hahn, C.-P. Heidel, and A. Scholz, *Medizin und Judentum* (Dresden: Verlag des Vereins für regionale Geschichte und Politik Dresden e.V., 1994), pp. 43f.

6. O. Nietz, "Herausbildung der Dermatologie als eigenständiges Fachgebiet in der Stadt Halle sowie Leben und Wirken der Direktoren der Hautklinik der Martin-Luther-Universität Halle-Wittenberg von 1894 bis 1949" (M.D. diss., Martin Luther-University, Halle, 1986), pp. 10ff; E. Hoffmann, *Ringen um Vollendung: Lebenserinnerungen aus einer Wendezeit der Heilkunde, 1933–1946* (Hannover: Schmorl & von Seefeld Nachf., Verlagsbuchhandlung, 1949), p. 22.

7. M.H. Kater, *Doctors Under Hitler* (Chapel Hill, NC: University of North Carolina Press, 1989), p. 221.

8. L.S. Dawidowicz, *The War Against the Jews, 1933–1945* (10th anniversary ed.) (New York: CBS Educational & Professional Publishing, 1986), p. 55.

9. H.J. Böhles, P. Chroust, R. Fieberg, et al., *Frontabschnitt Hochschule. Die Giessener Universität im Nationalsozialismus* (Giessen: Anabas–Verlag and Focus–Verlag, 1982), p. 126.

10. C. Schmidt, "Dermato-Venerologie im Nationalsozialismus—Die Neuordnung des Fachgebietes durch personelle Veränderungen im akademischen Bereich, in den Fachgesellschaften und Herausgeberkollegien der Fachzeitschriften" (M.D. diss., Carl Gustav Carus Medical Academy, Dresden, Germany, 1990), p. 32.

11. A. Hollander, "The tribulations of Jewish dermatologists under the Nazi regime" in *American Journal of Dermatopathology* 5(1983):19–26.

12. U. Saalfeld. "Ernst Sklarz zum 70. Geburtstag" in *Dermatologische Wochenschrift* 150(1964):369–371.

13. Secret Archives of the State of Preussen, I HA Rep 76, Nr. 261.

14. E. Hoffmann, "Franz Blumenthal zum 75. Geburtstag" in *Hautarzt* 4(1953):394–395.

15. A. Scholz, "Ludwig Halberstaedter (1876–1949)" in *Dermatologische Monatsschrift* 162(1976):1015–1025.

16. Archives of the University of Heidelberg, Germany, personnel file of Fritz Stern, PHA Stern.

17. Archives of the University of Heidelberg, personnel file of Siegfried Bettmann, PHA Bettmann.

18. The term *Jew* was applied by the Nazis to anybody who had a Jewish parent or grandparent, without regard for that particular person's religious belief. As a result, many citizens who did not consider themselves to be Jewish at all were suddenly designated Jews. Among dermatologists, some, like Abraham Buschke, were observant Jews, whereas others, like Siegfried Bettmann, were committed Christians. In this work, those like Bettmann are referred to as being "of Jewish descent." The religious and cultural inclinations of many dermatologists who were classified as Jews by the Nazis are not known.

19. D. Mussgnug, "Siegfried Bettmann 1869–1939" in *Aktuelle Dermatologie* 17(1991):25–27.

20. A. Hollander, "Oscar Gans (1888–1983)" in *American Journal of Dermatopathology* 6(1984):87–88; E. Landes and I. Menzel, *Geschichte der Universitätshautklinik in Frankfurt am Main* (Berlin: Grosse–Verlag, 1989), pp. 27ff.

21. T. Nasemann, "In memoriam Franz Herrmann 1898–1977" in *Hautarzt* 29(1978):506–507; Landes and Menzel, *Geschichte der Universitätshautklinik*, pp. 43ff.

22. Hollander, "Tribulations of Jewish dermatologists."

23. R.N. Proctor, *Racial Hygiene: Medicine Under the Nazis* (Cambridge, MA: Harvard University Press, 1988), p. 253.

24. Ibid., p. 252.

25. A. Proppe, *Ein Leben für die Dermatologie* (Berlin: Diesbach-Verlag, 1993).

26. W. Doerr, *Semper Apertus. Sechshundert Jahre Ruprecht-Karls-Universität Heidelberg, 1386–1986*, vol. 2: *Das zwanzigste Jahrhundert, 1918–1985* (Berlin: Springer–Verlag, 1985), p. 469.

27. Schmidt, "Dermato-Venerologie im Nationalsozialismus," pp. 27f.

28. A. Scholz, "Rudolph Leopold Mayer. Werk und Persönlichkeit" in *Dermatologische Monatsschrift* 167(1981):582–586.

29. W.N. Goldsmith, "Wilhelm Siegmund Frei" in *British Journal of Dermatology* 56(1944):187.

30. L. Büchner, A. Scholz, and H. Jacobi H, "In memoriam Walter Freudenthal 1893–1952" in *Der deutsche Dermatologe* 3(1994):350–352.

31. A.H. Mehregan and R.J. Schoenfeld. "Hermann K.B. Pinkus, M.D., 1905–1985" in *Journal of Cutaneous Pathology* 12(1995):453–455; A.B. Ackerman, "Remembering Hermann Pinkus" in *Journal of Cutaneous Pathology* 12(1985):456–458.

32. W.F. Schorr, "Stephan Epstein, M.D., 1900–1973" in *Archives of Dermatology* 108(1973):736.

33. O. Hornstein, "Zur Erinnerung an Ernst Melkersson (1898–1932) und Curt Rosenthal (1892–1937)" in *Hautarzt* 15(1964):515–516.

34. Schmidt, "Dermato-Venerologie im Nationalsozialismus," p. II/31.

35. Secret Archives of the State of Prussia, I HA Rep 90, Nr. 1770.

36. F. Herrmann, "Hans Biberstein" in *Dermatologische Wochenschrift* 150(1964): 617–618.

37. M.B. Sulzberger, "Max Jessner zum 70. Geburtstag" in *Hautarzt* 8(1957):478–479.

38. W. Schneider, "Paul Linser zum 90. Geburtstag" in *Hautarzt* 12(1961):430–431.

39. Archives of the University of Tübingen, personnel file of Paul Linser, PHA Linser.

40. O. Grütz, "In memoriam Franz Koch" in *Hautarzt* 7(1956):191–192.

41. Archives of the University of Tübingen, personnel file of Karl Hermann Vohwinkel, PHA Vohwinkel.

42. W. Knoth, "In memoriam Wilhelm Sevin, 1900–1976" in *Hautarzt* 28(1977):58–59.

43. I. Ehrenberg, "Leo Ritter von Zumbusch (1874–1940): Biobibliographie eines Münchner Dermatologen" (M.D. diss., Ludwig-Maximilians-University, Munich, Germany, 1987), p. 109.

44. Archives of the University of Munich, personnel file of Rudolf Maximilian Bohnstedt, PHA Bohnstedt.

45. Ibid.

46. W. Meyhöfer, "In memoriam Prof. Dr. R. M. Bohnstedt" in *Zeitschrift für Haut- und Geschlechtskrankheiten* 45(1970):187–188; Archives of the University of Munich, personnel file of Rudolf Maximilian Bohnstedt.

47. Ehrenberg, "Leo Ritter von Zumbusch (1847–1940)," pp. 16ff, 108ff.

48. K.H. Leven, *100 Jahre klinische Dermatologie an der Universität Freiburg im Breisgau, 1890–1990* (Freiburg: Albert-Ludwigs-University, Institute for the History of Medicine, 1990), p. 96.

49. Ibid., pp. 92f.

50. Archives of the University of Freiburg, personnel file of Georg Alexander Rost, PA Nr. B 24, 3045.

51. Leven, *100 Jahre klinische Dermatologie*, pp. 97f.

52. Archives of the University of Freiburg, personnel file of Berta Ottenstein, PA Nr. B 101, 3397.

53. Wilhelm Lutz was chair of dermatology at the University of Basel from 1934 to 1956. He also served as president and secretary of the Swiss Dermatological Society and editor of the journal *Dermatologica*. Lajos Nékám was the most prominent Hungarian dermatologist of the mid-twentieth century. He was director of the department of dermatology of the University of Budapest and chair of the International Congress

of Dermatology that convened in Budapest in 1935. Hulusi Behçet was professor of dermatology at the University of Istanbul from 1933 until his death in 1948.

54. G. Schmidt and F.M.Thurmon, "Zum Tode von Bertha Ottenstein (17. Juni 1956)" in *Hautarzt* 11(1956):527–528; Leven, *100 Jahre klinische Dermatologie*, pp. 102ff.

55. Archives of the University of Freiburg, personnel file of Erich Uhlmann, PA Nr. B24, 3828.

56. Leven, *100 Jahre klinische Dermatologie*, pp. 100f.

57. Archives of the University of Freiburg, personnel file of Philipp Keller, PA Nr. B24, 3316.

58. W. Gahlen, "In memoriam Philipp Keller 1891–1973" in *Hautarzt* 25(1974):361–362; Leven, *100 Jahre klinische Dermatologie*, pp. 106ff.

59. Leven, *100 Jahre klinische Dermatologie*, p. 111.

60. Archives of the University of Freiburg, personnel file of Alfred Marchionini, PA Nr. B24, 2290.

61. S. Jablonska, "Alfred Marchionini zum 65. Geburtstag" in *Hautarzt* 15(1964):47–49; Leven, *100 Jahre klinische Dermatologie*, pp. 109–116.

62. J. Bleker and N. Jachertz N (eds.), *Medizin im "Dritten Reich"* (Cologne: Deutscher Ärzte–Verlag, 1989), pp. 39f.

63. Böhles, Chroust, Fieberg, et al., *Frontabschnitt Hochschule*, p. 62.

64. Kater, *Doctors Under Hitler*, p. 150.

65. W. Schmidt, *Leben an Grenzen: Autobiographischer Bericht eines Mediziners aus dunkler Zeit* (Frankfurt: Suhrkamp Taschenbuch Verlag, 1993), p. 31.

66. Archives of the University of Giessen, personnel file of Robert Feulgen, PHA Feulgen.

67. R. Hilberg, *Die Vernichtung der europäischen Juden* (Frankfurt: Fischer Taschenbuch Verlag, 1990), p. 182.

68. R. Jäckle, *Schicksale jüdischer und "staatsfeindlicher" Ärztinnen und Ärzte nach 1933 in München* (Munich: Liste Demokratischer Ärztinnen und Ärzte München, 1988), p. 13.

69. Böhles, Chroust, Fieberg, et al., *Frontabschnitt Hochschule*, p. 73.

70. Kater, *Doctors Under Hitler*, p. 170.

71. R. Baer, personal communication, 1993.

72. Pross and Winau, *Nicht misshandeln*, pp. 30ff.

73. Jäckle, *Schicksale jüdischer*, p. 20.

74. H.M. Hanauske-Abel, "Not a slippery slope or sudden subversion: German medicine and National Socialism in 1933" in *British Medical Journal* 313(1996):1453–1463.

75. Kater, *Doctors Under Hitler*, pp. 186ff.

76. A. Scholz, "Eugen Galewsky (1864–1935)" in *Dermatologische Monatsschrift* 158(1972):53–68.

77. Ibid.

78. Schmidt, "Dermato-Venerologie im Nationalsozialismus," p. II/4.

NOTES TO CHAPTER 5:
THE NEW LEADERS OF GERMAN DERMATOLOGY

1. A. Beyerchen, R. Bollmus, J. Caplan, et al., *Erziehung und Schulung im Dritten Reich*, vol. 2, *Hochschule, Erwachsenenbildung* (Stuttgart: Klett-Cotta, 1980).

2. M.H. Kater, *Doctors Under Hitler* (Chapel Hill, NC: University of North Carolina Press, 1989), pp. 54ff.

3. R.N. Proctor, *Racial Hygiene: Medicine Under the Nazis* (Cambridge, MA: Harvard University Press, 1988), pp. 157ff; Kater, *Doctors Under Hitler*, pp. 13, 69, 85.

4. Kater, *Doctors Under Hitler*, p. 133.

5. Archives of the University of Würzburg, personnel file of Karl Hoede, PHA Hoede.

6. Ibid.

7. H. Röckl, "Karl Hoede zum 75. Geburtstag." *Hautarzt* 23(1972):382–383.

8. G. Grau and P. Schneck (eds.), *Akademische Karrieren im "Dritten Reich"* (Berlin: Medical Faculty of Humboldt-University, Institute for the History of Medicine, 1993), p. 4.

9. A. Scholz, S. Eppinger, S. Löscher, et al. "Dermatologie im Nationalsozialismus," as part of the poster presentation at the 39th Congress of the German Dermatological Society in Karlsruhe, Germany, 1997.

10. Beyerchen, Bollmus, Caplan, et al., *Erziehung und Schulung im Dritten Reich*, p. 12.

11. Kater, *Doctors Under Hitler*, pp. 126ff; Grau and Schneck, *Akademische Karrieren*, p. 5f.

12. Grau and Schneck, *Akademische Karrieren*, p. 26.

13. In fact, only 10 percent of the judgments rendered on political suitability were either definitely positive or negative. The Reich's leader of the National Socialist Lecturers' League, Walter Schultze, was disappointed with the vagueness of many of those judgments. In a series of circulars in 1937, he reminded his subordinates that "it cannot be the rule that people are suggested for advancement who are qualified only as politically reliable or who are said to be 'also nationalistic'; we need, instead, comrades who are committed to our ideology with their hearts. . . . Mere information about membership in the party and the divisions of it is necessary, but insufficient: The ideological attitude and the political activity must be specified"; Beyerchen, Bollmus, Caplan, et al., *Erziehung und Schulung im Dritten Reich*, p. 71.

14. Public Record Office of Hamburg, personnel file of Egon Keining (Hochschulwesen, Dozenten- und Personalakten IV, 477).

15. C. Schmidt, "Dermato-Venerologie im Nationalsozialismus—Die Neuordnung des Fachgebietes durch personelle Veränderungen im akademischen Bereich, in den Fachgesellschaften und Herausgeberkollegien der Fachzeitschriften" (M.D. diss., Carl Gustav Carus Medical Academy, Dresden, 1990), pp. 48f.

16. Ibid., pp. 60f.

17. Proctor, *Racial Hygiene*, p. 19.

18. Schmidt, "Dermato-Venerologie im Nationalsozialismus," p. 61.

19. Ibid., p. 66.

20. J. Krutmann, *Die Geschichte der Universitäts-Hautklinik in Münster in Westfalen* (Herzogenrath: Verlag Murken–Altrogge, 1987), pp. 65f; Archives of the University of Munich, personnel file of Julius Mayr, PHA Mayr.

21. Archives of the University of Munich, personnel file of August Poehlmann, PHA Poehlmann.

22. H. Götz, "In memoriam August Poehlmann" in *Hautarzt* 5(1954):384.

23. J. Geier, "Die Geschichte der dermatologischen Universitätsklinik in Göttingen von ihrer Gründung bis zum Umzug in das jetzige Kliniksgebäude" (M.D. diss., Georg-August-University, Göttingen, Germany, 1987), p. 39; Archives of the University of Göttingen, personnel file of Walther Krantz, PHA Krantz.

24. Secret Archives of the State of Preussen, I HA Rep 76, Nr. 700.

25. Archives of the University of Jena, personnel file of Josef Hämel, PHA Hämel, Bestand D, Nr. 2653.

26. A. Greither, "In memoriam Walther Schönfeld (1888–1977)" in *Hautarzt* 28(1977):504–505; Archives of the University of Jena, personnel file of Josef Hämel.

27. I. Eichert, personnel communication, 1993.

28. Archives of the University of Giessen, personnel file of Walther Schultze, PHA Schultze.

29. Ibid.

30. A. Stühmer, "In memoriam P.W. Schmidt" in *Hautarzt* 1(1950):191–192.

31. H. Jakobi, P. Chroust, and M. Hamann, *Aeskulap und Hakenkreuz: Zur Geschichte der Medizinischen Fakultät in Giessen zwischen 1933 und 1945* (Frankfurt: Mabuse–Verlag, 1989).

32. Eichert, personal communication, 1993; Archives of the University of Giessen, personnel file of Walther Schultze.

33. Archives of the University of Tübingen, personnel file of Willy Engelhardt, PHA Engelhardt; F. Mergenthal, "Die Klinik für Haut—und Geschlechtskrankheiten—und ein merkwürdiger Entnazifizierungsfall," Düsseldorf, 1995.

34. W. Schneider, "Prof. Dr. Wilhelm Engelhardt zum 70. Geburtstag." *Dermatologische Wochenschrift* 152(1966):689–691.

35. Archives of the University of Frankfurt, personnel file of Martin Schubert, PHA Schubert.

36. E. Landes, I. Menzel, *Geschichte der Universitäts-hautklinik in Frankfurt am Main* (Berlin: Grosse–Verlag, 1989), p. 36.; Archives of the University of Frankfurt, personnel file of Martin Schubert.

37. Archives of the University of Halle, personnel file of Julius Dörffel, PA Nr. 5460.

38. O. Nietz, "Herausbildung der Dermatologie als eigenständiges Fachgebiet in der Stadt Halle sowie Leben und Wirken der Direktoren der Hautklinik der Martin-Luther-Uni-

versität Halle-Wittenberg von 1894 bis 1949" (Thesis, Martin-Luther-University, Halle, 1986), pp. 34–39. Archives of the University of Halle, personnel file of Julius Dörffel.

39. G. Polemann, "Josef Vonkennel" in *Dermatologische Wochenschrift* 148(1963): 349–351; Schmidt, "Dermato-Venerologie im Nationalsozialismus," pp. 62ff.

40. Archives of the University of Greifswald, personnel file of Wilhelm Richter; Schmidt, "Dermato-Venerologie im Nationalsozialismus," pp. 46–48.

41. Archives of the University of Heidelberg, personnel file of Walther Schönfeld, PHA Schönfeld.

42. A. Greither, "In memoriam Walther Schönfeld (1888–1977)" in *Hautarzt* 28(1977):504–505.

43. Archives of the University of Giessen, personnel file of Walther Schultze.

44. K.H. Leven, *100 Jahre klinische Dermatologie an der Universität Freiburg im Breisgau, 1880–1900* (Freiburg: Albert-Ludwigs-University, Institute for the History of Medicine, 1990), p. 117.

45. I. Ehrenberg, "Leo Ritter von Zumbusch (1874–1940): Biobibliographie eines Münchner Dermatologen" (M.D. diss., Ludwig-Maximilians-University, Munich, 1987), p. 112.

46. On May 2, 1933, Kurt Strauss took over the department of surgery at the Moabit Hospital in Berlin. As a consequence, the death toll from surgical procedures rose in an unprecedented fashion. Nevertheless, Strauss maintained his position and, in 1940, was appointed full professor of surgery at the University of Prague. Because of corruption attributed to him, he was forced by the Nazis to commit suicide on September 8, 1944. Werner Forssmann described Strauss in his autobiography in these words: "He operated without restraints. I provoked his disgust by my careful preparation during surgery of fractures of the humerus: 'Now just look at him, gentlemen, how the assistant professor picks around. I do a single large cut straight down to the bone.' And that is what he did. However, there were already three liability charges against him because of his having cut through the radial nerve. Nevertheless, he was obstinate. The First and the Second Medical Departments sent their entire surgical material to other hospitals. Strauss did not receive a single patient from them. He commented repeatedly: 'Those reactionary pigs sabotage my National Socialist clinic.'" C. Pross and R. Winau, *Nicht misshandeln: Das Krankenhaus Moabit* (Berlin: Edition Hentrich im Verlag Frölich & Kaufmann, 1984), pp. 206ff.

47. A. Thom and G.I. Caregorodcev, *Medizin unterm Hakenkreuz* (Berlin: VEB Verlag Volk und Gesundheit, 1989), p. 258.

48. P. Milde and A.B. Ackerman, "A critical analysis of textbooks of dermatopathology in historical perspective. Part 8" in *American Journal of Dermatopathology* 15(1993):388–397.

49. Kater, *Doctors Under Hitler*, p. 173.

NOTES TO CHAPTER 6:
NEW MANNERS, MORALS, AND SUBJECTS IN MEDICINE

1. W. Weyers, "Dermatology under the Swastika: Die Entwicklung der Dermatologie im Nationalsozialismus" (Thesis for habilitation, Justus-Liebig-University, Giessen, 1997), p. S33.

2. In fact, Abraham Buschke was an observant Jew, but Paul Unna, Jr. did not regard himself as Jewish at all. His father, Paul Gerson Unna, had already left the Jewish community and considered himself a Monist, even publishing a journal devoted to that particular philosophy.

3. C. Schmidt, "Dermato-Venerologie im Nationalsozialismus—Die Neuordnung des Fachgebietes durch personelle Veränderungen im akademischen Bereich, in den Fachgesellschaften und Herausgeberkollegien der Fachzeitschriften" (M.D. diss., Carl Gustav Carus Medical Academy, Dresden, Germany, 1990), p. II/95.

4. Ibid., p. II/85.

5. Archives of the University of Tübingen, personnel file of Karl Hermann Vohwinkel, PHA Vohwinkel.

6. H. Götz, "In memoriam Alois Memmesheimer 1894–1973" in *Hautarzt* 24(1973): 508–509; Schmidt, "Dermato-Venerologie im Nationalsozialismus," pp. 92f.

7. Schmidt, "Dermato-Venerologie im Nationalsozialismus," p. II/85.

8. Ibid., p. II/86.

9. Ibid., pp. II/86f.

10. E. Hoffmann, *Ringen um Vollendung: Lebenserinnerungen aus einer Wendezeit der Heilkunde, 1933–1946* (Hannover: Schmorl & von Seefeld Nachf., Verlagsbuchhandlung, 1949), p. 65.

11. Schmidt, "Dermato-Venerologie im Nationalsozialismus," pp. II/111f.

12. Weyers, "Dermatology under the Swastika," pp. S27–S32.

13. K.H. Leven, *100 Jahre klinische Dermatologie an der Universität Freiburg im Breisgau, 1880–1900* (Freiburg: Albert-Ludwigs-University, Institute for the History of Medicine, 1990), pp. 121f; Archives of the University of Bonn, personnel file of Erich Hoffmann.

14. Schmidt, "Dermato-Venerologie im Nationalsozialismus," pp. II/115f.

15. Public Record Office of Hamburg, personnel file of Paul Mulzer, Hochschulwesen, Dozenten- und Personalakten IV, 721.

16. L.S. Dawidowicz, *The War Against the Jews, 1933–1945* (10th anniversary ed.) (New York: CBS Educational & Professional Publishing, 1986), pp. 381ff.

17. M.H. Kater, *Doctors Under Hitler* (Chapel Hill, NC: University of North Carolina Press, 1989), p. 114.

18. A. Hollander, "Geschichtliches aus vergangener Zeit: Politische Bekämpfung der Geschlechtskrankheiten?" in *Fortschritte der Medizin* 99(1981):928.

19. J. Bleker and N. Jachertz N (eds.), *Medizin im "Dritten Reich"* (Cologne: Deutscher Ärzte–Verlag, 1989).

20. Schmidt, "Dermato-Venerologie im Nationalsozialismus," p. 88.

21. B. Spiethoff, Editorial in *Mitteilungen der Deutschen Gesellschaft zur Bekämpfung der Geschlechtskrankheiten* 31(1933):73.

22. Schmidt, "Dermato-Venerologie im Nationalsozialismus," pp. 130ff.

23. J. Geier, "Die Geschichte der dermatologischen Universitätsklinik in Göttingen von ihrer Gründung bis zum Umzug in das jetzige Kliniksgebäude" (M.D. diss., Georg-August-University, Göttingen, 1987), p. 33.

24. W. Schultze, "Das Vorgehen gegen asoziale Geschlechtskranke" in *Dermatologische Wochenschrift* 36(1936):1227–1229.

25. L. Alexander, "Medical science under dictatorship" in *New England Journal of Medicine* 241(1949):39–47.

26. A. Thom and G.I Caregorodcev, *Medizin unterm Hakenkreuz* (Berlin: VEB Verlag Volk und Gesundheit, 1989), pp. 167ff; Weindling, *Health, Race and German Politics Between National Unification and Nazism, 1870–1945* (Cambridge: Cambridge University Press, 1989), p. 454.

27. R.N. Proctor, *Racial Hygiene: Medicine Under the Nazis* (Cambridge, MA: Harvard University Press, 1988), pp. 97ff.

28. Weindling, *Health, Race and German Politics, 1870–1945*, p. 454.

29. Kater, *Doctors Under Hitler*, pp. 114ff.

30. E. Klee, *Auschwitz, die NS-Medizin und ihre Opfer* (Frankfurt: Fischer, 1997), pp. 288ff.

31. B. Gebhard, "Hans Reiter" in *Journal of the American Medical Association* 212(1970):323.

32. H.M. Hanauske-Abel, "Not a slippery slope or sudden subversion: German medicine and National Socialism in 1933" in *British Medical Journal* 313(1996):1453–1463.

33. K. Hoede, "Hautarzt und Erbpflege" in *Archiv für Dermatologie und Syphilis* 172(1935):25–29.

34. Ibid.

35. Ibid.

36. Ibid.

37. A. Thom and G.I Caregorodcev, *Medizin unterm Hakenkreuz*, pp. 71ff.

38. H.F. Späte and A. Thom, "Psychiatrie im Faschismus: Bilanz einer historischen Analyse" in *Zeitschrift für die gesamte Hygiene und ihre Grenzgebiete* 26(1980): 553–560; Kater, *Doctors Under Hitler*, pp. 106ff; Thom and Caregorodcev, *Medizin unterm Hakenkreuz*, p. 75.

39. Bleker and Jachertz, *Medizin im "Dritten Reich,"* pp. 80ff; Alexander, "Medical science."

40. Ibid.; Hanauske-Abel, "Not a slippery slope."

41. Kater, *Doctors Under Hitler*, pp. 177ff.

42. G. Sticker, "Erblichkeit, Rassenhygiene und Bevölkerungspolitik." *Münchner Medizinische Wochenschrift* 80(1933):1931–1936, 1975–1980.

43. Weindling, *Health, Race and German Politics*, pp. 141ff.

44. Ibid., pp. 361ff.

45. Hanauske-Abel, "Not a slippery slope."

46. Kater, *Doctors Under Hitler*, p. 115.

47. H.W. Siemens, "Referate. Gottron H.: Ausgewählte Kapitel zur Frage von Konstitution und Hauterkrankungen" in *Zentralblatt für Haut- und Geschlechtskrankheiten* 52(1936):71–72.

48. K. Zieler, "Rede zur Eröffnung des 18. Kongresses der Deutschen Dermatologischen Gesellschaft am 18.9.1937 in Stuttgart." *Archiv für Dermatologie und Syphilis* 177(1938):2–7.

49. W. Jaensch (ed.), *Konstitutions- und Erbbiologie in der Praxis der Medizin* (Leipzig: Johann Ambrosius Barth Verlag, 1934).

50. Kater, *Doctors Under Hitler*, p. 236.

51. Ibid., pp. 25f.

52. A. Brauchle and L.R. Grote, *Ergebnisse aus der Gemeinschaftsarbeit von Naturheilkunde und Schulmedizin*, vol. 2 (Leipzig: Reclam, 1939), pp. 15f.

53. Weyers, "Dermatology Under the Swastika," pp. S21–S26.

54. Kater, *Doctors Under Hitler*, p. 122.

55. C. Steffen, "Max Borst (1869–1946)" in *American Journal of Dermatopathology* 7(1985):25–27.

56. H. Stroink, "Borst and the Von Brehmer incident" in *American Journal of Dermatopathology* 8(1986):522–524.

57. Jaensch, *Konstitutions- und Erbbiologie in der Praxis der Medizin*.

58. Kater, *Doctors Under Hitler*, p. 122.

59. E.H. Brill, "Rede zur Eröffnung des 17. Kongresses der Deutschen Dermatologischen Gesellschaft am 8.10.1934 in Berlin" in *Archiv für Dermatologie und Syphilis* 172(1935):6–8.

60. Kater, *Doctors Under Hitler*, p. 122.

NOTES TO CHAPTER 7:
COOPERATION WITH THE NAZIS

1. A. Holitscher and A. Turek (eds.), *Internationales ärztliches Bulletin: Zentralorgan der Internationalen Vereinigung Sozialistischer Ärzte*, reprint, vol. 1, no. 1 (Berlin: Rothbuch Verlag, 1989), p. 3.

2. C. Schmidt, "Dermato-Venerologie im Nationalsozialismus—Die Neuordnung des Fachgebietes durch personelle Veränderungen im akademischen Bereich, in den Fachgesellschaften und Herausgeberkollegien der Fachzeitschriften" (M.D. diss., Carl Gustav Carus Medical Academy, Dresden, Germany, 1990), p. 31.

3. W. Johe, *Hitler in Hamburg* (Hamburg: Ergebnisse Verlag, 1996), pp. 43–74.

4. G. Stresemann, *Wie konnte es geschehen? Hitlers Aufstieg in der Erinnerung eines Zeitzeugen* (Berlin: Ullstein, 1987), p. 69.

5. S. Haffner, *Anmerkungen zu Hitler* (Frankfurt: Fischer Taschenbuch Verlag GmbH, 1981), pp. 136f.

6. R. Hilberg, *Die Vernichtung der europäischen Juden* (Frankfurt: Fischer Taschenbuch Verlag, 1990), p. 340.

7. Ibid., p. 1085.

8. Haffner, *Anmerkungen zu Hitler*, pp. 31ff.

9. H.M. Hanauske-Abel, "Not a slippery slope or sudden subversion: German medicine and National Socialism in 1933" in *British Medical Journal* 313(1996):1453–1463.

10. M.H. Kater, *Doctors Under Hitler* (Chapel Hill, NC: University of North Carolina Press, 1989), pp. 31ff.

11. V. Klemperer, *Ich will Zeugnis ablegen bis zum letzten: Tagebücher 1933–1941*, vol. 1 (Berlin: Aufbau Verlag, 1995), p. 67.

12. Archives of the University of Freiburg, personnel file of Paul Wilhelm Schmidt, PA Nr. B 24, 3316.

13. E. Hiemer, *Der Giftpilz: Ein Stürmerbuch für Jung u. Alt* (Nuremberg: Verlag Der Stürmer, 1938), pp. 77ff.

14. Ibid.

15. In the story "How Inge fared at the Jew doctor," nothing really happens. Inge goes to the doctor's office, sits in the waiting room for a while, and leaves before being examined. The Jewish physician, "Dr. Bernstein," is not accused of maltreatment or offensive behavior. All accusations are general, vague, and implied ("Many a girl who sought healing from a Jewish physician found lingering illness and shame!"), but the story conveys nonetheless an ill-defined, but palpable, sense of horror. This style—that is, by implication—was found by the Nazis to be most effective in fostering anti-Semitism. Ibid., p. 33.

16. C. Pross and R. Winau, *Nicht misshandeln: Das Krankenhaus Moabit* (Berlin: Edition Hentrich im Verlag Frölich & Kaufmann, 1984), p. 203.

17. Public Record Office of Hamburg, personnel file of Paul Mulzer.

18. Archives of the University of Würzburg, personnel file of Karl Hoede.

19. W. Weyers, "Dermatology under the Swastika: Die Entwicklung der Dermatologie im Nationalsozialismus." (Thesis for habilitation, Justus-Liebig-University, Giessen, 1997), p. S34.

20. E. Hoffmann, *Ringen um Vollendung: Lebenserinnerungen aus einer Wendezeit der Heilkunde, 1933–1946* (Hannover: Schmorl & von Seefeld Nachf., Verlagsbuchhandlung, 1949), p. 14.

21. Archives of the University of Bonn, personnel file of Erich Hoffmann.

22. Archives of the University of Bonn, personnel file of Carl Ludwig Karrenberg.

23. Schmidt, "Dermato-Venerologie im Nationalsozialismus," p. 34.

24. K. Schlenzka and B. Junge, "Schicksale Magdeburger jüdischer Dermatologen im Nazi-Reich. Carl Lennhoff und Otto Schlein" in *Dermatologische Monatsschrift* 175(1989):307–312; H. Gollnick and K.H. Kühne, "Zum Gedenken an Dr. Otto Schlein (1895–1944), Arzt für Dermatologie und Venerologie in Magdeburg" in *Hautarzt* 47(1996):395.

25. B. Bromberger, H. Mausbach, and K.D. Thomann, *Medizin, Faschismus und Widerstand* (Frankfurt: Mabuse–Verlag, 1990), pp. 292–300.

26. Pross and Winau, *Nicht misshandeln*, pp. 240f.

27. P. Milde and A.B. Ackerman, "A critical analysis of textbooks of dermatopathology in historical perspective. Part 5" in *American Journal of Dermatopathology* 15(1993): 85–95.

28. I. Ehrenberg, "Leo Ritter von Zumbusch (1874–1940): Biobibliographie eines Münchner Dermatologen" (M.D. diss., Ludwig-Maximilians-University, Munich, Germany, 1987), p. 111.

29. K.H. Leven, *100 Jahre klinische Dermatologie an der Universität Freiburg im Breisgau, 1880–1900* (Freiburg: Albert-Ludwigs-University, Institute for the History of Medicine, 1990), p. 126.

30. Klemperer, *Ich will Zeugnis*, p. 296.

31. H. Götz, "In memoriam Theodor Grüneberg 1901–1979" in *Hautarzt* 31(1980): 465–466; Schmidt, "Dermato-Venerologie im Nationalsozialismus," pp. 51f.

32. Leven, *100 Jahre klinische Dermatologie*, p. 127.

33. E. Klee, *Auschwitz, die NS-Medizin und ihre Opfer* (Frankfurt: Fischer, 1997), pp. 199ff.

34. J.J. Herzberg, "In memoriam Heinrich Löhe 1877–1961" in *Hautarzt* 12(1951):334–335.

35. A.U. Gindele, "Die Düsseldorfer Hautklinik und ihre historische Entwicklung von 1896–1982 (M.D. diss., Heinrich Heine University, Düsseldorf, Germany, 1991); F. Mergenthal, "Die Klinik für Haut—und Geschlechtskrankheiten—und ein merkwürdiger Entnazifizierungsfall.

36. Archives of the University of Tübingen, personnel file of Heinrich Adolf Gottron, PHA Gottron.

37. F. Leyh and V. Wendt, "Heinrich A. Gottron (1890–1974)" in *American Journal of Dermatopathology* 5(1983):241–243.

38. A. Scholz, personal communication, 1997.

39. Schmidt, "Dermato-Venerologie im Nationalsozialismus," p. 34.

40. Hoffmann, *Ringen um Vollendung*, p. 30.

41. Archives of the University of Bonn, personnel file of Erich Hoffmann.

NOTES TO CHAPTER 8:
THE ESCALATION OF SUPPRESSION

1. L.S. Dawidowicz, *The War Against the Jews, 1933–1945* (10th anniversary ed.) (New York: CBS Educational & Professional Publishing, 1986), pp. 172ff.

2. Ibid., pp. 182f.

3. R.L. Baer, personal communication, 1993.

4. H. Freund and A. Berg (eds.), *Geschichte der Mikroskopie: Leben und Werk großer Forscher*, vol. 2 (Frankfurt: Umschau–Verlag, 1964), pp. 221ff.

5. Baer, personal communication, 1993.

6. A.B. Ackerman, personal communication, 1995.

7. P. Milde and A.B. Ackerman, "A critical analysis of textbooks of dermatopathology in historical perspective. Part 8" in *American Journal of Dermatopathology* 15(1993): 388–397.

8. Public Record Office of the city of Erfurt, resident registration list of 1938, 1-2/370-21396.

9. The denial of Jewish descent by Walter Lever is not an exception. Another more recent and prominent example is U.S. Secretary of State Madeleine K. Albright, who was raised as a Christian. When she was informed that both of her parents had been Jewish and that three of her grandparents had died in German concentration camps, she chose to ignore that fact and refused to respond to letters by relatives of Jewish descent still residing in the Czech Republic. Almost unbelievably, Albright, a graduate of the prestigious Wellesley College, claimed that she had no knowledge of any Jewish heritage before her nomination as secretary of state, at nearly age 60. L. Begley, "In Patriotism's Name" in *The New York Times* (Feb 12, 1997), p. A25.

10. Baer, personal communication, 1993.

11. O. Braun-Falco, "Rudolf Baer, 1910–1997" in *Hautarzt* 48(1997):771–772; Ackerman, personal communication, 1997.

12. I. Silberberg-Sinakin, personal communication, 1997.

13. Ackerman, personal communication, 1997; Silberberg-Sinakin, personal communication, 1997.

14. I. Fischer (ed.), *Biographisches Lexikon der hervorragenden Ärzte der letzten fünfzig Jahre*, 3rd ed., vol. 2 (Berlin: Urban & Schwarzenberg, 1962); Notice about Fritz Juliusberg in *Braunschweiger Werkstücke, vol. 35: Brunsvicensia Judaica* (Braunschweig, 1966); Registration Office of the city of Braunschweig, resident registration list of 1938.

15. F. Goldmann and G. Wolff, *Tod und Todesursachen unter den Berliner Juden* (Berlin: Zentralwohlfahrtsstelle der Reichsvertretung der Juden in Deutschland, 1937).

16. Dawidowicz, *The War Against the Jews*, p. 173.

17. Ibid., p. 175.

18. Ibid.

19. Ibid., p. 173.

20. A. Hollander, "The tribulations of Jewish dermatologists under the Nazi regime" in *American Journal of Dermatopathology* 5(1983):19–26.

21. M.H. Kater, *Doctors Under Hitler* (Chapel Hill, NC: University of North Carolina Press, 1989), pp. 193f.

22. H. Lautsch and H. Dornedden, *Verzeichnis der deutschen Ärzte und Heilanstalten: Reichs-Medizinal-Kalender für Deutschland*, part 2 (Leipzig: Georg Thieme Verlag, 1937), p. 358.

23. H. Biberstein, "In memoriam Kurt Wiener" in *Hautarzt* 11(1960):561.

24. C. Schmidt, "Dermato-Venerologie im Nationalsozialismus—Die Neuordnung des Fachgebietes durch personelle Veränderungen im akademischen Bereich, in den Fachgesellschaften und Herausgeberkollegien der Fachzeitschriften" (M.D. diss., Carl Gustav Carus Medical Academy, Dresden, Germany, 1990), pp. 51f; Secret Archives of the State of Prussia, I HA Rep 76, Nr. 700.

25. D.J. Goldhagen, *Hitler's Willing Executioners: Ordinary Germans and the Holocaust* (New York: Vintage, 1997), pp. 80–128.

26. Archives of the University of Munich, personnel file of Rudolf Maximilian Bohnstedt, PHA Bohnstedt; R. Jahn, personal communication, 1996.

27. Schacht criticized encroachments on Jews at a meeting with leading representatives of the party and the government on August 20, 1935. The only reason for his criticism were economic considerations. R. Hilberg, *Die Vernichtung der europäischen Juden* (Frankfurt: Fischer Taschenbuch Verlag, 1990), pp. 41ff.

28. The appearance of moderation for the Olympic Games was partially achieved by prophylactic compulsory measures. Potential troublemakers were arrested before the international guests arrived. An example is the incarceration of prostitutes in Berlin hospitals that was carried out on the order of Leonardo Conti. L. Conti, "Gesundheitspflicht und Geschlechtskrankheiten: Bilanz einer erfolgreichen Bekämpfung" in *Archiv für Dermatologie und Syphilis* 184(1943):7–21.

29. Dawidowicz, *The War Against the Jews, 1933–1945*, p. 96.

30. C. Pross and R. Winau, *Nicht misshandeln: Das Krankenhaus Moabit* (Berlin: Edition Hentrich im Verlag Frölich & Kaufmann, 1984), p. 43.

31. Ibid., p. 119.

32. Kater, *Doctors Under Hitler*, pp. 192ff.

33. Archives of the University of Frankfurt, personnel file of Karl Altmann, PHA Altmann.

34. Kater, *Doctors Under Hitler*, p. 196.

35. R.N. Proctor, *Racial Hygiene: Medicine Under the Nazis* (Cambridge, MA: Harvard University Press, 1988), p. 153.

36. W. Schönfeld, "Paul Richter" in *Dermatologische Wochenschrift* 132(1955):1149–1155; R. Synnatzschke, "Paul Caesar Richter" in *Dermatologische Wochenschrift* 136(1957):1055–1056.

37. Kater, *Doctors Under Hitler*, pp. 200f.

38. P. Milde and A.B. Ackerman, "A critical analysis of textbooks of dermatopathology in historical perspective. Part 12" in *American Journal of Dermatopathology* 16(1994):201–220; Hollander, "The tribulations of Jewish dermatologists."

39. E. Hoffmann, *Ringen um Vollendung: Lebenserinnerungen aus einer Wendezeit der Heilkunde, 1933–1946* (Hannover: Schmorl & von Seefeld Nachf., Verlagsbuchhandlung, 1949), pp. 149, 178.

40. Hilberg, *Die Vernichtung der europäischen Juden*, pp. 43ff.

41. T. Nasemann, "In memoriam Franz Herrmann 1898–1977" in *Hautarzt* 29(1978): 506–507.

42. R.L. Baer, "In memoriam Alfred Hollander" in *Hautarzt* 38(1987):58.

43. H. Ollendorff Curth, "Erich Kuznitzky" in *Hautarzt* 11(1960):288.

44. H. Beerman, "In memoriam Emil Meirowsky" in *Hautarzt* 11(1960):335–336.

45. P. Milde, A.B. Ackerman, "A critical analysis of textbooks .... Part 12."

46. H. Gentele, "In memoriam Carl Lennhoff" in *Hautarzt* 16(1965):96; Schlenzka and Junge, "Schicksale Magdeburger jüdischer Dermatologen im Nazi-Reich: Carl Lennhoff und Otto Schlein."

47. Hilberg, *Die Vernichtung der europäischen Juden*, pp. 140ff.

48. Proctor, *Racial Hygiene: Medicine Under the Nazis*, p. 167.

49. Ibid., p. 166.

50. P.A. Johnson, *A History of the Jews* (New York: Harper/Perennial, 1987), p. 504.

51. Ibid., pp. 459ff, 503f.

52. J. Bleker and N. Jachertz (eds.), *Medizin im "Dritten Reich"*: Deutscher Ärzte–Verlag, 1989), pp. 78ff; Kater, *Doctors Under Hitler*, pp. 210ff.

53. M.B. Sulzberger, "In memoriam George Miller MacKee 1875–1955" in *Hautarzt* 6(1955):431–432.

54. I. Rosen, "Fred Wise" in *Hautarzt* 2(1951):95–96.

55. R.L. Baer, J. Epstein, B. Epstein, et al., "A memorial to Marion Baldur Sulzberger" in *Archives of Dermatology* 120(1984):857–858; M. Leider (ed.), "Sulzberger! Biography, autobiography, iconography: A posthumous festschrift" in *American Journal of Dermatopathology* 6(1984):345–370.

56. Kater, *Doctors Under Hitler*, pp. 211f.

57. N. Goldenbogen, S. Hahn, C.-P. Heidel, and A. Scholz, *Medizin und Judentum* (Dresden: Verlag des Vereins für regionale Geschichte und Politik Dresden e.V., 1994), p. 11.

58. Dawidowicz, *The War Against the Jews*, pp. 190f.

NOTES TO CHAPTER 9:
WAR AND ANNIHILATION

1. R.N. Proctor, *Racial Hygiene: Medicine Under the Nazis* (Cambridge, MA: Harvard University Press, 1988), pp. 168f.

2. E. Ernst, "A leading medical school seriously damaged: Vienna 1938" in *Annals of Internal Medicine* 122(1995):789–792.

3. K. Holubar, C. Schmidt, and K. Wolff, *Challenge Dermatology: Vienna 1841–1992* (Vienna: Verlag der Österreichischen Akademie der Wissenschaften, 1993), pp. 77ff.

4. W.L. Shirer, *The Rise and Fall of the Third Reich: A History of Nazi Germany* (30th anniversary ed.). (New York: Touchstone, 1990), pp. 322ff.

5. Ibid.

6. A. Scholz, "Der Suizid von Dermatologen in Abhängigkeit von politischen Veränderungen" in *Hautarzt* 48(1997):929–935.

7. L.S. Dawidowicz, *The War Against the Jews, 1933–1945* (10th anniversary ed.). (New York: CBS Educational & Professional Publishing, 1986), pp. 104f.

8. M. Hubenstorf, "Der Wahrheit ins Auge sehen" in *Wiener Arzt* 5(1995):14–27.

9. Holubar, Schmidt, and Wolff, *Challenge Dermatology*, p. 79.

10. M. Tobis, "Die bisherige Organisation der österreichischen Ärzteschaft" in *Deutsches Ärzteblatt* 68(1938):270.

11. W.E. Seidelman, "Nuremberg lamentation: For the forgotten victims of medical science" in *British Medical Journal* 313(1996):1463–1467; H.A. Israel, "Nazi origins of an anatomy text: The Pernkopf atlas" in *Journal of the American Medical Association* 276(1996):1633.

12. Ernst, "A leading medical school."

13. Ibid.

14. J. Bleker and N. Jachertz (eds.), *Medizin im "Dritten Reich"* (Cologne: Deutscher Ärzte–Verlag, 1989), p. 40; Ernst, "A leading medical school."

15. Ernst, "A leading medical school."

16. Hubenstorf, "Der Wahrheit."

17. K. Holubar, personal communication, 1995.

18. Ernst, "A leading medical school."

19. Holubar, Schmidt, and Wolff, *Challenge Dermatology*, p. 79.

20. S.R. Brunauer, "Maurice Oppenheim, 1876–1949" in *British Journal of Dermatology* 62(1950):93–94; G. Riehl, "Gedenkworte für Moritz Oppenheim" in *Hautarzt* 1(1950):95–96.

21. K. Holubar and K. Wolff, "The genesis of American investigative dermatology from its roots in Europe" in *Journal of Investigative Dermatology* 92(1989):14S–21S; W.B. Shelley, J.T. Crissey JT, and J.H. Stokes, *Classics in Clinical Dermatology* (Springfield, IL: Charles C. Thomas, 1953), pp. 433–436.

22. K. Holubar and K. Wolff, "The genesis of American investigative dermatology from its roots in Europe" in *Journal of Investigative Dermatology* 92(1989):14S–21S; E. Lesky, *Meilensteine der Wiener Medizin: Große Ärzte Österreichs in drei Jahrhunderten* (Vienna: Verlag Wilhelm Maudrich, 1981).

23. A. Wiedmann, "Stephan Robert Brunauer zum 75. Geburtstag!" in *Hautarzt* 13(1962):382.

24. L. Arzt, "In memoriam Hans Königstein" in *Hautarzt* 5(1954):336.

25. A. Wiedmann, "Zum 70. Geburtstag von R.O. Stein" in *Hautarzt* 1(1950):567.

26. V. Klemperer, *Ich will Zeugnis ablegen bis zum letzten*, vol. 2 (Berlin: Aufbau Verlag, 1995), pp. 491, 563.

27. H. Weiss (Israelite Cultural Community of Vienna), personal communication 1995; Wiedmann, "Zum 70. Geburtstag von R.O. Stein."

28. Hubenstorf, "Der Wahrheit."

29. Ibid.

30. K.H. Leven, *100 Jahre klinische Dermatologie an der Universität Freiburg im Breisgau, 1890–1990* (Freiburg: Albert-Ludwigs-University, Institute for the History of Medicine, 1990), p. 127.

31. C. Schmidt, "Dermato-Venerologie im Nationalsozialismus—Die Neuordnung des Fachgebietes durch personelle Veränderungen im akademischen Bereich, in den Fachgesellschaften und Herausgeberkollegien der Fachzeitschriften" (M.D. diss., Carl Gustav Carus Medical Academy, Dresden, Germany, 1990), p. 85.

32. A. Marchionini, "Abschied von Leopold Arzt" in *Hautarzt* 6(1955):335–336; J. Tappeiner, "Prof. Dr. Leopold Arzt" in *Dermatologische Wochenschrift* 132(1955):761–763.

33. Holubar, Schmidt, and Wolff, *Challenge Dermatology*, p. 83; Holubar, personal communication, 1995.

34. J. Konrad, "Leo Kumer 1886–1951" in *Dermatologische Wochenschrift* 125(1952): 97–98.

35. H. Kresbach, "Anton Musger, 1898–1983" in *Hautarzt* 35(1984):272–273.

36. A. Musger, "Albert Wiedmann zum 65. Geburtstag" in *Hautarzt* 17(1966):190–191.

37. K. Holubar, "Hans von Hebra (1847–1902) zum 150. Geburtstag: Ein Epitaph" in *Hautarzt* 48(1997):276–277.

38. J.A. Gammel, "Hugo Hecht" in *Hautarzt* 14(1963):383–384.

39. E.J. Feuerman, "In memoriam Felix Sagher" in *Hautarzt* 34(1983):101.

40. C. Calnan, "Henry Haber (1900–1962)" in *American Journal of Dermatopathology* 7(1985):537–539; P.D. Samman, "Henry Haber" in *American Journal of Dermatopathology* 7(1985):541–542; K.V. Sanderson, "Henry Haber" in *American Journal of Dermatopathology* 7(1985):543–545.

41. J. Kanopik, "In memoriam Karel Gawalowski (1890–1965)" in *Hautarzt* 17(1966):192; A. Scholz, G. Sebastian, and J. Trnka, "Prager Dermatologie und der 1. Kongreß der Deutschen Dermatologischen Gesellschaft 1889" in *Hautarzt* 40(1989):652–659.

42. F. Kogoj, "In memoriam Anton Tryb (1884–1960)" in *Hautarzt* 12(1961):144.

43. F. Zaruba, "In memoriam Jan Kanopik" in *Hautarzt* 37(1986):689.

44. Scholz, "Der Suizid von Dermatologen."

45. S. Lorant, *Sieg Heil! Eine deutsche Bildergeschichte von Bismarck zu Hitler* (Frankfurt: Zweitausendeins, 1979), p. 263.

46. G. Stresemann, *Wie konnte es geschehen? Hitlers Aufstieg in der Erinnerung eines Zeitzeugen* (Berlin: Ullstein, 1987), p. 215.

47. Lorant, *Sieg Heil!*, p. 263.

48. Dawidowicz, *The War Against the Jews*, p. 91.

49. W. Weyers, "Dermatology under the Swastika: Die Entwicklung der Dermatologie im Nationalsozialismus" (Thesis for habilitation, Justus-Liebig-University, Giessen, 1997), p. 535.

50. Bleker and Jachertz, *Medizin im "Dritten Reich,"* pp. 122ff.

51. A. Marchionini, "Lucien Marie Pautrier zum 80. Geburtstag" in *Hautarzt* 7(1956):382–384.

52. L. Arzt, "In memoriam Franz Walter" in *Hautarzt* 2:(1951)94–95.

53. A. Vasiljevic, "In memoriam Josip Fleger" in *Hautarzt* 18(1967):95.

54. A. Brnobic, "In memoriam Franjo Kogoj, 1894–1983" in *Hautarzt* 35:(1984)270–271.

55. U.W. Schnyder, "Tibor Salamon, 1914–1995" in *Hautarzt* 47(1996):69.

56. T. Nasemann, "Der Morphologe Hermann Werner Siemens und seine Bemühungen um eine 'Allgemeine Dermatologie'" in *Hautarzt* 34(1983):569–573.

57. Klemperer, *Ich will Zeugnis*.

58. Scholz, "Der Suizid von Dermatologen."

59. Klemperer, *Ich will Zeugnis*, pp. 681f.

60. N. Goldenbogen, S. Hahn, C.-P. Heidel, and A. Scholz, *Medizin und Judentum* (Dresden: Verlag des Vereins für regionale Geschichte und Politik Dresden e.V., 1994), pp. 15ff.

61. C. Pross and R. Winau, *Nicht misshandeln: Das Krankenhaus Moabit* (Berlin: Edition Hentrich im Verlag Frölich & Kaufmann, 1984), pp. 23f.

62. Dawidowicz, *The War Against the Jews*, pp. 112f.

63. Ibid., pp. 357ff.

64. Christoforos Doucas was director of dermatology at the Evangelismos Hospital in Athens from 1935 to 1955. I. Capetanakis, "Christopher Doucas zum 70. Geburtstag" in *Hautarzt* 11(1960):560.

65. C.E. Orfanos, "Haim A. Cohen zum 75. Geburtstag" in *Hautarzt* 40(1989):466–467; C.A. Cohen, personal communication, 1995.

66. K. Schlenzka and B. Junge, "Schicksale Magdeburger jüdischer Dermatologen im Nazi-Reich. Carl Lennhoff und Otto Schlein" in *Dermatologische Monatsschrift* 175(1989):307–312.

67. A. Marchionini, "Viktor Kafka zum 70. Geburtstag" in *Hautarzt* 2(1951):478–479.

68. The order concerning exploitation of Jewish workers was issued by Fritz Sauckel, head of the Allocation of Labour Office, who was sentenced to death in the Nuremberg trials. P.A. Johnson, *A History of the Jews* (New York: Harper/Perennial, 1987), p. 490.

69. Dawidowicz, *The War Against the Jews*, p. 115.

70. D.J. Goldhagen, *Hitler's Willing Executioners: Ordinary Germans and the Holocaust* (New York: Vintage 1996), pp. 180–280.

71. Haffner, *Anmerkungen zu Hitler*, p. 114.

72. Dawidowicz, *The War Against the Jews*, p. 106.

73. Hilberg, *Die Vernichtung der europäischen Juden*, pp. 422ff.

74. H. Jakobi, P. Chroust, and M. Hamann, *Aeskulap und Hakenkreuz: Zur Geschichte der Medizinischen Fakultät in Giessen zwischen 1933 und 1945* (Frankfurt: Mabuse–Verlag, 1989), pp. 54f; Scholz, "Der Suizid."

75. P.-M. Seiffert, *Die Hamburger Dermatologische Gesellschaft* (Berlin: Grosse, 1985), pp. 21ff; Scholz, "Der Suizid."

76. Ibid.

77. F. Golczewski, *Kölner Universitätslehrer und der Nationalsozialismus* (Köln: Böhlau-Verlag, 1988).

78. Calnan, "Henry Haber (1900–1962);" Samman, "Henry Haber"; Sanderson, "Henry Haber."

79. Dawidowicz, *The War Against the Jews*, p. 403.

80. L. Chagoll, *Im Namen Hitlers: Kinder hinter Stacheldraht* (Cologne: Pahl-Rugenstein Verlag, 1979), p. 134.

81. P. Dejas-Eckertz, D. Ruckhaberle, A. Tebbe, et al., *Faschismus* (Berlin: Elefanten Press Verlag GmbH, 1976), pp. 17ff.

82. Ibid., p. S68.

83. P. Weindling, *Health, Race and German Politics Between National Unification and Nazism, 1870–1945* (Cambridge, England: Cambridge University Press, 1989), pp. 167ff and 485ff; J. Vollmann, R. Winau, "Informed consent in human experimentation before the Nuremberg code" in *British Medical Journal* 313(1996):1445–1447.

84. E. Klee, *Auschwitz, die NS-Medizin und ihre Opfer* (Frankfurt: Fischer, 1997), p. 335.

85. E. Klee, *Was sie taten - was sie wurden. Ärzte: Juristen und andere Beteiligte am Kranken- oder Judenmord* (Frankfurt: Fischer Taschenbuch Verlag, 1986), p. 280; Klee, *Auschwitz*, p. 156.

86. A.U. Gindele, "Die Düsseldorfer Hautklinik und ihre historische Entwicklung von 1896–1982" (M.D. diss., Heinrich Heine University, Düsseldorf, Germany, 1991); F. Mergenthal, "Die Klinik für Haut- und Geschlechtskrankheiten - und ein merkwürdiger Entnazifizierungsfall," Düsseldorf, 1995.

87. Klee, *Auschwitz*, pp. 199ff.

88. Dejas-Eckertz, Ruckhaberle, Tebbe, et al., *Faschismus*, p. 119.

89. O. Gans, "Zum 100. Geburtstag von Karl Herxheimer" in *Hautarzt* 12(1961): 241–242.

90. E. Landes and I. Menzel, *Geschichte der Universitätshautklinik in Frankfurt am Main* (Berlin: Grosse–Verlag, 1989), pp. 26f.

91. Gans, "Zum 100. Geburtstag von Karl Herxheimer"; F. Schmidt-La Baume. "In memoriam Karl Herxheimer" in *Hautarzt* 4(1953):444.

92. Gans, "Zum 100. Geburtstag von Karl Herxheimer."

93. N. Hammerstein, *Die Johann Wolfgang Goethe-Universität Frankfurt am Main: Von der Stiftungsuniversität zur staatlichen Hochschule*, vol. 1, 1914–1950 (Frankfurt: Alfred Metzner Verlag, 1989), p. 226.

94. Gans, "Zum 100. Geburtstag von Karl Herxheimer."

95. J.A. Gold and F.G. Nürnberger, "A tribute to Abraham Buschke" in *Journal of the American Academy of Dermatology* 26(1992):1019–1022.

96. W. Curth and H. Ollendorff Curth, "Remembering Abraham Buschke" in *American Journal of Dermatopathology* 5(1983):27–29; Gold and Nürnberger, "A tribute to Abraham Buschke."

NOTES TO CHAPTER 10:
THE END AND THE YEARS AFTER

1. W. Weyers, "Dermatology under the Swastika: Die Entwicklung der Dermatologie im Nationalsozialismus" (Thesis for habilitation, Justus-Liebig-University, Giessen, 1997), p. S45.

2. J. Krutmann, *Die Geschichte der Universitäts-Hautklinik in Münster in Westfalen* (Herzogenrath: Verlag Murken–Altrogge, 1987), pp. 95f.

3. L. Conti, "Gesundheitspflicht und Geschlechtskrankheiten: Bilanz einer erfolgreichen Bekämpfung" in *Archiv für Dermatologie und Syphilis* 184(1943):7–21.

4. K. Zieler, "Rede zur Eröffnung des 20. Kongresses der Deutschen Dermatologischen Gesellschaft am 28.10.1942 in Würzburg" in *Archiv für Dermatologie und Syphilis* 184(1943):3–6, 21–22.

5. P.J. Unna, personal communication, 1992.

6. K. Jakstat, *Geschichte der Dermatologie in Hamburg*, Bibliotheca Diesbach, vol. 1 (Berlin: Diesbach Verlag, 1987), pp. 112f.

7. M.H. Kater, *Doctors Under Hitler* (Chapel Hill, NC: University of North Carolina Press, 1989), pp. 45f.

8. Ibid., p. 41.

9. Ibid., pp. 42ff.

10. Ibid., p. 12.

11. Ibid., pp. 47ff.

12. A.B. Ackerman, "Doctors may yet save the world" in *American Journal of Dermatopathology* 6(1984):315–316.

13. R.L. Baer, "Otto Braun-Falco zum 60. Geburtstag" in *Hautarzt* 33(1982):242–243.

14. Archives of the University of Frankfurt, personnel file of Karl Altmann, PHA Altmann.

15. C. Schmidt, "Dermato-Venerologie im Nationalsozialismus—Die Neuordnung des Fachgebietes durch personelle Veränderungen im akademischen Bereich, in den Fachgesellschaften und Herausgeberkollegien der Fachzeitschriften" (M.D. diss., Carl Gustav Carus Medical Academy, Dresden, Germany, 1990), p. 68.

16. Krutmann, *Die Geschichte der Universitäts-Hautklinik*, pp. 79f.

17. Kater, *Doctors Under Hitler*, p. 47f; Weyers, *Dermatology Under the Swastika*, pp. S44ff.

18. S. Haffner, *Anmerkungen zu Hitler* (Frankfurt: Fischer Taschenbuch Verlag GmbH, 1981), p. 141.

19. W.L. Shirer, *The Rise and Fall of the Third Reich: A History of Nazi Germany* (30th anniversary ed.). (New York: Touchstone, 1990), p. 1104.

20. P. Milde and A.B. Ackerman, "A critical analysis of textbooks of dermatopathology in historical perspective. Part 5" in *American Journal of Dermatopathology* 15(1993):85–95.

21. A. Scholz, "Der Suizid von Dermatologen in Abhängigkeit von politischen Veränderungen" in *Hautarzt* 48(1997):929–935.

22. Public Record Office of Hamburg, personnel file of Paul Mulzer, Hochschulwesen, Dozenten- und Personalakten IV, 721.

23. G. Grau and P. Schneck (eds.), *Akademische Karrieren im "Dritten Reich."* (Berlin: Medical Faculty of Humboldt-University, Institute for the History of Medicine, 1993), p. 30.

24. B. Bromberger, H. Mausbach, and K.D. Thomann, *Medizin, Faschismus und Widerstand* (Frankfurt: Mabuse-Verlag, 1990), pp. 319ff.

25. Jakstat, *Geschichte der Dermatologie*, p. 117; Public Record Office of Hamburg, personnel file of Paul Mulzer, Hochschulwesen, Dozenten- und Personalakten IV, 721.

26. Archives of the University of Giessen, personnel file of Walther Schultze, PHA Schultze.

27. Weyers, "Dermatology under the Swastika," pp. S42ff.

28. Archives of the University of Giessen, personnel file of Walther Schultze, PHA Schultze.

29. Public Record Office of Marburg, personnel file of Alfred Ruete, PHA Ruete.

30. Archives of the University of Göttingen, personnel file of Walther Krantz, PHA Krantz.

31. A. Scholz, S. Eppinger, S. Löscher, S. Scholz, and W. Weyers, "Dermatologie im Nationalsozialismus" as part of the poster presentation at the 39th Congress of the German Dermatological Society in Karlsruhe, Germany, 1997.

32. K.H. Leven, *100 Jahre klinische Dermatologie an der Universität Freiburg im Breisgau, 1890–1990* (Freiburg: Albert-Ludwigs-University, Institute for the History of Medicine,1990), pp. 131f.

33. J. Schreier, U.F. Haustein, and K.H. Karbe, "Zur Geschichte der Dermatologie an der Universität Leipzig" in *Dermatologische Monatsschrift* 170(1984):1–14; G. Polemann, "Josef Vonkennel" in *Dermatologische Wochenschrift* 148(1963):349–351; Schmidt, "Dermato-Venerologie im Nationalsozialismus."

34. E. Klee, *Auschwitz, die NS-Medizin und ihre Opfer* (Frankfurt: Fischer, 1997), p. 335.

35. M. Meyhöfer, personal communication, 1993.

36. Archives of the University of Tübingen, personnel file of Heinrich Adolf Gottron, PHA Gottron.

37. Meyhöfer, personal communication, 1993.

38. R.L. Baer, personal communication, 1993.

39. W. Gertler, "Heinrich A. Gottron, 10.3.1890–23.6.1974" in *Dermatologische Wochenschrift* 160(1974):962–963; F. Leyh and V. Wendt, "Heinrich A. Gottron (1890–1974)" in *American Journal of Dermatopathology* 5(1983):241–243.

40. Leyh and Wendt, "Heinrich A. Gottron (1890–1974)."

41. A recent (1997) example of failure to come to grips with the past is the rejection by a current chair of the University of Giessen of a poster about the role physicians of that university played in Nazi Germany. On the occasion of the 800th anniversary of the city of Giessen, an exhibition about the history and future of medicine in Giessen was to be presented in the spacious atrium of his clinic. The chair, who was born in 1940, allowed that exhibition only on the condition that the poster regarding the involvement of the medical faculty in the Third Reich be excluded.

42. M. Franzblau, "Nazi medical cronies unpunished 50 years later" in *Dermatopathology: Practical and Conceptual* 2(1996):83–86; W.E. Seidelman, "Nuremberg lamentation: For the forgotten victims of medical science" in *British Medical Journal* 313(1996):1463–1467.

43. Kater, *Doctors Under Hitler*, p. 223.

44. Kater, *Doctors Under Hitler*, p. 224; Proctor, *Racial Hygiene: Medicine Under the Nazis* (Cambridge, MA: Harvard University Press, 1988), pp. 299ff; G. Aumüller, H. Lauer, and H. Remschmidt (eds.), *Kontinuität und Neuanfang in der Hochschulmedizin nach 1945* (Marburg: Schüren, 1997), pp. 37–53.

45. Kater, *Doctors Under Hitler*, pp. 202, 233.

46. Aumüller, *Kontinuität und Neuanfang in der Hochschulmedizin nach 1945*, pp. 37–53.

47. Ibid.; Proctor, *Racial Hygiene*, pp. 307f.

48. Proctor, *Racial Hygiene*, p. 306.

49. P. Diepgen, *Die Heilkunde und der ärztliche Beruf*, 2nd ed. (Berlin: Urban & Schwarzenberg, 1947), p. VI.

50. Proctor, *Racial Hygiene*, pp. 303ff.

51. Klee, *Auschwitz*, pp. 199f.

52. Ibid., pp. 241f.

53. Aumüller, *Kontinuität und Neuanfang in der Hochschulmedizin nach 1945*, pp. 102–107.

54. Archives of the University of Bonn, personnel file of Erich Hoffmann.

55. Aumüller, *Kontinuität und Neuanfang in der Hochschulmedizin nach 1945*, p. 110.

56. Scholz, Eppinger, Löscher, Scholz, and Weyers, "Dermatologie im Nationalsozialismus."

57. Ibid.

58. H. Köhler, "Zum 60. Geburtstag von Rudolf Maximilian Bohnstedt" in *Hautarzt* 11(1960):334–335; W. Meyhöfer, "In memoriam Prof. Dr. R. M. Bohnstedt" in *Zeitschrift für Haut- und Geschlechtskrankheiten* 45(1970):187–188.

59. R. Frühwald, "Oskar Kieß" in *Hautarzt* 6(1955):96; W. Gertler, "In memoriam Oskar Kiess" in *Dermatologische Wochenschrift* 131(1955):16; Schmidt, "Dermato-Venerologie," pp. 61ff.

60. Archives of the University of Munich, personnel file of Heinrich Höcker, PHA Höcker.

61. K. Halter, "In memoriam Erich Langer" in *Hautarzt* 9(1958):47–48; Scholz, Eppinger, Löscher, Scholz, and Weyers, "Dermatologie im Nationalsozialismus."

62. E. Landes and I. Menzel, *Geschichte der Universitätshautklinik in Frankfurt am Main* (Berlin: Grosse–Verlag, 1989), pp. 36f.

63. I. Niemand-Anderssen, "G.A.Rost zum 80. Geburtstag" in *Dermatologische Wochenschrift* 135(1957);257–259; I. Niemand, "In memoriam Georg Alexander Rost, 1877–1970" in *Hautarzt* 22(1971):229.

64. A. Wiedmann, "In memoriam Johann Heinrich Rille (1864–1956)" in *Hautarzt* 8(1957):95–96.

65. E. Ernst, "A leading medical school seriously damaged: Vienna 1938" in *Annals of Internal Medicine* 122(1995):789–792.

66. J. Bleker and N. Jachertz (eds.), *Medizin im "Dritten Reich"* (Cologne: Deutscher Ärzte–Verlag, 1989), p. 44.

67. Archives of the University of Cologne, personnel file of Emil Meirowsky (UAK 27/55, 17/3694, UAK67/1.088).

68. Archives of the University of Frankfurt, personnel file of Franz Herrmann, PHA Herrmann.

69. Jakstat, *Geschichte der Dermatologie*, pp. 118–129.

70. A. Marchionini, Editorial. *Hautarzt* 1(1950):1.

71. S. Jablonska, "Alfred Marchionini zum 65. Geburtstag" in *Hautarzt* 15(1964):47–49.

GLOSSARY

Words that appear often in this glossary are common parlance in dermatology: A macule is a small, flat, discolored lesion; a patch is a broad, flat, discolored lesion; a papule is a small slightly elevated lesion; a nodule is a big papule; a tumor is a big nodule.

Acne is an inflammatory condition that chiefly affects adolescents and young adults. The most characteristic lesions are comedones—that is, hair follicles whose upper parts are dilated and whose openings to the skin surface are either widened (appearing as black spots, or blackheads) or occluded (appearing as white spots, or whiteheads). Other characteristic lesions are pustules, "zits" (papules), and, in severe cases, "goobers" (nodules), which may heal with scars. Acne involves hair follicles in regions of the skin in which sebaceous glands are abundant, such as the forehead, cheeks, and chin. The condition is so common that some students of the subject regard mild cases of acne as physiologic rather than pathologic.

Acrodermatitis chronica atrophicans is a cutaneous manifestation of infection by *Borrelia burgdorferi* that occurs months to years after transmission of that spirochete from deer or mice to humans via bites by ticks of the species *Ixodes dammini.* The disease starts with redness tinged with violet on the extensor aspects of extremities, especially the legs. After many months and sometimes years, the skin becomes so severely thinned that blood vessels positioned superficially in it are readily visible.

Acrodermatitis continua suppurativa is an uncommon pustular variant of psoriasis characterized by redness, scaling, and pustules situated at the tips of fingers and toes. When the pustular process is long-term, it may result in atrophy of fingertips and destruction of nails.

Adenoma sebaceum is a condition in which many tiny papules are situated in the center of the face. Each consists of a mixture of mature tissues (fibrous tissue, blood vessels, and distorted hair follicles) arranged in a disorganized fashion. The lesions appear early in childhood and persist for life. They are a sure sign of tuberous sclerosis, a hereditary disease associated with lesions in the brain (tubers), retina (phakomas), and viscera, as well as with mental retardation and seizures.

Alopecia mucinosa is typified by plaques punctuated by accentuation of ostia of hair follicles and by loss of hair. The name derives from the combination of loss of hair (alopecia) and presence within follicles of abundant mucin (mucinosis).

Amyloidosis designates a heterogeneous group of diseases characterized by accumulation of insoluble proteins with particular tinctorial and ultrastructural properties (amyloid) that are deposited in various tissues of the body. The source of amyloid varies; it may be derived from immunoglobulins (in patients with multiple myeloma) or from other proteins such as keratin (in persons with macular and papular lesions of amyloidosis in the skin). Accumulation of amyloid in internal organs may result in morbidity and even mortality (for example, renal failure, cardiomyopathy, and Alzheimer's disease).

Amyloidosis nodularis atrophicans (nodular localized cutaneous amyloidosis) is a manifestation of extramedullary plasmacytoma characterized by single or multiple papules or nodules in a circumscribed area of the skin. Amyloid is derived from immunoglobulin light chains produced by neoplastic plasma cells at the site of the lesion.

Anthralin (dithranol, Cignolin) is a synthetic derivation of chrysarobin that, for many years, was considered to be the best topical treatment of psoriasis vulgaris. The mechanism of its beneficial effects has never been elucidated, but anthralin has been shown to influence several enzymes that are involved with the regulation of inflammation and epidermal proliferation. When applied to the skin, anthralin has an irritating and staining effect that diminishes its applicability on an outpatient basis. Because of its irritating effects, treatment with anthralin has to be monitored carefully.

Apocrine glands release a product into the lumen of the gland by pinching off the distal part of their glandular cells' cytoplasm. In humans, apocrine glands are found in the axillae, areolae, perineal and circumanal regions, prepuce, scrotum, mons pubis, and labia minora. Ceruminous glands of the ear canals, Moll's glands of the eyelids, and mammary glands of the breasts are all characterized by apocrine secretion. Except for the mammary gland, which secretes colostrum (milk) during lactation, the function of apocrine glands in humans has yet to be determined. In lower animals, the products of apocrine glands serve as a pheromone.

Aschoff's bodies, a sign of rheumatic myocarditis, are collections of macrophages (histiocytes) in the muscle of the heart.

Atopic dermatitis is a skin disease of persons who have a diathesis to allergies such as allergic rhinitis (hay fever) and allergic asthma. The skin of patients with these allergies sometimes is extraordinarily itchy, and in response to the maddening pruritus, furious scratching and vigorous rubbing ensue, the result being disease in the form of erosions, ulcerations, and crusts, all of which are secondary to scratching, and marked thickening of the skin consequent to rubbing. The lesions are found mostly on the neck and the flexural aspects of knees and elbows of children and young adults, but other sites and age groups may be affected.

Auspitz phenomenon denotes the appearance of bleeding points on the surface of a lesion of psoriasis after scales have been yanked from it.

Behçet's disease consists of multiple, recurrent aphthous ulcers in the mouth and on genital skin, and lesions in the eye, especially the retina, and the brain. The cause of this multisystem disorder is not known.

Borrelia are a genus of spirochetes—that is, motile, unicellular, spiral-shaped bacteria that cause Lyme borreliosis, a chronic multisystem disease that follows transmission of *Borrelia burgdorferi* from deer or mice to humans by way of the bite of a tick. At the site of the bite, a centrifugally expanding red ring (erythema chronicum migrans) may develop within a few days or weeks. After weeks or months, a bluish-red nodule (lymphocytoma cutis) may appear at the site of the bite or at another location. Cutaneous signs that tend to develop months or years after the bite are acrodermatitis chronica atrophicans and morphea (circumscribed scleroderma). Extracutaneous manifestations of borreliosis, known also as Lyme disease and Lyme borreliosis, are enlarged lymph nodes, arthritis, pericarditis, polyneuropathy, meningitis, and encephalitis.

Borst-Jadassohn phenomenon refers to nests of abnormal epithelial cells that are sharply demarcated from epithelial cells of the surrounding normal epidermis. Formerly thought to represent a specific neoplasm, i.e., the Borst-Jadassohn intraepidermal epithelioma, the condition is now regarded as a nonspecific pattern that may be observed in a variety of epithelial neoplasms—for example, the benign seborrheic keratosis and the malignant Bowen's disease.

Bullous pemphigoid, a disease of the elderly, consists of widespread blisters that develop as a consequence of the effects of autoantibodies against components of the epidermal basement membrane. The blisters may be small (vesicles), but more often are large (bullae). They often appear on red urticarial plaques.

Buschke-Löwenstein tumor is a type of warty-appearing squamous cell carcinoma caused by carcinogenic human papillomavirus. It usually occurs on the uncircumcised penis but also can be seen elsewhere in the anogenital region, such as near the anus and on the vulva. It presents itself as a large, verrucous or fungating, cauliflower-like mass that penetrates slowly but persistently, eventually destroying deeper tissues. Rarely does it metastasize.

Busse-Buschke disease is an eponymic designation for cryptococcosis, an infection caused by the encapsulated yeast *Cryptococcus neoformans*. The organism has a marked predilection for the brain and meninges, but the lungs and other tissues also may be affected. In the skin, cryptococcosis usually presents itself as an ulcerated nodule or plaque. The infection tends to occur in persons who are immunosuppressed.

Cicatricial pemphigoid is a blistering disease that affects the conjunctivae and oral mucous membranes as well as the skin. It results from the effects of autoantibodies directed against a component of the epidermal basement membrane. As a consequence, the epidermis becomes detached from the dermis. The scarring that results from injury to the dermis may lead to blindness when eyes are affected and death when the gastrointestinal tract is severely involved.

Contact dermatitis is an inflammatory response of the skin to substances applied externally and is manifested by redness and formation of blisters that vary from tiny to large. Irritant contact dermatitis results from the direct effects of external substances (toxicity), whereas allergic contact dermatitis is mediated by immunologic mechanisms (allergy).

Darier's disease is a hereditary disorder in which keratotic papules and plaques appear mostly on the chest, back, ears, nasolabial folds, forehead, scalp, and groin. Nails and mucous membranes may also be affected. The lesions begin to develop at the end of the first decade of life.

Dermabrasion is planing of the skin by mechanical means for purposes of removal of superficial scars and other pathologic conditions, such as superficial benign and malignant neoplasms. Motor-driven abraders are equipped with a rotating wire brush or diamond fraise. If dermabrasion is not confined to removal of tissue in the epidermis and uppermost part of the dermis, it causes scars to form.

Dermatitis bullosa praetensis, also known as phytophotodermatitis, is a phototoxic dermatitis usually encountered in persons who lie in grass after swimming (*pratum* is Latin for grass). Contact with wet skin enables substances of grass and weeds to penetrate into the uppermost part of the epidermis—that is, the horny layer. Under the influence of ultraviolet light, the toxic substances react with proteins in the epidermis, thereby inducing an inflammatory response characterized by redness and blisters.

Dermatofibrosarcoma protuberans is a malignant neoplasm—a sarcoma—capable of infiltrative and destructive growth, but with little tendency for metastases. It usually presents itself as a nodule, plaques, or tumor on the upper part of the trunk or the proximal part of the extremities.

Dermatomyositis is an uncommon autoimmune disease characterized by the combination of muscle weakness and distinctive skin lesions, among them lividity resulting from widely dilated superficial blood vessels on swollen eyes, forehead, and cheeks, and flat-topped papules with central atrophy over the dorsal surfaces of joints of fingers (Gottron's papules), as well as strikingly dilated vessels in the skin of the proximal margin of fingernails. Apart from skin and muscles, the joints, heart, lungs, and other organs may be affected by the inflammatory process. The result may be potentially fatal complications, such as cardiac arrhythmias and pulmonary fibrosis.

Dowling-Degos disease is a hereditary disorder in which numerous brown macules appear, especially in the axilla and groin. Lesions begin to develop in adult life and extend slowly in symmetrical fashion.

Eczematoid purpura is a variant of progressive pigmented purpuric dermatosis characterized by more pronounced inflammation and scaling than other clinical variants of the disease. The condition consists of macules and papules, which at first are red and purple and later become yellow and brown, on the skin of the anterior surface of the legs. The purple color results from extravasation of red blood cells from small blood vessels in the upper part of the dermis. Eventually, the color of skin lesions changes because of an accumulation of siderophages (macrophages containing brown hemosiderin that is derived from ingested red blood cells).

Epidermolysis bullosa dystrophica Hallopeau-Siemens is a hereditary disease in which blisters on the skin and mucous membranes are induced by slight trauma and heal with scars. The disease presents itself at birth and persists thereafter, eventually leading to atrophic scars that cause contractions of the knees, elbows, and wrists; fusion of fingers and toes in mitten-like encasements and, in time, loss of them; and oral, pharyngeal, and esophageal strictures that impair eating. Death often ensues within the first three decades of life.

Epidermolysis bullosa simplex of Köbner is a hereditary disease in which blisters form and heal without scarring. The blisters begin to develop early in infancy and appear especially on the extensor surfaces of extremities, hands, and feet. The disease lasts for a lifetime, but tends to improve after puberty.

Epilepsy refers to any transient disturbance of electrical activity in the brain that is manifested as episodic impairment or loss of consciousness, abnormal motor activity, and psychic or sensory disturbances. A single episode is called a *seizure*. Most types of epilepsy are not inherited.

Erysipeloid is an acute infection by the bacterium *Erysipelothrix rhusiopathiae* and occurs in fishermen, butchers, and others who handle raw meat, poultry, and fish. The bacteria usually are inoculated from those contaminated products through a tiny break in the skin of the hands. After a few days, a violaceous, swollen, sharply circumscribed lesion develops at the site of inoculation. Lymphangitis, enlarged lymph nodes, fever, malaise, and, rarely, bacteremia and endocarditis may ensue.

Erythema chronicum migrans is a cutaneous manifestation early in the course of infection by the spirochete *Borrelia burgdorferi*. It usually occurs a few weeks after transmission of *Borrelia* at the site of the bite of a tick. It is characterized by a red patch that slowly spreads centrifugally, sometimes covering a large part of the body. Erythema chronicum migrans disappears after a few weeks, even in the absence of treatment. It may, however, be followed by signs of systemic infection by the spirochete.

Erythema infectiosum, known also as fifth disease, is an infectious disease caused by a parvovirus. It affects children mostly and leaves them with lifelong immunity. The disease usually begins with headache, cough, and low-grade fever. After about two days a rash develops, usually beginning on the cheeks and conveying the impression of their having been slapped. As the facial rash fades over a period of one to four days, a lacy, reticulate eruption of pink erythematous macules and papules develops on the trunk, neck, and extensor surfaces of the extremities. The disease usually resolves in one to two weeks, but may recur or persist for months.

Fibroepithelial tumor of Pinkus is a variant of basal-cell carcinoma that presents itself, usually on the trunk, as a smooth, sessile nodule.

Finkelstein's disease is a distinctive expression of allergic vasculitis that occurs in children up to two years of age, usually after an infection of the upper respiratory tract. It manifests itself, often on the face, as swollen, purple, rosette-shaped lesions that usually resolve without treatment.

Frei test has been used to establish the diagnosis of lymphogranuloma venereum, a venereal disease that is caused by *Chlamydia trachomatis* and that manifests itself as one or more ulcers on genital skin. The test is positive if a papule develops forty-eight hours after intradermal injection of material prepared from the causative organisms grown on chick embryo yolk sacs. The Frei test, introduced in 1930, has been replaced by diagnostic tests for lymphogranuloma venereum that are more sensitive and more specific.

Gaucher's disease is a lipidosis caused by deficient activity of an enzyme necessary for degradation of the lipid molecule, glucocerebroside. As a consequence of the deficiency, that lipid accumulates in various organs. The liver and spleen become enlarged, and thrombocytes and erythrocytes become reduced in number. There is also jaundice, bone lesions, and impairment of the central nervous system.

Gonorrhea is a sexually transmitted bacterial infection caused by the gram-negative diplococcus *Neisseria gonorrhoeae*. Men and women usually develop an acute urethritis with pain on urination and a purulent discharge from the urethra. Women may also develop signs of acute inflammation of the fallopian tubes. Some infected women, and less often men, may remain asymptomatic and be carriers of the bacteria, capable of spreading the disease.

Gottron's papules, characteristic clinical signs of dermatomyositis, are purple, flat-topped papules that occur over the dorsal surfaces of the joints of fingers. Eventually they develop central atrophy, which is expressed as white depressions in the skin.

Grenz rays are poorly penetrating ionizing rays that were used to treat a host of superficial skin diseases, ranging from palmoplantar psoriasis to mycosis fungoids, because they are effective without causing damage to deeper structures. Better treatments for those disease are now available, and Grenz rays are no longer used.

Haber's syndrome is a rare familial disease in which the cheeks, nose, forehead, and chin are flushed permanently and show a combination of redness, dilation of small superficial blood vessels, widened ostia of hair follicles, small scaly papules, and tiny atrophic pits. It is probably a variant of rosacea.

Hair disc is reputed to be a type of nerve ending positioned at the junction of epidermis and dermis. It is thought to be a slow-adapting touch receptor present in mammalian skin, but it is not visible in sections of human skin stained conventionally and viewed by light microscopy.

Huntington's chorea is a hereditary disease characterized by a wide variety of ceaseless, rapid, complex, jerky, dyskinetic movements that appear to be coordinated but that are involuntary. The disease, which usually begins in the fourth decade of life, takes a chronic progressive course, terminating in dementia. Death usually follows within fifteen years.

Hydroa vacciniformia is a rare photodermatosis characterized by the development of crops of blisters after exposure to ultraviolet light. The blisters tend to recur and resolve with tiny superficial scars. The disease usually begins in childhood, occurs only during the summer, and generally improves or disappears in adolescence. Its cause is unknown.

Hyperkeratosis denotes thickening of the uppermost part of the epidermis—to wit, the stratum corneum. On palpation, hyperkeratotic lesions usually feel rough.

Incontinentia pigmenti is a hereditary disease linked to the female sex (X) chromosome. Males do not have the disease because carriers of it die in utero. The disease presents itself at birth with rows of blisters on the extremities that, after a few months, eventuate in verrucous keratoses that eventually regress, leaving behind whorled streaks of brown pigmentation. Mental retardation, seizures, microcephaly, and other disorders of the central nervous system occur in about one-third of patients.

Jarisch-Herxheimer reaction is a transient immunologic reaction that commonly occurs in patients being treated for secondary syphilis with antibiotics. It is typified by fever, chills, headache, myalgias, and exacerbation of the skin lesions. The reaction has been attributed to liberation of substances released from the dead or dying spirochetes, but its precise mechanism is unclear.

Kaposi's sarcoma is a proliferation of abnormal small blood vessels that results in formation of blue-red, purple, or dark brown macules, papules, and nodules. Kaposi's sarcoma is probably caused by a virus. It occurs in three different clinical settings: in elderly patients of Mediterranean background; on the legs of Africans, especially children, in widespread fashion; and in patients who are immunosuppressed, such as those with acquired immunodeficiency syndrome in whom lesions are widespread on the skin and in other organs.

Keratoacanthoma is a distinctive type of squamous cell carcinoma that usually has a domed shape with a central keratinous crater. When solitary, it is typified by rapid growth from papule to nodule to tumor. Unlike other types of squamous cell carcinoma, keratoacanthoma of the solitary type tends to involute without therapy. In some immunosuppressed patients, however, it may metastasize. There are other variants of keratoacanthoma, all of which are squamous cell carcinomas and none of which involute spontaneously.

Keratoderma is the name applied to a heterogeneous group of diseases marked by hyperkeratoses of the palms and soles. Some keratodermas are hereditary, whereas others are not.

Keratosis lichenoides chronica (Nékám's disease) is characterized by violaceous papules and nodules arranged in a linear and reticulate pattern on the extremities, especially the hands and feet. It is probably one of the many clinical patterns that results from scratching vigorously for many years.

Langerhans' cells are derived from bone marrow from whence they home to stratified epithelia, among them the epidermis, as well as to other sites such as the dermis, thymus, tonsils, and lymph nodes. At those sites, they take up antigens, process them, and present them to specifically sensitized T lymphocytes, resulting in proliferation of those lymphocytes in preparation for their destroying threats to the host, such as infectious agents and allergens. Langerhans' cells are crucial for generation of immune responses by the epidermis, and in that capacity, they represent the most distant outpost of the immune system.

Leishmaniasis is an infection with *Leishmania*, parasites of worldwide distribution. *Leishmania* multiply in the gastrointestinal tract of female sandflies and are injected into mammalian hosts as the flies enjoy a blood meal from them. Different species of *Leishmania* are pathogenic for humans and may produce a variety of diseases that include plaques on the skin and mucous membranes, and lesions in viscera.

Leprosy is a chronic, slowly progressive infectious disease caused by *Mycobacterium leprae* and typified by the development of lesions on the skin, mucous membranes, nerves, bones, and viscera. It is manifested by a spectrum of clinical pictures that range from diffuse lesions teeming with bacteria in patients with poor immune response (lepromatous leprosy) to discrete lesions with only a few or no bacteria in patients with well-developed immunity (tuberculoid leprosy). Because cutaneous nerves often are involved by the bacteria, skin lesions of tuberculoid leprosy often are anesthetic.

Lichen amyloidosis is one of many different responses to long-standing scratching and rubbing. Clinically, it is characterized by densely aggregated, uniform, dome-shaped papules situated mostly on the legs. It is called *amyloidosis* because globules of amyloid accumulate in the uppermost part of the dermis. The amyloid is derived from cells of the epidermis that die secondary to the effects of animated scratching and then drop into the dermis.

Lichen nitidus is an uncommon eruption of tiny, sharply defined, skin-colored papules that affects the penis, arms, and abdomen, especially of children. The disease usually resolves after several years. Its cause is unknown.

Lipoid proteinosis (hyalinosis cutis et mucosae, Urbach-Wiethe disease) is an uncommon hereditary disease characterized by the accumulation of basement membrane–like material in various connective tissues, among them those of skin and mucous membranes, where they appear as papules. The nature of the material has not yet been clarified. When the papules in the respiratory tract become larger, they can compromise breathing and result in death.

Lupus erythematosus tumidus is a variant of discoid lupus erythematosus characterized by smooth-surfaced plaques that are replete with mucin.

Lymphangioma is a benign proliferation of lymphatic vessels that in the skin presents itself as many tiny blister-like lesions in a circumscribed zone. The appearance of the lesions has been likened to the eggs of frogs.

Lymphocytic infiltration of Jessner is a smooth-surfaced plaque made up largely of mucin and dense infiltrates of lymphocytes around dermal blood vessels. It probably is synonymous with the tumid variant of discoid lupus erythematosus.

Lymphogranuloma venereum is a sexually transmitted disease caused by *Chlamydia trachomatis*. After inoculation of the micro-organism, a soft, painless erosion develops. One or two weeks after the appearance of the primary lesion, lymph nodes in the inguinal regions enlarge. Rupture of fluctuant lymph nodes may result in formation of sinuses. Systemic symptoms often accompany involvement of skin and lymph nodes by the organisms of lymphogranuloma venereum.

Mantle of the hair follicle is a cloak-like cord of undifferentiated epithelial cells that emanates from the follicle and gives rise at puberty to the entire sebaceous unit, namely, sebaceous glands and ducts.

Mastocytosis is a neoplastic process characterized by infiltrates of mast cells in the skin, bone marrow, liver, spleen, lymph nodes, and gastrointestinal tract. It often is accompanied by flushing, wheels, abdominal pain, nausea, and diarrhea. The cutaneous manifestation of mastocytosis is known as urticaria pigmentosa. Although the condition usually is benign, a rare malignant analogue exists.

Meirowsky phenomenon is a darkening of already existing epidermal melanin beginning within seconds and completed within minutes to a few hours after exposure to long-wave ultraviolet radiation. It was observed originally in cadavers, thereby excluding active synthesis of melanin as a cause of the pigmentation.

Melanocytes are cells that synthesize melanin, a substance that scatters and absorbs light and that thereby protects the skin from the damaging effects of ultraviolet light. Melanocytes are found chiefly in the basal layer of the epidermis, but also at sites such as the iris and the retina of the eyes. The amount of melanin in the epidermis determines the degree of color of the normal skin.

Melkersson-Rosenthal syndrome is the triad of severely wrinkled tongue, paralysis of the muscles of expression on one side of the face, and swelling of the lips and cheek of that side of the face. The cause of Melkersson-Rosenthal syndrome is unknown, but at times it may be associated with Crohn's disease.

Microsporum is one of three genera of superficial fungi (dermatophytes), the two others being *Trichophyton* and *Epidermophyton.* Dermatophytes live only in cornified (fully mature) epithelial cells of the epidermis and its appendages, hairs and nails. Because skin lesions of dermatophytes are usually circular with raised borders and tend to expand centrifugally, the condition is known colloquially as ringworm.

Mycosis fungoides is a lymphoma that usually is manifest first in the skin as ill-defined patches and, in most patients, persists as slowly expanding patches for the lifetime of the patient. In some patients, however, plaques, nodules, and tumors develop. Signs of systemic lymphoma appear in some patients, usually those with nodules and tumors, and systemic involvement may lead to death.

Necrobiosis lipoidica is a chronic inflammatory disease of the skin that is observed especially in patients with diabetes mellitus. It is characterized by yellow plaques on the skin of the anterior aspects of the legs. In time, the plaques resolve as atrophic patches.

Neurofibromatosis generalisata of von Recklinghausen is a relatively common hereditary disease characterized by developmental changes in the nervous system, muscles, bones, and skin. The most common clinical manifestations are café-au-lait spots (sharply defined, hyperpigmented patches), neurofibromas (benign neoplasms of Schwann cells), glioma of the optic nerve, reddish-white spots on the iris, and skeletal changes such as thinning of long bones.

Nevus sebaceus is a mixture of elements found normally in the skin but that are flawed either in appearance and/or in arrangement. It presents itself as a single lesion on the face or scalp, usually at birth or in early childhood. At that beginning stage it is a slightly raised, sometimes linear, hairless patch or plaque. With the efflorescence of sebaceous glands at puberty, the lesion becomes yellow because those glands are filled with lipid. In time, a variety of benign and malignant neoplasms may arise in a nevus sebaceus. An extensive lesion of nevus sebaceus may be accompanied by other types of skin lesions, neurologic defects, and skeletal deformities.

Nonbullous ichthyosiform erythroderma is a rare hereditary disease that presents itself at birth with redness of the entire skin. Newborns with the condition are often enveloped by a colloidionlike membrane that restricts movement. When the membrane is shed soon after birth, large, closely approximated scales appear, especially in the flexures and on palms and soles. Redness and scaling persist throughout life, although they may fade somewhat in some patients.

Nummular dermatitis is an inflammatory skin disease of unknown cause in which tiny blisters congregate in coin-shaped lesions on the trunk and extremities. In time, the itchy blisters are scratched away, leaving behind oozing, crusted, red plaques. The disease usually comes and goes episodically, and the lesions tend to recur for years.

Pachyonychia congenita is a hereditary disease in which increased nail thickness progresses to onychogryphosis, a clawlike deformity. Other signs of the disease are excessive sweating of palms and soles; hyperkeratosis of palms, soles, knees, and elbows; widespread tiny keratoses; white plaques on mucous membranes; and blisters, which sometimes follow trauma, on palms and soles.

Patch test is a method for validating a diagnosis of allergic contact sensitization and for identifying the causative agent. The test duplicates the events that lead to development of allergic contact dermatitis by exposing small zones of healthy skin to the presumed sensitizers in the form of small patches. The patches are removed after forty-eight hours, and if a person is sensitive to the applied agent, redness and vesicles occur at those sites.

Pautrier's microabscesses are collections of abnormal lymphocytes within the epidermis of a patient with mycosis fungoids. For years, these collections, which are not true abscesses, were thought to be specific to mycosis fungoids, but they are known now to occur in other lymphomas and to be seen in only a minority of lesions of mycosis fungoides.

Pemphigus vegetans is an expression of pemphigus vulgaris, a blistering disease of skin and mucous membranes caused by antibodies directed against an antigen on the membrane of cells of surface epithelium. Sometimes, especially in intertriginous regions, lesions of pemphigus do not resolve in the usual fashion, but become strikingly heaped up..

Perifolliculitis capitis abscedens et suffodiens (dissecting cellulitis of the scalp), an uncommon variant of acne vulgaris, is characterized by follicular pustules on the scalp that rupture to form sinus tracts that heal with scarring. The condition is often accompanied by other manifestations of severe acne, such as conglobate lesions on the face, keloidal lesions over the occiput of the scalp, and lesions of hydradenitis suppurativa in the axillae and groin.

Pityriasis lichenoides is an inflammatory skin disease of unknown cause in which lesions may evolve rapidly as red or purple papules and papulovesicles (pityriasis lichenoides acuta or Mucha-Habermann disease) or slowly as scaly papules (pityriasis lichenoides chronica). The lesions come and go for many months and sometimes years, but usually disappear completely.

Poroma is a benign cutaneous neoplasm consisting of ductal cells like those of the ducts of eccrine and apocrine glands. It presents itself as a solitary, firm papule or nodule, usually on a sole or the side of a foot, a hand, or a finger.

Psoriasis is a common, chronic hereditary skin disease that is influenced by a variety of factors—for example, environmental and emotional ones—thereby causing it to have a fluctuating course with remissions and exacerbations of variable duration. Psoriasis manifests itself as sharply circumscribed red papules and plaques covered by prominent white scales. If the psoriatic process is accelerated, sterile pustules appear. Nails may be pitted, the tongue may show figurate lesions (geographic tongue), and arthritis may develop, especially in patients whose skin involvement is severe.

Pustular psoriasis of von Zumbusch is a caricature of the psoriatic process characterized by the sudden, explosive, widespread eruption of small, sterile pustules that emerge from bright red skin. The condition is usually accompanied by fever and lasts for days or weeks before resolving, only to recur again without warning.

Reiter's disease is a genetically determined condition characterized by arthritis, conjunctivitis, urethritis, and psoriasis, the latter being manifested as pustular and keratotic lesions on the feet, well-demarcated erosions with a slightly raised border on the glans penis, onychodystrophy, and typical psoriatic plaques on the extremities. Reiter's disease is often preceded by an infection of the gastrointestinal or genitourinary tract. It begins abruptly and follows a persistent course.

Rosacea is a chronic disease of the face of middle-aged and elderly persons, characterized by redness, dilated superficial blood vessels, papules, and pustules. It especially affects the chin, nose, perinasal regions, and central parts of the forehead. A distinctive feature of rosacea is remarkable enlargement of the nose, known medically as rhinophyma and colloquially as "rummy nose." The cause of rosacea is not known.

Sarcoidosis is a systemic inflammatory disease of unknown cause in which accumulations of tissue macrophages—that is, histiocytes—appear in various organs. In the skin, those collections manifest themselves as papules and plaques, often in annular configuration and widespread distribution, with a predilection for the periocular, paranasal, and perioral regions. The disease often involves lymph nodes, eyes, and lungs.

Schizophrenia is a heterogeneous group of mental disorders characterized by disturbances in form and content of thought (e.g., loosening of associations, hallucinations), mood (blunt, flattened, or inappropriate affect), decreased sense of self and of relationship to the external world (loss of boundaries of the ego and autistic withdrawal, etc.), and aberrant behavior (bizarre, apparently purposeless, and stereotyped activity or inactivity such as catatonia).

Scleredema of Buschke is a rare disease of connective tissue of unknown cause, characterized by symmetrical, poorly circumscribed, nonpitting induration of thickened skin that usually is most prominent on the neck and upper part of the back. The skin has a wooden consistency and may be red, waxy, and shiny. The condition affects all races, occurs in children and adults, and commonly is associated with diabetes mellitus.

Scleroderma unmodified refers to systemic sclerosis, a multisystem disease of unknown cause that affects connective tissue of the skin, lungs, gastrointestinal tract, kidneys, and heart. The most common cutaneous changes are purplish discoloration of fingers after exposure to cold, chronic swelling of hands and fingers eventuating in hardening of the skin, ulceration of fingertips, radial furrows around the mouth, loss of normal lines of facial expression resulting in a masklike appearance, and mats of dilated superficial blood vessels. In most patients, the disease is slowly progressive, but extensive cardiopulmonary and renal involvement may prove to be fatal. Sometimes, the disease progresses in fulminating fashion to death. So-called circumscribed scleroderma (morphea) and linear scleroderma are completely unrelated to systemic sclerosis. In some instances, they may represent a late manifestation of an infection by *Borrelia*.

Scleromyxedema is an uncommon, chronic disease characterized by tiny papules composed of an increased amount of mucin and collagen in conjunction with an increased number of fibrocytes. The papules are seen especially on the neck, lateral aspects of the face, forehead, and behind the ears. Scleromyxedema is commonly associated with an abnormality of serum proteins. The cause of the disease is unknown.

Sebaceous glands are lipid-producing glands that connect through ducts to the upper part of the hair follicle. The material manufactured by sebaceous glands is sebaceous secretion, which is conveyed by sebaceous ducts to the upper part of hair follicles and through the ostia of them onto the surface of the skin. When sebaceous secretion is joined by yeasts, bacteria, and mites housed within the upper part of a hair follicle, it is then termed *sebum*. The function of sebum is not known.

Seborrhea is considered conventionally to be overproduction of sebum and is most pronounced in areas with an abundance of large sebaceous glands, especially the nose and forehead.

Solar keratosis is an incipient squamous cell carcinoma induced by years of prolonged exposure to ultraviolet light. It presents itself as a keratotic papule or plaque on sun-damaged skin of adults, usually of pale-skinned older persons. If left untreated, a solar keratosis tends to progress slowly over years, but sometimes it may grow rapidly and become a nodule or tumor, in time even metastasizing as the squamous cell carcinoma that it is. Usually more than one solar keratosis is present in a particular individual.

Spirochetes are motile, unicellular, spiral-shaped bacteria that, when examined by dark-field microscopy, are seen to have a characteristic motility—namely, apparent rotation around their long axis in a boring corkscrew motion. Three genera of spirochetes are pathogenic for men: *Treponema*, which cause syphilis, yaws, and pinta; *Borrelia*, which cause relapsing fever and Lyme disease; and *Leptospira*, which cause Weil's disease.

Spongiform pustules are collections of neutrophils in sponge-like fashion in the upper part of the epidermis. They are distinctive histopathologically but are not specific, being seen in such disparate diseases as psoriasis, syphilis, and superficial fungal infections.

Sulzberger-Garbe disease was diagnosed often in the 1940s, when Sulzberger was the dominant force in American dermatology, but now it is considered to be a mere variant of nummular dermatitis that involves the penis and scrotum of adult Jews mostly.

Syphilis is a sexually transmitted disease caused by a spirochete, *Treponema pallidum*. If left untreated, the disease tends to progress in sequence from a firm ulcer at the site of infection (chancre of primary syphilis) to an exanthem after a few weeks secondary to systemic spread of spirochetes (secondary syphilis), to crusted nodules and ulcers on the skin, as well as involvement of the cardiovascular and central nervous systems after a latent period of many years (tertiary syphilis). Tertiary syphilis often is fatal.

Touton giant cells are multinucleated histiocytic giant cells with a central dark-staining core surrounded by nuclei in a rim and a periphery of pale foamy appearance. The cells can be found in a variety of inflammatory diseases, the best known of which is juvenile xanthogranuloma.

Trachoma is a chronic infectious disease of the conjunctiva and cornea manifested by photophobia, pain, and lacrimation. It is caused by a strain of the bacterium *Chlamydia trachomatis*. The severity of the disease ranges from slight inflammation to severe contractions and scarring that may result in blindness.

Trichodiscoma is a condition consisting of structures that resemble mantles of a normal hair follicle, but those structures, which represent undifferentiated sebaceous cells, are distorted and arranged in a peculiar fashion. When only undifferentiated sebocytes are present in cords within a lesion, it is called *fibrofolliculoma*; when sebaceous lobules are present, the same condition is termed *trichodiscoma*. Fibrofolliculomas and trichodiscomas usually present themselves as numerous, tiny, smooth-surfaced papules on the face, neck, trunk, and extremities.

Trichophyton schoenleinii is a major cause of favus, a severe form of fungal infection of the scalp that leads to destruction of hair follicles and permanent loss of hair. *Trichophyton schoenleini* was the first microbial pathogen of man to be identified, isolated, and established as a pathogen through experimental infection of an animal host.

Trypanosomes are flagellated parasites transmitted to vertebrates, including humans, by bloodsucking insects. Depending on the species of trypanosome, different diseases may result, including African trypanosomiasis (also known as African sleeping sickness) and American trypanosomiasis (also known as Chagas' disease).

Vohwinkel's syndrome, known also as mutilating keratoderma, is a hereditary disorder characterized by palmar and plantar keratoses arranged in a honeycomb fashion and by verrucous lesions on the dorsa of hands and feet. By the second decade of life, the keratotic lesions on fingers and toes compress underlying tissues and cause them to become constricted, eventuating in amputation of phalanges.

Xeroderma pigmentosum is a hereditary disease typified by markedly enhanced sensitivity to sunlight, with resultant development on sun-exposed sites of malignant neoplasms, especially basal cell carcinomas, squamous cell carcinomas, and melanomas.

BIBLIOGRAPHY

Ackerman, A.B. "Doctors may yet save the world." *American Journal of Dermatopathology* 6(1984):315–316.

———. "Remembering Hermann Pinkus." *Journal of Cutaneous Pathology* 12(1985):456–458.

Alexander, L. "Medical science under dictatorship." *New England Journal of Medicine* 241(1949):39–47.

Arzt, L. "In memoriam Franz Walter." *Hautarzt* 2(1951):94–95.

———. "In memoriam Hans Königstein." *Hautarzt* 5(1954):336.

———. "In memoriam Hofrat Professor Gustav Riehl anlässlich seines 100. Geburtstages." *Hautarzt* 6(1955):239–240.

Atermann, K., W. Remmele, and M. Smith. "Karl Touton and His 'Xanthelasmatic Giant Cell.'" *American Journal of Dermatopathology* 10(1988):257–269.

Aumüller, G., H. Lauer, and H. Remschmidt (eds.). *Kontinuität und Neuanfang in der Hochschulmedizin nach 1945*. Marburg: Schüren, 1997.

Baader, G., and U. Schultz (eds.). *Medizin und Nationalsozialismus: Tabuisierte Vergangenheit—ungebrochene Tradition? Dokumentation des Gesundheitstages. Berlin 1980*. 4th ed. Frankfurt: Mabuse-Verlag, 1989.

Baer, R.L. "In memoriam Alfred Hollander." *Hautarzt* 38(1987):58.

———. "Otto Braun-Falco zum 60. Geburtstag." *Hautarzt* 33(1982):242–243.

———. "Stephan Epstein zum 60. Geburtstag." *Hautarzt* 11(1960):431–432.

———. Personal communication, 1993.

Baer, R.L., J. Epstein, B. Epstein, et al. "A memorial to Marion Baldur Sulzberger." *Archives of Dermatology* 120(1984):857–858.

Baló-Banga, J.M. "Ludwig Nékám: 1868–1957. Ein verspäteter Nekrolog." *Hautarzt* 44(1993):54–55, 857–858.

Baumgartner, W. "Alfred Ruete: 1882–1951." *Dermatologische Wochenschrift* 124(1951):905–906.

Berenbaum, M. *The World Must Know: The History of the Holocaust as Told in the United States Holocaust Memorial Museum*. Boston: Little, Brown, 1993.

Beerman, H. "Alfred Hollander zum 75. Geburtstag." *Hautarzt* 25(1974):261.

————. "In memoriam Emil Meirowsky." *Hautarzt* 11(1960):335–336.

Benedum, J., and C. Giese. *375 Jahre Medizin in Giessen.* Giessen: Wilhelm Schmitz Verlag, 1983.

Betetto, M. "Franjo Kogoj zum 75. Geburtstag." *Hautarzt* 20(1969):477.

Beutelspacher, M.H., U. Brändle, A. Eberhardt, H. Haith, F. Mammel, H. Mausbach, B. Mausbach-Bromberger, A. Oesterle, M. Opielka, A. Panzer, J. Schübelin, M. Stahl, I. Stefanska, K. Wild, E. Wolff, and W. Wuttke. *Volk und Gesundheit: Heilen und Vernichten im Nationalsozialismus.* Frankfurt: Mabuse-Verlag, 1988.

Beyerchen, A., R. Bollmus, J. Caplan, J. Erger, A. Faust, G. Fischer, G.J. Giles, R.C. Kelly, A.F. Kleinberger, H. Küppers, V. Losemann, M. Messerschmidt, G. Miller, H. Scholtz, J. Stephenson, and E. Stranz. *Erziehung und Schulung im Dritten Reich. Vol. 2, Hochschule, Erwachsenenbildung.* Stuttgart: Klett-Cotta, 1980.

Biberstein, H.H. "In memoriam Kurt Wiener." *Hautarzt* 11(1960):561.

Bleker, J., and N. Jachertz (eds.). *Medizin im Dritten Reich.* Cologne: Deutscher Ärzte-Verlag, 1989.

Blumenthal, F., and H. Löhe. "Edmund Lesser zum 100. Geburtstag." *Dermatologische Wochenschrift* 125(1952):457–459.

Böhles, H.J., P. Chroust, R. Fieberg, U. Jordan, E. Meredig, W. Pusch, B. Reifenrath, B.W. Reimann, and C. Schröder. *Frontabschnitt Hochschule: Die Giessener Universität im Nationalsozialismus.* Giessen: Anabas-Verlag and Focus-Verlag, 1982.

Brauchle, A., and L.R. Grote. *Ergebnisse aus der Gemeinschaftsarbeit von Naturheikunde und Schulmedizin,* vol. 2. Leipzig: Reclam, 1939.

Braun-Falco, O. "Egon Keining zum 70. Geburtstag." *Hautarzt* 13(1962):477–479.

————."Walter F. Lever zum 60. Geburtstag." *Hautarzt* 20(1969):565–566.

Brill, E.H. "Rede zur Eröffnung des 17. Kongresses der Deutschen Dermatologischen Gesellschaft am 8.10.1934 in Berlin." *Archiv für Dermatologie und Syphilis* 172(1935):6–8.

Brnobic, A. "In memoriam Franjo Kogoj: 1894–1983." *Hautarzt* 35(1984):270–271.

Brockhaus Enzyklopädie in 20 Bänden. 7th ed. Wiesbaden: F.A. Brockhaus, 1966–1974.

Bromberger, B., H. Mausbach, and K.D. Thomann. *Medizin, Faschismus und Widerstand.* Frankfurt: Mabuse-Verlag, 1990.

Brunauer, S.R. "Maurice Oppenheim: 1876–1949." *British Journal of Dermatology* 62(1950):93–94.

Büchner, L., A. Scholz, and H. Jacobi. "In memoriam Walter Freudenthal: 1893–1952." *Der deutsche Dermatologe* 3(1994):350–352.

Bürger, M., G. Domagk, A. Leinbrock, and A. Marchionini. "In memoriam, Gedenkworte der Freunde für Otto Grütz." *Hautarzt* 15(1964):272–274.

Busch, W. *Die schönsten Bildergeschichten in Farbe*. Cologne: Buch und Zeit Verlagsgesellschaft GmbH, 1974.

Calnan, C. "Henry Haber (1900–1962)." *American Journal of Dermatopathology* 7(1985):537–539.

Capetanakis, J. "Christopher Doucas zum 70. Geburtstag." *Hautarzt* 11(1960):560.

Chagoll, L. *Im Namen Hitlers: Kinder hinter Stacheldraht*. Cologne: Pahl-Rugenstein Verlag, 1979.

Cohen, H.A. Personal communication, 1995.

Conti, L. "Gesundheitspflicht und Geschlechtskrankheiten. Bilanz einer erfolgreichen Bekämpfung." *Archiv für Dermatologie und Syphilis* 184(1943):7–21.

Crissey, J.T., and L.C. Parish. *The Dermatology and Syphilology of the Nineteenth Century*. New York: Praeger, 1981.

Curth, W., and H. Ollendorff Curth. "Remembering Abraham Buschke." *American Journal of Dermatopathology* 5(1983):27–29.

Dawidowicz, L.S. *The War Against the Jews, 1933–1945*. 10th anniversary ed. New York: CBS Educational and Professional Publishing, 1986.

Dejas-Eckertz, P., D. Ruckhaberle, A. Tebbe, K. Tebbe, and C. Ziesecke. *Faschismus*. Berlin: Elefanten Press Verlag GmbH, 1976.

Diepgen, P. *Die Heilkunde und der ärztliche Beruf*, 2nd ed. Berlin: Urban & Schwarzenberg, 1947.

Doerr, W. *Semper Apertus*. Sechshundert Jahre Ruprecht-Karls-Universität Heidelberg: 1386–1986. *Vol. 2, Das zwanzigste Jahrhundert: 1918–1985*. Berlin: Springer Verlag, 1985.

Drexler, S., S. Kalinski, and H. Mausbach. *Ärztliches Schicksal unter der Verfolgung 1933–1945 in Frankfurt am Main und Offenbach: Eine Denkschrift*. Frankfurt: VAS Verlag für Akademische Schriften, 1990.

Ehrenberg, I. "Leo Ritter von Zumbusch (1874–1940): Biobibliographie eines Münchner Dermatologen." Dissertation for the degree of Doctor of Medicine, Ludwig-Maximilians-University, Munich, 1987.

Ehring, F. *Hautkrankheiten: 5 Jahrhunderte wissenschaftlicher Illustration*. Stuttgart: Gustav Fischer Verlag, 1989.

Eichert, I. Personal communication, 1993.

Ernst, E. "A leading medical school seriously damaged: Vienna 1938." *Annals of Internal Medicine* 122(1995):789–792.

Fest, J.C. *Hitler*. 3rd ed. Frankfurt: Verlag Ullstein GmbH, 1992.

Feuerman, E.J. "In memoriam Felix Sagher," *Hautarzt* 34(1983):101.

Fischer, I. (ed.). *Biographisches Lexikon der hervorragenden Ärzte der letzten fünfzig Jahre*. 3rd ed. Vol. 2. Munich: Urban and Schwarzenberg, 1962.

Franzblau, M. "Nazi medical crimes unpunished 50 years later." *Dermatopathology: Practical and Conceptual* 2(1996):83–86.

Freund, H., and A. Berg (eds.). *Geschichte der Mikroskopie: Leben und Werk grosser Forscher*. Vol. 2. Frankfurt: Umschau-Verlag, 1964.

Frühwald, R. "Oskar Kiess." *Hautarzt* 6(1955):96.

Funk, C. "Heinrich Löhe zum 75. Geburtstag." *Hautarzt* 3(1952):382–383.

Gahlen, W. "In memoriam Philipp Keller: 1891–1973." *Hautarzt* 25(1974):361–362.

Gammel, J.A. "Hugo Hecht." *Hautarzt* 14(1963):383–384.

Gans, O. "Zum 100. Geburtstag von Karl Herxheimer." *Hautarzt* 12(1961):241–242.

———. "Zum 70. Geburtstag von Prof. Otto Grütz in Bonn." *Hautarzt* 7(1956):239–240.

Gebhard, B. "Hans Reiter." *Journal of the American Medical Association* 212(1970):323.

Geier, J. "Die Geschichte der dermatologischen Universitätsklinik in Göttingen von ihrer Gründung bis zum Umzug in das jetzige Kliniksgebäude." Dissertation for the degree of Doctor of Medicine, Georg-August-University, 1987.

Gentele, H. "In memoriam Carl Lennhoff." *Hautarzt* 16(1965):96.

Gertler, W. "Heinrich A. Gottron, 10.3.1890–3.6.1974." *Dermatologische Wochenschrift* 160(1974):962–963.

———. "In memoriam Oskar Kiess." *Dermatologische Wochenschrift* 131(1955):16.

Gindele, A.U. "Die Düsseldorfer Hautklinik und ihre historische Entwicklung von 1896–1982." Dissertation for the degree of Doctor of Medicine, Heinrich-Heine-University, 1991.

Golczewski, F. *Kölner Universitätslehrer und der Nationalsozialismus*. Köln: Böhlau-Verlag, 1988.

Gold, J.A., and F.G. Nürnberger. "A tribute to Abraham Buschke." *Journal of the American Academy of Dermatology* 26(1992):1019–1022.

Goldenbogen, N., S. Hahn, C.-P. Heidel, and A. Scholz. *Medizin und Judentum*. Dresden: Verlag des Vereins für regionale Geschichte und Politik Dresden e.V., 1994.

Goldhagen, D.J. *Hitler's Willing Executioners: Ordinary Germans and the Holocaust*. New York: Knopf, 1996.

Goldmann, F., and G. Wolff. *Tod und Todesursachen unter den Berliner Juden*. Berlin: Zentralwohlfahrtsstelle der Reichsvertretung der Juden in Deutschland, 1937.

Goldsmith, W.N. "Dr. Walter Freudenthal, 6th May 1893–27th March 1952." *Journal of Pathology and Bacteriology* 68(1954):649–650.

―――. "Wilhelm Siegmund Frei." *British Journal of Dermatology* 56(1944):187.

Gollnick, H., and K.H. Kühne. "Zum Gedenken an Dr. Otto Schlein (1895–1944), Arzt für Dermatologie und Venerologie in Magdeburg." *Hautarzt* 47(1996):395.

Gottlieb, G., and A.B. Ackerman. *Kaposi's Sarcoma: A Text and Atlas*. Philadelphia: Lea & Febiger, 1988.

Gottron, H.A. "Josef Vonkennel zum 60. Geburtstag am 9. August 1957." *Dermatologische Wochenschrift* 136(1957):869–872.

―――. "Karl Linser zum 70. Geburtstag am 10. September 1965." *Dermatologische Wochenschrift* 151(1965):1063–1068.

Götz, H. "In memoriam Alois Memmesheimer: 1894–1973." *Hautarzt* 24(1973):508–509.

―――. "In memoriam August Poehlmann." *Hautarzt* 5(1954):384.

―――. "In memoriam Theodor Grünberg: 1901–1979." *Hautarzt* 31(1980):465–466.

Grau, G., and P. Schneck (eds.). *Akademische Karrieren im "Dritten Reich."* Berlin: Medizinische Fakultät der Humboldt-Universität zu Berlin, Universitätsklinikum Charité, Institut für Geschichte der Medizin, 1993.

Greither, A. "In memoriam Josef Hämel." *Hautarzt* 20(1969):336–337.

―――. "In memoriam Walther Schönfeld (1888–1977)." *Hautarzt* 28(1977):504–505.

Grote, H. "Bestallungsentziehung der jüdischen Ärzte." *Deutsches Ärzteblatt* 68(1938):545–547.

Grüneberg, T. "Sigwald Bommer: 1893–1963." *Hautarzt* 14(1963):528.

Grütz, O. "In memoriam Franz Koch." *Hautarzt* 7(1956):191–192.

Haffner, S. *Anmerkungen zu Hitler*. Frankfurt: Fischer Taschenbuch Verlag GmbH, 1981.

Halter, K. "In memoriam Erich Langer." *Hautarzt* 9(1958):47–48.

Hamann, B. *Hitler's Wien: Lehrjahre eines Diktators*. Munich: Piper, 1996.

Hammerstein, N. *Die Johann Wolfgang Goethe-Universität Frankfurt am Main: Von der Stiftungsuniversität zur staatlichen Hochschule*. Vol. 1, 1914–1950. Neuwied: Alfred Metzner Verlag, 1989.

Hanauske-Abel, H.M. "Not a slippery slope or sudden subversion: German medicine and national socialism in 1933." *British Medical Journal* 313(1996):1453–1463.

Heinemann, M. (ed.). *Erziehung und Schulung im Dritten Reich*. Vol. 2, Hochschule, Erwachsenenbildung. Stuttgart: Klett-Cotta, 1980.

Hentschel, V. *So kam Hitler: Schicksalsjahre 1932–1933*. Düsseldorf: Droste Verlag, 1990.

Hermann, F. "Hans Biberstein." *Dermatologische Wochenschrift* 150(1964):617–618.

Herzberg, J. J. "In memoriam Heinrich Löhe: 1877–1961." *Hautarzt* 12(1951):334–335.

Herzberg, J. J., and G. W. Korting (eds.). *Zur Geschichte der deutschen Dermatologie: Zusammengestellt aus Anlass des XVII. Congressus Mundi Dermatologiae*. Berlin: Grosse Verlag, 1987.

Hiemer, E. *Der Giftpilz: Ein Stürmerbuch für Jung u. Alt.* Nuremberg: Verlag Der Stürmer, Nürnberg, 1938.

Hilberg, R. *Die Vernichtung der europäischen Juden.* Vol. 1. Frankfurt: Fischer Taschenbuch Verlag, 1990.

Hoede, K. "*Hautarzt* und Erbpflege." *Archiv für Dermatologie und Syphilis* 172(1935):25–29.

Hoffmann, E. "Alois Memmesheimer zum 60. Geburtstag am 14. Juli 1954." *Dermatologische Wochenschrift* 130(1954):767–768.

———. "Franz Blumenthal zum 75. Geburtstag." *Hautarzt* 4(1953):394–395.

———. "In memoriam Karl Herxheimer, Carl Touton und Friedrich Hammer." *Hautarzt* 1(1950):238–239.

———. Ringen um Vollendung: *Lebenserinnerungen aus einer Wendezeit der Heilkunde, 1933–1946.* Hannover: Schmorl and von Seefeld Nachf., Verlagsbuchhandlung, 1949.

———. "Zum X. Internationalen Dermatologenkongress in London: Über die bisherigen 9 Internationalen Dermatologenkongresse von 1889–1935." *Hautarzt* 3(1952):289–293.

Holitscher, A., and A. Turek. *Internationales ärztliches Bulletin: Zentralorgan der Internationalen Vereinigung Sozialistischer Ärzte.* Reprint, Jahrgang I-VI (1934–1939). Berlin: Rothbuch Verlag, 1989.

Hollander, A. "Development of dermatopathology and Paul Gerson Unna." *Journal of the American Academy of Dermatology* 15(1986):727–734.

———. "Geschichtliches aus vergangener Zeit: Politische Bekämpfung der Geschlechtskrankheiten?" *Fortschritte der Medizin* 99(1981):927–928.

———. "Das Lebenswerk von Paul Gerson Unna." *Dermatologische Monatsschrift* 160(1974):1–5.

———. "Oscar Gans (1888–1983)." *American Journal of Dermatopathology* 6(1984):87–88.

———. "The tribulations of Jewish dermatologists under the Nazi regime." *American Journal of Dermatopathology* 5(1983):19–26.

Holmsten, G. *Kriegsalltag 1939–1945 in Deutschland.* Düsseldorf: Droste Verlag, 1982.

Holubar, K. "Hans von Hebra (1847–1902) zum 150. Geburtstag: Ein Epitaph." *Hautarzt* 48(1997):276–277.

———. "Remembering Heinrich Auspitz." *American Journal of Dermatopathology* 8(1986):83–85.

———. Personal communication, 1995.

Holubar, K., C. Schmidt, and K. Wolff. *Challenge Dermatology: Vienna 1841–1992.* Vienna: Verlag der Österreichischen Akademie der Wissenschaften, 1993.

Holubar, K., and K. Wolff. "The genesis of American investigative dermatology from its roots in Europe." *Journal of Investigative Dermatology* 92(1989):14S–21S.

Hornstein, O. "Zur Erinnerung an Ernst Melkersson (1898–1932) und Curt Rosenthal (1892–1937)." *Hautarzt* 15(1964):515–516.

Hubenstorf, M. "Der Wahrheit ins Auge sehen." *Wiener Arzt* 5(1995):14–27.

Jablonska, S. "Alfred Marchionini zum 65. Geburtstag." *Hautarzt* 15(1964):47–49.

Jäckle, R. *Schicksale jüdischer und "staatsfeindlicher" Ärztinnen und Ärzte nach 1933 in München.* Munich: Liste Demokratischer Ärztinnen und Ärzte München, 1988.

Jadassohn, W. "In memoriam Wilhelm Lutz." *Hautarzt* 9(1958):527–528.

———. "Max Jessner zum 75. Geburtstag." *Hautarzt* 13(1962):562.

Jaensch, W. (ed.). *Konstitutions- und Erbbiologie in der Praxis der Medizin.* Leipzig: Johann Ambrosius Barth Verlag, 1934.

Jahn, R. Personal communication.

Jakobi, H., P. Chroust, and M. Hamann. *Aeskulap und Hakenkreuz: Zur Geschichte der MedizinischenFakultät in Giessen zwischen 1933 und 1945.* Frankfurt: Mabuse-Verlag, 1989.

Jakstat, K. *Geschichte der Dermatologie in Hamburg. Bibliotheca Diesbach.* Vol. 1. Berlin: Diesbach Verlag, 1987.

Johe, W. *Hitler in Hamburg.* Hamburg: Ergebnisse Verlag, 1996.

Johnson, P. *A History of the Jews.* New York: Harper/Perennial, 1987.

Jordan, P. "In memoriam W. Freudenthal." *Hautarzt* 3(1952):383–384.

Kalkoff, K.W. "In memoriam Carl Moncorps." *Hautarzt* 3(1952):143–144.

———. "Theodor Grüneberg zum 60. Geburtstag." *Dermatologische Wochenschrift* 143(1961):217–219.

Kanopik, J. "In memoriam Karel Gawalowski (1890–1965)." *Hautarzt* 17(1966):192.

Kater, M.H. *Doctors Under Hitler.* Chapel Hill, NC: University of North Carolina Press, 1990.

Keilig, W. "Zur Geschichte der Dermatologie in München." *Hautarzt* 3(1952):273–278.

Keller, P. "G. A. Rost zum 75. Geburtstag." *Dermatologische Wochenschrift* 125(1952):241–243.

———. "In memoriam Rudolf Leopold Mayer: 1895–1962." *Hautarzt* 14(1963):526–527.

Kimmig, J. "Walther Schönfeld zum 65. Geburtstag." *Hautarzt* 4(1953):239–240.

Kisch, B. "Forgotten leaders in modern medicine." *Transactions of the American Philosophical Society* 44(1954):227–296.

Klee, E. *Auschwitz, die NS-Medizin und ihre Opfer* Frankfurt: Fischer, 1997, pp. 288ff.

Klee, E. *Was sie taten—was sie wurden: Ärzte, Juristen und andere Beteiligte am Kranken— oder Judenmord.* Frankfurt: Fischer Taschenbuch Verlag, 1986.

Klemperer, V. *Ich will Zeugnis ablegen bis zum letzten.* Berlin: Aufbau Verlag, 1995.

Klüken, N. "In memoriam Rudolf Strempel: 1891–1981." *Hautarzt* 33(1982):49.

———. "Rudolf Strempel zum 65. Geburtstag." *Hautarzt* 7(1956):336.

Knierer, W. "In memoriam Julius Mayr." *Dermatologische Wochenschrift* 152(1966):817–818.

———. "Julius Mayr zum 75. Geburtstag." *Dermatologische Wochenschrift* 148(1963):169–170.

Knoth, W. "In memoriam Wilhelm Sevin: 1900–1976." *Hautarzt* 28(1977):58–59.

Koch, F. "In memoriam Friedrich Bering." *Hautarzt* 1:(1950)567–568.

Köhler, H. "Zum 60. Geburtstag von Rudolf Maximilian Bohnstedt." *Hautarzt* 11(1960):334–335.

Kogoj, F. "In memoriam Anton Tryb (1884–1960)." *Hautarzt* 12(1961):144.

———. "K. Gawalowski—70 Jahre." *Hautarzt* 12(1961):94–95.

Konrad, J. "Leo Kumer 1886–1951." *Dermatologische Wochenschrift* 125(1952):97–98.

Korting, G.W. "H.A. Gottron—Octogesimus." *Hautarzt* 21(1970):145–147.

Kresbach, H. "Anton Musger: 1898–1983." *Hautarzt* 35(1984):272–273.

Krutmann, J. *Die Geschichte der Universitäts-Hautklinik in Münster in Westfalen.* Herzogenrath: Verlag Murken-Altrogge, 1987.

Küster, W. "90 Jahre Düsseldorfer Hautklinik." *Hautarzt* 39(1988):114–116.

Kyrle. J. *Histo-Biologie der menschlichen Haut und ihrer Erkrankungen.* Vol. 1. Vienna: Verlag von Julius Springer, 1925.

Landes, E. "In memoriam Oscar Gans (1888–1983)." *Hautarzt* 34(1983):527–528.

Landes, E., and I. Menzel. *Geschichte der Universitätshautklinik in Frankfurt am Main.* Berlin: Grosse-Verlag, 1989.

Lautsch, H., and H. Dornedden. *Verzeichnis der deutschen Ärzte und Heilanstalten: Reichs-Medizinal-Kalender für Deutschland.* Part 2. Leipzig: Georg Thieme Verlag, 1937.

Leider, M. (ed.). "Sulzberger! Biography, autobiography, iconography: A posthumous festschrift." *American Journal of Dermatopathology* 6(1984):345–370.

Lesky, E. *Meilensteine der Wiener Medizin: Grosse Ärzte Österreichs in drei Jahrhunderten.* Vienna: Verlag Wilhelm Maudrich, 1981.

Leven, K.H. *100 Jahre klinische Dermatologie an der Universität Freiburg im Breisgau, 1890–1990.* Freiburg: Albert-Ludwigs-Universität Freiburg, Institut für Geschichte der Medizin, 1990.

Lever, W.F. "In memoriam Siegfried J. Thannhauser: 1885–1962." *Hautarzt* 14(1963):335–336.

Lever, W.F., and G. Schaumburg-Lever. *Histopathology of the Skin.* 7th ed. Philadelphia: Lippincott, 1990.

Leyh, F., and V. Wendt. "Heinrich A. Gottron (1890–1974)." *American Journal of Dermatopathology* 5(1983):241–243.

Lifton, R.J. *The Nazi Doctors: Medical Killing and the Psychology of Genocide.* New York: Harper Collins, 1986.

Lindemayr, W. "Alfred Wiedmann zum 60. Geburtstag." *Dermatologische Wochenschrift* 143(1961):321–322.

Löhe, H. "Josef Hämel zum 60. Geburtstag." *Dermatologische Wochenschrift* 130(1954): 1424–1425.

Long, E.R. *A History of Pathology*. New York: Dover Publications, 1965.

Lorant, S. *Sieg Heil! Eine deutsche Bildergeschichte von Bismarck zu Hitler*. Frankfurt: Zweitausendeins, 1979.

Lorincz, A.L. "In memoriam Stephen Rothman." *Hautarzt* 20(1969):429–430.

Lyell, A. "Hermann Pinkus (1905–1985)." *British Journal of Dermatology* 115(1986): 507–509.

Mann, G., A. Heuss, and A. Nitschke (eds.). *Weltgeschichte: Eine Universalgeschichte*. Gütersloh: Prisma Verlag, 1979–1980.

Marchionini, A. "Abschied von Leopold Arzt." *Hautarzt* 6(1955):335–336.

———. "Berta Ottenstein zum 60. Geburtstag." *Hautarzt* 2(1951):94.

———. "Fr. Kogoj zum 60. Geburtstag." *Hautarzt* 6(1955):479.

———. "Lucien Marie Pautrier zum 80. Geburtstag." *Hautarzt* 7(1956):382–384.

———. "Marion B. Sulzberger zum 60. Geburtstag." *Hautarzt* 6(1955):142–143.

———. "Persönliche Erinnerungen an Fritz T. Callomon." *Hautarzt* 16(1965):47–48.

———. "Viktor Kafka zum 70. Geburtstag." *Hautarzt* 2(1951):478–479.

Mayer, H. *Der Widerruf: Über Juden und Deutsche*. Frankfurt: Suhrkamp Verlag, 1994.

Mehregan, A.H,. and R.J. Schoenfeld. "Hermann K.B. Pinkus, M.D.: 1905–1985." *Journal of Cutaneous Pathology* 12(1985):453–455.

Memmesheimer, A. "Erich Hoffmann (1868–1959) zur Wiederkehr seines 110. Geburtstags." *Hautarzt* 29(1978):242–243.

———. "Ernst Sklarz 70 Jahre." *Hautarzt* 15(1964):577.

———. "Oscar Gans 75 Jahre." *Hautarzt* 14(1963):49.

Mergenthal, F. "Die Klinik für Haut- und Geschlechtskrankheiten- und ein merkwürdiger Entnazifizierungsfall." Düsseldorf, 1995.

Meyhöfer, W. "In memoriam Prof. Dr. R.M. Bohnstedt." *Zeitschrift für Haut- und Geschlechtskrankheiten* 45(1970):187–188.

———. Personal communication, 1993.

Michelson, H.E. "Felix Pinkus, M.D.: 1868–1947." *Archives of Dermatology and Syphilology (Chicago)* 57(1948):92–94.

———. "Forty-five years in the Chicago Dermatological Society." *Archives of Dermatology and Syphilogy (Chicago)* 85(1962):167–185.

Milde, P., and A.B. Ackerman. "A critical analysis of textbooks of dermatopathology in historical perspective." Parts 5, 8, and 12. *American Journal of Dermatopathology* 15(1993):85–95, 388–397; 16(1994):201–220.

Möhrle, A. "Der Weg zum Nürnberger Ärzteprozess und die Folgerungen daraus." *Deutsches Ärzteblatt* 93(1996):B-2170–2176.

Moncorps, C. "Leo Ritter von Zumbusch." *Münchener Medizinische Wochenschrift* 86(1940):516–517.

Montgomery, H. "Die Bedeutung von Oscar Gans für die amerikanische Dermatologie, zugleich eine persönliche Erinnerung." *Hautarzt* 14(1963):49–51.

Musger, A. "Albert Wiedmann zum 65. Geburtstag." *Hautarzt* 17(1966):190–191.

———. "Franz Kogoj zum 70. Geburtstag." *Hautarzt* 15(1964):577–578.

Mussgnug, D. "Siegfried Bettmann: 1869–1939." *Aktuelle Dermatologie* 17(1991):25–27.

Nasemann, T. "In memoriam Franz Herrmann: 1898–1977." *Hautarzt* 29(1978):506–507.

———. "Der Morphologe Hermann Werner Siemens und seine Bemühungen um eine 'Allgemeine Dermatologie.'" *Hautarzt* 34(1983):569–573.

Nékám, L. (ed.). Deliberationes Congressus Dermatologorum Internationalis IX–I. Vol. 4. Budapest, 1935.

Niemand, I. "In memoriam Georg Alexander Rost: 1877–1970." *Hautarzt* 22(1971):229.

Niemand-Anderssen, I. "G.A. Rost zum 80. Geburtstag." *Dermatologische Wochenschrift* 135(1957):257–259.

Nietz, O. "Herausbildung der Dermatologie als eigenständiges Fachgebiet in der Stadt Halle sowie Leben und Wirken der Direktoren der Hautklinik der Martin-Luther-Universität Halle-Wittenberg von 1894 bis 1949." Diploma thesis, Martin-Luther-University, 1986.

Ollendorff, C.H. "Erich Kuznitzky." *Hautarzt* 11(1960):288.

Orfanos, C.E. "Haim A. Cohen zum 75. Geburtstag." *Hautarzt* 40(1989):466–467.

Pinkus, H. "Etiology of an anatomist's discoveries in dermatology." *American Journal of Dermatopathology* 4(1982):127–135.

———. "Remembering Joseph Jadassohn." *American Journal of Dermatopathology* 7(1985):29–30.

Pleticha, H. *Deutsche Geschichte.* Gütersloh: Prisma Verlag, 1983–1984.

Polano, M.K. "H.W. Siemens zum 60. Geburtstage!" *Hautarzt* 2(1951):431–432.

Polemann, G. "Josef Vonkennel." *Dermatologische Wochenschrift* 148(1963):349–351.

Pospisil, L. "Zum 100. Geburtstag von Prof. Antonin Tryb." *Dermatologische Monatsschrift* 170(1984):349–350.

Proctor, R.N. *Racial Hygiene: Medicine Under the Nazis.* Cambridge, MA: Harvard University Press, 1988.

Proppe, A. *Ein Leben für die Dermatologie.* Berlin: Diesbach-Verlag, 1993.

———. "Erich Langer zum 65. Geburtstag." *Hautarzt* 7(1956):143–144.

————. "Hans Theo Schreus zum 60. Geburtstage." *Hautarzt* 3(1951):431–432.

————. "Horst-Günther Bode zum 60. Geburtstag." *Hautarzt* 15(1964):463–464.

————. "Prof. Dr. H. Th. Schreus zum 70. Geburtstag." *Dermatologische Wochenschrift* 146(1962):265–269.

Pross, C., and R. Winau. *Nicht misshandeln: Das Krankenhaus Moabit.* Berlin: Edition Hentrich im Verlag Frölich and Kaufmann, 1984.

Reiter, C. "Albert Jesionek—Sein Leben und wissenschaftliches Werk zur Tuberkulose der Haut unter besonderer Berücksichtigung seiner lichtbiologischen Forschung." D.D.S. diss., Justus-Liebig University, 1992.

Riecke, E. (ed.). *Deutsches Dermatologen-Verzeichnis: Lebens- und Leistungsschau.* 2nd ed. Leipzig: Johann Ambrosius Barth Verlag, 1939.

Riehl, G. "Gedenkworte für Moritz Oppenheim." *Hautarzt* 1(1950):95–96.

Röckl, H. "Karl Hoede zum 75. Geburtstag." *Hautarzt* 23(1972):382–383.

Roeder, W., and H.A. Strauss (eds.). *Biographisches Handbuch der deutschsprachigen Emigration nach 1933.* Vol. 1, Politik, Wirtschaft, Öffentliches Leben. Munich: Saur-Verlag, 1980.

Rook, A. "Ernst Sklarz zum 75. Geburtstag." *Hautarzt* 20(1969):478.

Rosen, I. "Fred Wise." *Hautarzt* 2(1951):95–96.

Rost, G.A. "Alfred Stühmer zum Gedächtnis." *Dermatologische Wochenschrift* 136(1957):1033–1035.

————. "Philipp Keller 65 Jahre alt." *Hautarzt* 7(1956):562.

Rüther, M. "Mit windigen Paragraphen wider die ärztliche Ethik." *Deutsches Ärzteblatt* 94(1997):A511–A515.

————. "Zucht und Ordnung in den eigenen Reihen." *Deutsches Ärzteblatt* 94(1997):A434–A439.

Saalfeld, U. "Ernst Sklarz zum 70. Geburtstag." *Dermatologische Wochenschrift* 150(1964):369–371.

Samman, P.D. "Henry Haber." *American Journal of Dermatopathology* 7(1985):541–542.

Sanderson, K.V. "Henry Haber." *American Journal of Dermatopathology* 7(1985):543–545.

Sarkowski, H. *Der Springer Verlag: Stationen seiner Geschichte.* Vol. 1, 1842–1945. Berlin: Springer-Verlag, 1992.

Schirren, C., and N. Reinhard. *Geschichte der Dermatologie in Norddeutschland.* Berlin: Grosse-Verlag, 1980.

Schlenzka, K., and B. Junge. "Schicksale Magdeburger jüdischer Dermatologen im Nazi-Reich: Carl Lennhoff und Otto Schlein." *Dermatologische Monatsschrift* 175(1989):307–312.

Schmidt, C. "Dermato-Venerologie im Nationalsozialismus—Die Neuordnung des Fachge-bietes durch personelle Veränderungen im akademischen Bereich, in den Fachgesellschaften und Herausgeberkollegien der Fachzeitschriften." M.D. diss., Carl Gustav Carus Medical Academy, 1990.

Schmidt, G., and F.M. Thurmon. "Zum Tode von Bertha Ottenstein (17. Juni 1956)." *Hautarzt* 11(1956):527–528.

Schmidt, W. *Leben an Grenzen: Autobiographischer Bericht eines Mediziners aus dunkler Zeit.* Frankfurt: Suhrkamp Taschenbuch Verlag, 1993.

Schmidt-La Baume, F. "In memoriam Karl Herxheimer." *Hautarzt* 4(1953):444.

Schneider, W. "Paul Linser zum 90. Geburtstag." *Hautarzt* 12(1961):430–431.

———. "Prof. Dr. Walter Schultze zum 70. Geburtstag am 1. Februar 1963." *Dermatologische Wochenschrift* 147(1962):257–259.

———. "Prof. Dr. Wilhelm Engelhardt zum 70. Geburtstag." *Dermatologische Wochenschrift* 152(1966):689–691.

———. "Wilhelm Sevin zum 60. Geburtstag." *Hautarzt* 11(1960):46–47.

Schnyder, U.W. "Tibor Salomon. 1914–1995." *Hautarzt* 47(1996):69.

Schoeps, J.H., and J. Schlör (eds.). *Antisemitismus: Vorurteile und Mythen.* Munich: Piper, 1995.

Scholz, A. "Der Suizid von Dermatologen in Abhängigkeit von politischen Veränderungen." *Hautarzt* 48(1997):929–935.

———. "Eugen Galewsky (1864–1935)." *Dermatologische Monatsschrift* 158(1972):53–68.

———. "Ludwig Halberstaedter (1876–1949)." *Dermatologische Monatsschrift* 162(1976):1015–1025.

———. "Rudolph Leopold Mayer. Werk und Persönlichkeit." *Dermatologische Monatsschrift* 167(1981):582–586.

———. "Zum 150. Geburtstag von Heinrich Köbner." *Dermatologische Monatsschrift* 175(1989):111–117.

Scholz, A., F. Ehring, and H. Zaun. *Exlibris berühmter Dermatologen.* Dresden: Institut für Geschichte der Medizinischen Fakultät "Carl Gustav Carus," 1995.

Scholz, A., S. Eppinger, S. Löscher, S. Scholz, and W. Weyers. "Dermatologie im Nationalsozialismus." Part of the poster presentation at the 39th Congress of the German Dermatological Society, Karlsruhe, 1997.

Scholz, A., and C. Schmidt. "Decline of German dermatology under the Nazi regime." *International Journal of Dermatology* 32(1993):71–74.

Scholz, A., and G. Sebastian. "Erinnerungen an Heinrich Auspitz zum 150. Geburtstag." *Dermatologische Monatsschrift* 172(1986):37–43.

Scholz, A., G. Sebastian, and J. Trnka. "Prager Dermatologie und der 1. Kongress der Deutschen Dermatologischen Gesellschaft 1889." *Hautarzt* 40(1989):652–659.

Schönfeld, W. "Die Beteiligung Heidelbergs an der Entwicklung der Dermatologie und Venerologie und die Heidelberger Hautklinik von 1904–1935." *Hautarzt* 6(1955):469–473.

———. "Die Geschichte der Würzburger Hautklinik bis 1939." *Hautarzt* 7(1956):134–137.

———. "Paul Richter." *Dermatologische Wochenschrift* 132(1955):1149–1155.

Schorr, W.F. "Stephan Epstein, M.D.: 1900–1973." *Archives of Dermatology* 108(1973):736.

Schreier, J., U.F. Haustein, and K.H. Karbe. "Zur Geschichte der Dermatologie an der Universität Leipzig." *Dermatologische Monatsschrift* 170(1984):1–14.

Schulze, W. "Alfred Stühmer zum 70. Geburtstag." *Dermatologische Wochenschrift* 131(1955):217–219.

Schultze, W. "Das Vorgehen gegen asoziale Geschlechtskranke" in *Dermatologische Wochenschrift* 36(1936):39–47.

———. "Die dermatologische Klinik der Universität Rostock: Ein Rückblick auf ihre Gründung und Entwicklung." *Hautarzt* 6(1955):84–88.

———. "In memoriam Alfred Stühmer." *Dermatologische Wochenschrift* 136(1957):1035–1037.

———. "Das Vorgehen gegen asoziale Geschlechtskranke." *Dermatologische Wochenschrift* 36(1936):1227–1229.

Sebastian, G., and A. Scholz. "Zum 150. Geburtstag von Filip Josef Pick." *Dermatologische Monatsschrift* 171(1985):123–127.

Seidelman, W.E. "Nuremberg lamentation: For the forgotten victims of medical science." *British Medical Journal* 313(1996):1463–1467.

Shelley, W.B., J.T. Crissey, and J.H. Stokes. *Classics in Clinical Dermatology*. Springfield, IL: Charles C. Thomas, 1953.

Shirer, W.L. *The Rise and Fall of the Third Reich: A History of Nazi Germany*. 30th anniversary ed. New York: Touchstone, 1990.

Siemens, H.W. "Referate. Gottron H.: Ausgewählte Kapitel zur Frage von Konstitution und Hauterkrankungen." *Zentralblatt für Haut- und Geschlechtskrankheiten* 52(1936):139–140.

———. "Referate. Gottron H.: Hautkrankheiten unter dem Gesichtspunkt der Vererblichkeit." *Zentralblatt für Haut- und Geschlechtskrankheiten* 52(1936):71–72.

Späte, H.F., and A. Thom. "Psychiatrie im Faschismus: Bilanz einer historischen Analyse." *Zeitschrift für die gesamte Hygiene und ihre Grenzgebiete* 26(1980):553–560.

Spier, H.W. "In memoriam Stephan Rothman (1894–1963)." *Hautarzt* 15(1964):145–146.

Spiethoff, B. Editorial in *Mitteilungen der Deutschen Gesellschaft zur Bekämpfung der Geschlechtskrankheiten* 31(1933):73.

Steffen, C. "Max Borst (1869–1946)." *American Journal of Dermatopathology* 7(1985):25–27.

Steigleder. G.K. "Franz Herrmann als Geburtstagsgruss." *Hautarzt* 14(1963):334–335.

Sticker, G. "Erblichkeit, Rassenhygiene und Bevölkerungspolitik." *Münchner Medizinische Wochenschrift* 80(1933):1931–1936, 1975–1980.

Stokes, J.H. "Erich Urbach, M.D.: 1893–1946." *Archives of Dermatology and Syphilology (Chicago)* 55(1947):545–547.

Strauss, H.A., and W. Roeder (eds.). *International Biographical Dictionary of Central European Emigres, 1933–1945.* Vol. 2, The Arts, Sciences, and Literature. Munich: Saur-Verlag, 1983.

Stresemann, G. *Wie konnte es geschehen? Hitler's Aufstieg in der Erinnerung eines Zeitzeugen.* Berlin: Ullstein, 1987.

Stroink, H. "Borst and the Von Brehmer incident." *American Journal of Dermatopathology* 7(1985):25–27.

Stühmer, A. "Erinnerungen an Paul Ehrlich." *Hautarzt* 5(1954):127–134.

———. "In memoriam P.W. Schmidt." *Hautarzt* 1(1950):191–192.

———. "Georg A. Rost zum 75. Geburtstag." *Hautarzt* 3(1952):141–143.

Sulzberger, M.B. "Hans Biberstein zum 70. Geburtstag." *Hautarzt* 10(1959):561–562.

———. "In memoriam George Miller MacKee: 1875–1955." *Hautarzt* 6(1955):431–432.

———. "Joseph Jadassohn: A personal appreciation." *American Journal of Dermatopathology* 7(1985):31–36.

———. "Max Jessner zum 70. Geburtstag." *Hautarzt* 8(1957):478–479.

———. "Rudolf L. Baer zum 60. Geburtstag." *Hautarzt* 21(1970):339–340.

Synnatzschke, R. "Paul Caesar Richter." *Dermatologische Wochenschrift* 136(1957):1055–1056.

Tappeiner, J. "Leopold Arzt zum 70. Geburtstag." *Dermatologische Wochenschrift* 127(1953):265–267.

———. "Prof. Dr. Leopold Arzt." *Dermatologische Wochenschrift* 132(1955):761–763.

Thom, A., and G.I. Caregorodcev. *Medizin unterm Hakenkreuz.* Berlin: VEB Verlag Volk und Gesundheit, 1989.

Tobis, M. "Die bisherige Organisation der österreichischen Ärzteschaft." *Deutsches Ärzteblatt* 68(1938):270.

Toellner, R. (ed.). *Illustrierte Geschichte der Medizin.* Salzburg: Andreas and Andreas, 1986.

Unna, P.G. "Ernst Delbanco." *Dermatologische Wochenschrift* 88(1929):260–261.

Unna, P.J. Personal communication, 1992.

Vasiljevic, A. "In memoriam Josip Fleger." *Hautarzt* 18(1967):95.

Vollmann, J., and R. Winau. "Informed consent in human experimentation before the Nuremberg code." *British Medical Journal* 313(1996):1445–1447.

Webster's New World Dictionary of the American Language. College Edition. Cleveland: The World Publishing Company, 1966.

Weindling, P. *Health, Race and German Politics Between National Unification and Nazism, 1870–1945*. Cambridge: Cambridge University Press, 1989.

Weiss, H. Personal communication.

Weyers, W. "Dermatology under the Swastika: Die Entwicklung der Dermatologie im Nationalsozialismus" (Thesis for habilitation, Justus-Liebig-University, Giessen, 1997), p. S33.

Wiedmann, A. "In memoriam Alfred Marchionini." *Hautarzt* 16(1965):193.

———. "In memoriam Johann Heinrich Rille (1864–1956)." *Hautarzt* 8(1957):95–96.

———. "J.H. Rille zum 90. Geburtstag." *Hautarzt* 5(1954):562.

———. "Stephan Robert Brunauer zum 75. Geburtstag!." *Hautarzt* 13(1962):382.

———. "Zum 70. Geburtstag von R. O. Stein." *Hautarzt* 1(1950):567.

Woringer, F. "In memoriam Lucien-Marie Pautrier (1876–1959)." *Hautarzt* 10(1959):431.

Zaruba, F. "In memoriam Jan Kanopik." *Hautarzt* 37(1986):689.

Zentner, C. *Illustrierte Geschichte des Dritten Reiches*. Eltville: Bechtermünz Verlag, 1990.

———. *Illustrierte Geschichte des Zweiten Weltkriegs*. Eltville: Bechtermünz Verlag, 1990.

Zentner, C., and F. Bedürftig. *Das grosse Lexikon des Dritten Reiches*. Munich: Südwest Verlag, 1985.

Zieler, K. "Rede zur Eröffnung des 17. Kongresses der Deutschen Dermatologischen Gesellschaft am 8.10.1934 in Berlin." *Archiv für Dermatologie und Syphilis* 172(1935):3–6.

———. "Rede zur Eröffnung des 18. Kongresses der Deutschen Dermatologischen Gesellschaft am 18.9.1937 in Stuttgart." *Archiv für Dermatologie und Syphilis* 177(1938):2–7.

———. "Rede zur Eröffnung des 20. Kongresses der Deutschen Dermatologischen Gesellschaft am 28.10.1942 in Würzburg." *Archiv für Dermatologie und Syphilis* 184(1943):3–6, 21–22.

Zierz, P. "Josef Vonkennel: 1897–1963." *Hautarzt* 14(1963):527.

———. "Walther Schönfeld zum 75. Geburtstag." *Dermatologische Wochenschrift* 147(1963):505–508.

NOTICES

Biberstein, Hans (notice). *Journal of the American Medical Association* 195(1966):333.

Blumenthal, Franz (notice). *Dermatologische Monatsschrift* 158(1972):244.

Brunauer, Stephan Robert (notice). *Journal of the American Medical Association* 208(1969):2171.

Callomon, Fritz Thomas (notice). *Journal of the American Medical Association* 190(1964):956.

Frei, Wilhelm Siegmund (notice). *British Journal of Dermatology* 56(1944):187.

Hecht, Hugo (notice). *Journal of the American Medical Association* 213(1970):478.

Hoede, Karl (notice). *Hautarzt* 24(1973):90.

Hoffmann, Erich (notice). *Zentralblatt für Haut- und Geschlechtskrankheiten* 48(1934):752.

Juliusberg, Fritz (notice). *Braunschweiger Werkstücke*. Vol. 35, Brunsvicensia Judaica. Braunschweig, 1966.

Reiter, Hans (notice). *Journal of the American Medical Association* 211(1970):821–823.

Sklarz, Ernst (notice). *British Medical Journal* 2(1975):449.

Uhlmann, Erich (notice). *Journal of the American Medical Association* 190(1964):798.

Wise, Fred (notice). *Journal of the American Medical Association* 144(1950):254.

ARCHIVES

Archives of the University of Bonn, personnel file of Otto Grütz.

Archives of the University of Bonn, personnel file of Erich Hoffmann.

Archives of the University of Bonn, personnel file of Carl Ludwig Karrenberg.

Archives of the University of Cologne, personnel file of Friedrich Bering, UAK 17/368a.

Archives of the University of Cologne, personnel file of Emil Meirowsky, UAK 27/55,
17/3694, UAK 67/1.088.

Archives of the University of Frankfurt, personnel file of Karl Altmann, PHA Altmann.

Archives of the University of Frankfurt, personnel file of Oscar Gans, PHA Gans 4/448, part 1.

Archives of the University of Frankfurt, personnel file of Franz Herrmann, PHA Herrmann.

Archives of the University of Frankfurt, personnel file of Martin Schubert, PHA Schubert.

Archives of the University of Freiburg, personnel file of Philipp Keller, PA Nr. B24, 3316.

Archives of the University of Freiburg, personnel file of Alfred Marchionini, PA Nr. B24, 2290.

Archives of the University of Freiburg, personnel file of Berta Ottenstein, PA Nr. B24, 2732;
PA Nr. B 101, 3397.

Archives of the University of Freiburg, personnel file of Georg Alexander Rost, PA Nr. B
24, 3045.

Archives of the University of Freiburg, personnel file of Paul Wilhelm Schmidt, PA Nr. B24,
3316.

Archives of the University of Freiburg, personnel file of Erich Uhlmann, PA Nr. B24, 3828.

Archives of the University of Giessen, personnel file of Rudolf Maximilian Bohnstedt, PHA
Bohnstedt.

Archives of the University of Giessen, personnel file of Robert Feulgen, PHA Feulgen.

Archives of the University of Giessen, personnel file of Walther Schultze, PHA Schultze.

Archives of the University of Göttingen, personnel file of Walther Krantz, PHA Krantz.

Archives of the University of Göttingen, personnel file of Erhard Riecke, PHA Riecke.

Archives of the University of Greifswald, personnel file of Wilhelm Richter.

Archives of the University of Halle, personnel file of Julius Dörffel, PA Nr. 5460.

Archives of the University of Heidelberg, personnel file of Siegfried Bettmann, PHA Bettmann.

Archives of the University of Heidelberg, personnel file of Walther Schönfeld, PHA Schönfeld.

Archives of the University of Heidelberg, personnel file of Fritz Stern, PHA Stern.

Archives of the University of Jena, personnel file of Josef Hämel, PHA Hämel, Bestand D, Nr. 2653.

Archives of the University of Jena, personnel file of Walther Schultze, PHA Schultze, Bestand D, Nr. 2653.

Archives of the University of Munich, personnel file of Rudolf Maximilian Bohnstedt, PHA Bohnstedt.

Archives of the University of Munich, personnel file of Heinrich Höcker, PHA Höcker.

Archives of the University of Munich, personnel file of Julius Mayr, PHA Mayr.

Archives of the University of Munich, personnel file of August Poehlmann, PHA Poehlmann.

Archives of the University of Tübingen, personnel file of Willy Engelhardt, PHA Engelhardt.

Archives of the University of Tübingen, personnel file of Heinrich Adolf Gottron, PHA Gottron.

Archives of the University of Tübingen, personnel file of Paul Linser, PHA Linser.

Archives of the University of Tübingen, personnel file of Karl Hermann Vohwinkel, PHA Vohwinkel.

Archives of the University of Würzburg, personnel file of Karl Hoede, PHA Hoede.

Archives of the University of Würzburg, personnel file of Karl Zieler, PHA Zieler.

Public Record Office of Braunschweig, resident registration list of 1938.

Public Record Office of Erfurt, resident registration list of 1938.

Public Record Office of Hamburg, personnel file of Egon Keining, Hochschulwesen, Dozenten- und Personnelakten IV,477.

Public Record Office of Hamburg, personnel file of Paul Mulzer, Hochschulwesen, Dozenten- und Personnelakten IV,721.

Public Record Office of Marburg, personnel file of Alfred Ruete, PHA Ruete.

Secret Archives of the State of Preussen, I HA Rep 76, Nr. 261.

Secret Archives of the State of Preussen, I HA Rep 76, Nr. 700.

Secret Archives of the State of Preussen, I HA Rep 90, Nr. 1770.

SOURCES OF ILLUSTRATIONS

Fig. 1   J.T. Crissey and L.C. Parish, *The Dermatology and Syphilology of the Nineteenth Century* (New York: Praeger, 1981), p. 255.

Fig. 2   Ibid.

Fig. 3   Ibid.

Fig. 4   G. Sebastian and A. Scholz, "Zum 150. Geburtstag von Filip Josef Pick" in *Dermatologische Monatsschrift* 171(1985):123.

Fig. 5   A. Scholz, "Zum 150. Geburtstag von Heinrich Köbner" in *Dermatologische Monatsschrift* 175(1989):112.

Fig. 6   A. Stühmer, "Erinnerungen an Paul Ehrlich" in *Hautarzt* 5(1954):127.

Fig. 7   F. Ehring, *Hautkrankheiten: 5 Jahrhunderte wissenschaftlicher Illustration* (Stuttgart: Gustav Fischer Verlag, 1989), p. 228.

Fig. 8   Ibid., p. 146.

Fig. 9   Original figure.

Fig. 10   C. Zentner, *Illustrierte Geschichte des Dritten Reiches* (Eltville: Bechtermünz Verlag, 1990), p. 336.

Fig. 11   Original figure.

Fig. 12   *Brockhaus Enzyklopädie* in 20 Bänden, 7th ed., vol. 13 (Wiesbaden: F.A. Brockhaus, 1966–1974), p. 302.

Fig. 13   Ibid., vol. 7, p. 288.

Fig. 14   Ibid., vol. 9, p. 267.

Fig. 15   R. Toellner (ed.), *Illustrierte Geschichte der Medizin* (Salzburg: Andreas & Andreas, 1986), p. 3220.

Fig. 16   B. Kisch, "Forgotten leaders in modern medicine" in *Transactions of the American Philosophical Society* 44(1954):193.

Fig. 17   Ibid., p. 227.

Fig. 18   H. Freund and A. Berg (eds.), *Geschichte der Mikroskopie: Leben und Werk großer Forscher*, vol. 2 (Frankfurt: Umschau–Verlag, 1964), p. 464a.

Fig. 19   H. Florey, *General Pathology*, 3rd ed. (London: Lloyd-Luke, 1962).

Fig. 20   Stühmer, "Erinnerungen an Paul Ehrlich," p. 127.

Fig. 21   C. Zentner, *Illustrierte Geschichte des deutschen Kaiserreichs* (Eltville: Bechter-münz Verlag, 1990), p. 14.

Fig. 22   Ibid., p. 213.

Fig. 23   *Brockhaus Enzyklopädie* in 20 Bänden, 7th ed., vol. 7, p. 271.

Fig. 24   J. Bleker and N. Jachertz (eds.), *Medizin im "Dritten Reich"* (Cologne: Deutscher Ärzte–Verlag, 1989), p. 29.

Fig. 25   G. Mann, A. Heuss, and A. Nitschke (eds.), *Weltgeschichte: Eine Universalgeschichte*, vol. 9 (Gütersloh: Prisma Verlag, 1979–1980), p. 759.

Fig. 26   Freund and Berg, *Geschichte der Mikroskopie*, vol. 2, p. 368a.

Fig. 27   Ibid., p. 360a.

Fig. 28   L. Nékám (ed.), *Deliberationes Congressus Dermatologorum Internationalis IX-I*, vol. 4 (Budapest, 1935), p. 247.

Fig. 29   B. Hamann, *Hitlers Wien. Lehrjahre eines Diktators* (München: Piper, 1996), p. 475.

Fig. 30   Hamann, *Hitlers Wien. Lehrjahre eines Diktators*, p. 492.

Fig. 31   Toellner, *Illustrierte Geschichte der Medizin*, p. 3135.

Fig. 32   M. Hubenstorf, "Der Wahrheit ins Auge sehen" in *Wiener Arzt* 5(1995):26.

Fig. 33   Nékám, *Deliberationes Congressus Dermatologorum Internationalis IX-I*, p. 366.

Fig. 34   J.E. Thiele, *Elisabeth: Das Buch ihres Lebens* (München: List, 1996), p. 400.

Fig. 35   *Brockhaus Enzyklopädie* in 20 Bänden, 7th ed., vol. 22, p. 147.

Fig. 36   Ibid., vol. 4, p, 71.

Fig. 37   B. Hausen, *Die Inseln des Paul Langerhans: Eine Biographie in Bildern und Dokumenten* (Vienna: Ueberreuther Wissenschaft, 1988).

Fig. 38   W. Busch, *Die schönsten Bildergeschichten in Farbe* (Cologne: Buch und Zeit Verlagsgesellschaft mbH, 1974), p. 119.

Fig. 39   Ibid., p. 120.

Fig. 40   Freund and Berg, *Geschichte der Mikroskopie*, vol. 2, p. 224a.

Fig. 41   S. Lorant, *Sieg Heil! Eine deutsche Bildergeschichte von Bismarck zu Hitler* (Frankfurt: Zweitausendeins, 1979), p. 54.

Fig. 42   Ibid., p. 121.

Fig. 43   E. Hoffmann, "In memoriam Karl Herxheimer, Carl Touton und Friedrich Hammer" in *Hautarzt* 1(1950):238.

Fig. 44   Zentner, *Illustrierte Geschichte des Dritten Reiches*, p. 10.

Fig. 45   Lorant, *Sieg Heil!*, p. 140.

Fig. 46   Ibid., p. 158.

Fig. 47   Ibid., p. 131.

Fig. 48   Ibid.

Fig. 49   Zentner, *Illustrierte Geschichte des deutschen Kaiserreichs*, p. 193.

Fig. 50   Zentner, *Illustrierte Geschichte des Dritten Reiches*, p. 136.

Fig. 51   J. Benedum and C. Giese, *375 Jahre Medizin in Giessen* (Giessen: Wilhelm Schmitz Verlag, 1983), p. 125.

Fig. 52   H.W. Spier, "In memoriam Stephan Rothman (1894–1963)" in *Hautarzt* 15(1964):145.

Fig. 53   Zentner, *Illustrierte Geschichte des Dritten Reiches*, p. 18.

Fig. 54   Ibid., p. 52.

Fig. 55   H. Pleticha, *Deutsche Geschichte*, vol. 6 (Gütersloh: Prisma Verlag, 1983–1984), p. 193.

Fig. 56   Lorant, *Sieg Heil!*, p. 200.

Fig. 57   Zentner, *Illustrierte Geschichte des Dritten Reiches*, p. 93.

Fig. 58   Lorant, *Sieg Heil!*, p. 155.

Fig. 59   Zentner, *Illustrierte Geschichte des Dritten Reiches*, p. 92.

Fig. 60   Lorant, *Sieg Heil!*, p. 212.

Fig. 61   V. Hentschel, *So kam Hitler: Schicksalsjahre 1932–1933* (Düsseldorf: Droste Verlag, 1990), p. 137.

Fig. 62   C. Zentner and F. Bedürftig, *Das große Lexikon des Dritten Reiches* (Munich: Südwest Verlag, 1985), p. 83.

Fig. 63   Bleker and Jachertz, *Medizin im "Dritten Reich,"* p. 192.

Fig. 64   Ibid., p. 193.

Fig. 65   G. Miescher, "In memoriam Joseph Jadassohn" in *Hautarzt* 5(1954):95–96.

Fig. 66   L. Arzt, "In memoriam Hofrat Professor Gustav Riehl anlässlich seines 100. Geburtstages" in *Hautarzt* 6(1955):239.

Fig. 67   Toellner, *Illustrierte Geschichte der Medizin*, p. 3227.

Fig. 68   *Archiv für Dermatologie und Syphilis* 173(1936).

Fig. 69   *Archiv für Dermatologie und Syphilis* 174(1936).

Fig. 70   J.H. Rille, "Fritz Th. Callomon zum 75. Geburtstag" in *Dermatologische Wochenschrift* 123(1951):433–435.

Fig. 71   P.G. Unna, "Ernst Delbanco" in *Dermatologische Wochenschrift* 88(1929):260.

Fig. 72   A. Hollander, "Development of dermatopathology and Paul Gerson Unna" in *Journal of the American Academy of Dermatology* 15(1986):727.

Fig. 73   *Dermatologische Wochenschrift* 96(1933).

Fig. 74   *Dermatologische Wochenschrift* 100(1935).

Fig. 75   J.J. Herzberg and G.W. Korting (eds.), *Zur Geschichte der deutschen Dermatologie: Zusammengestellt aus Anlass des XVII. Congressus Mundi Dermatologiae* (Berlin: Grosse Verlag, 1987), p. 91.

Fig. 76   C. Pross and R. Winau, *Nicht misshandeln: Das Krankenhaus Moabit* (Berlin: Edition Hentrich im Verlag Frölich & Kaufmann, 1984), p. 181.

Fig. 77   Herzberg and Korting, *Zur Geschichte der deutschen Dermatologie*, p. 55.

Fig. 78   O. Nietz, "Herausbildung der Dermatologie als eigenständiges Fachgebiet in der Stadt Halle sowie Leben und Wirken der Direktoren der Hautklinik der Martin-Luther-Universität Halle-Wittenberg von 1894 bis 1949" (M.D. diss., Martin Luther-University, Halle, 1986), p. 9.

Fig. 79   P. Dejas-Eckertz, D. Ruckhaberle, A. Tebbe, et al., *Faschismus* (Berlin: Elefanten Press Verlag GmbH, 1976), p. 17.

Fig. 80   Lorant, *Sieg Heil!*, p. 224.

Fig. 81   Ibid., p. 282.

Fig. 82   S. Drexler, S. Kalinski, and H. Mausbach. *Ärztliches Schicksal unter der Verfolgung 1933–1945 in Frankfurt am Main und Offenbach: Eine Denkschrift* (Frankfurt: VAS Verlag für Akademische Schriften, 1990), p. 10.

Fig. 83   W. Curth and H. Ollendorff Curth, "Remembering Abraham Buschke" in *American Journal of Dermatopathology* 5 (1983): 27.

Fig. 84   A. Memmesheimer, "Ernst Sklarz 70 Jahre" in *Hautarzt* 15(1964):577.

Fig. 85   E. Hoffmann. "Franz Blumenthal zum 75. Geburtstag" in *Hautarzt* 4(1953):394.

Fig. 86   A. Scholz, "Ludwig Halberstaedter (1876–1949)" in *Dermatologische Monatsschrift* 162(1976):1015.

Fig. 87   D. Mussgnug, "Siegfried Bettmann 1869–1939" in *Aktuelle Dermatologie* 17(1991):25.

Fig. 88   *Dermatologische Wochenschrift* 147(1963).

Fig. 89   G.K. Steigleder, "Franz Herrmann als Geburtstagsgruß" in *Hautarzt* 14(1963):334.

Fig. 90   W. Weyers, "Dermatology under the Swastika: Die Entwicklung der Dermatologie im Nationalsozialismus" (Thesis for habilitation, Justus-Liebig-University, Giessen, 1997), p. S102.

Fig. 91   *Brockhaus Enzyklopädie* in 20 Bänden, 7th ed., vol. 17, p. 87.

Fig. 92   "Jubiläumsbeilage" in *Münchener Medizinische Wochenschrift* 80(1933).

Fig. 93   Herzberg and Korting, *Zur Geschichte der deutschen Dermatologie*, p. 79.

Fig. 94   Ibid., p. 80.

Fig. 95   P. Keller, "In memoriam Rudolf Leopold Mayer 1895–1962" in *Hautarzt* 14(1963):526.

Fig. 96   P. Jordan, "In memoriam W. Freudenthal" in *Hautarzt* 3(1952):383.

Fig. 97   Courtesy of A.B. Ackerman, New York.

Fig. 98   R.L. Baer, "Stephan Epstein zum 60. Geburtstag" in *Hautarzt* 11(1960):431.

Fig. 99   O. Hornstein, "Zur Erinnerung an Ernst Melkersson (1898–1932) und Curt Rosenthal (1892–1937)" in *Hautarzt* 15(1964):515.

Fig. 100   W. Jadassohn, "Max Jessner zum 75. Geburtstag" in *Hautarzt* 13(1962):562.

Fig. 101   M.B. Sulzberger, "Hans Biberstein zum 70. Geburtstag" in *Hautarzt* 10(1959):561.

Fig. 102   *Dermatologische Wochenschrift* 124(1951).

Fig. 103   O. Grütz, "In memoriam Franz Koch" in *Hautarzt* 7(1956):191.

Fig. 104   "Jubiläumsbeilage" in *Münchener Medizinische Wochenschrift* 80(1933).

Fig. 105   Weyers, "Dermatology under the Swastika," p. 89.

Fig. 106   W. Schneider, "Wilhelm Sevin zum 60. Geburtstag" in *Hautarzt* 11(1960):46.

Fig. 107   W. Keilig, "Zur Geschichte der Dermatologie in München" in *Hautarzt* 3(1952):273.

Fig. 108   Zentner and Bedürftig, *Das große Lexikon des Dritten Reiches*, p. 515.

Fig. 109   H. Köhler, "Zum 60. Geburtstag von Rudolf Maximilian Bohnstedt" in *Hautarzt* 11(1960):334.

Fig. 110   "Jubiläumsbeilage" in *Münchener Medizinische Wochenschrift* 80(1933).

Fig. 111   A. Marchionini, "Berta Ottenstein zum 60. Geburtstag" in *Hautarzt* 2(1951):94.

Fig. 112   W. Jadassohn, "In memoriam Wilhelm Lutz" in *Hautarzt* 9(1958):527.

Fig. 113   J.M. Baló-Banga, "Ludwig Nékám, 1868–1957: Ein verspäteter Nekrolog" in *Hautarzt* 44(1993):54.

Fig. 114   K.H. Leven, *100 Jahre klinische Dermatologie an der Universität Freiburg im Breisgau, 1890–1990* (Freiburg: Albert-Ludwigs-University, Institute for the History of Medicine,1990), p. 88.

Fig. 115   G.A. Rost, "Philipp Keller 65 Jahre alt" in *Hautarzt* 7(1956):562.

Fig. 116   K. Jakstat, *Geschichte der Dermatologie in Hamburg*, Bibliotheca Diesbach, vol. 1 (Berlin: Diesbach Verlag, 1987) p. 119.

Fig. 117   Zentner and Bedürftig, *Das große Lexikon des Dritten Reiches*, p. 242.

Fig. 118   Weyers, "Dermatology under the Swastika," p. S115.

Fig. 119   "Jubiläumsbeilage" in *Münchener Medizinische Wochenschrift* 80(1933).

Fig. 120   H.J. Böhles, P. Chroust, R. Fieberg, et al., *Frontabschnitt Hochschule: Die Giessener Universität im Nationalsozialismus* (Giessen: Anabas-Verlag and Focus-Verlag, 1982), p. 62.

Fig. 121   Benedum and Giese, *375 Jahre Medizin in Giessen*, p. 195.

Fig. 122   M.B. Sulzberger, "Rudolf L. Baer zum 60. Geburtstag" in *Hautarzt* 21(1970):339.

Fig. 123   H.M. Hanauske-Abel, "Not a slippery slope or sudden subversion: German medicine and National Socialism in 1933" in *British Medical Journal* 313(1996):1456.

Fig. 124 R. Jäckle, *Schicksale jüdischer und "staatsfeindlicher" Ärztinnen und Ärzte nach 1933 in München* (Munich: Liste Demokratischer Ärztinnen und Ärzte München, 1988), p. 25.

Fig. 125 *Dermatologische Wochenschrift* 156(1970).

Fig. 126 A. Scholz, "Eugen Galewsky (1864–1935)" in *Dermatologische Monatsschrift* 158(1972):53.

Fig. 127 G. Baader and U. Schultz (eds.), *Medizin und Nationalsozialismus: Tabuisierte Vergangenheit - ungebrochene Tradition? Dokumentation des Gesundheitstages Berlin 1980*, 4th ed. (Frankfurt: Mabuse-Verlag, 1989), p. 61.

Fig. 128 R.N. Proctor, *Racial Hygiene: Medicine Under the Nazis* (Cambridge, MA: Harvard University Press, 1988), p. 162a.

Fig. 129 Pleticha, *Deutsche Geschichte*, vol. 6, p. 176.

Fig. 130 Ibid., p. 230.

Fig. 131 W. Schönfeld, "Die Geschichte der Würzburger Hautklinik bis 1939" in *Hautarzt* 7(1956):134.

Fig. 132 H. Röckl, "Karl Hoede zum 75. Geburtstag" in *Hautarzt* 23(1972):382.

Fig. 133 Original figure.

Fig. 134 Original figure.

Fig. 135 Original figure.

Fig. 136 *Dermatologische Wochenschrift* 126(1952).

Fig. 137 *Dermatologische Wochenschrift* 92(1931).

Fig. 138 "Jubiläumsbeilage" in *Münchener Medizinische Wochenschrift* 80(1933).

Fig. 139 M.K. Polano, "H.W. Siemens zum 60. Geburtstage!" in *Hautarzt* 2(1951):431.

Fig. 140 W. Schulze, "Die dermatologische Klinik der Universität Rostock: Ein Rückblick auf ihre Gründung und Entwicklung" in *Hautarzt* 6(1955):84.

Fig. 141 C. Schmidt, "Dermato-Venerologie im Nationalsozialismus - Die Neuordnung des Fachgebietes durch personelle Veränderungen im akademischen Bereich, in den Fachgesellschaften und Herausgeberkollegien der Fachzeitschriften" (M.D. diss., Carl Gustav Carus Medical Academy, Dresden, Germany, 1990), p. II/41.

Fig. 142 W. Knierer, "In memoriam Julius Mayr" in *Dermatologische Wochenschrift* 152(1966):817.

Fig. 143 Weyers, "Dermatology under the Swastika," p. S242.

Fig. 144 H. Götz, "In memoriam August Poehlmann" in *Hautarzt* 5(1954):384.

Fig. 145 "Jubiläumsbeilage" in *Münchener Medizinische Wochenschrift* 80(1933).

Fig. 146 C. Schirren and N. Reinhard, *Geschichte der Dermatologie in Norddeutschland* (Berlin: Grosse-Verlag, 1980), p. 33.

Fig. 147 Benedum and Giese, *375 Jahre Medizin in Giessen*, p. 215.

Fig. 148 Courtesy of H.-J. Roewert, Kiel.

Fig. 149 Böhles, Chroust P, Fieberg, et al., *Frontabschnitt Hochschule*, p. 142.

Fig. 150 W. Schneider, "Prof. Dr. Wilhelm Engelhardt zum 70. Geburtstag" in *Dermatologische Wochenschrift* 152(1966):689.

Fig. 151 E. Landes and I. Menzel, *Geschichte der Universitätshautklinik in Frankfurt am Main* (Berlin: Grosse-Verlag, 1989), p. 55.

Fig. 152 Nietz, "Herausbildung der Dermatologie," p. 27.

Fig. 153 Ibid., p. 33.

Fig. 154 *Dermatologische Wochenschrift* 148(1963).

Fig. 155 Courtesy of A. Scholz, Dresden.

Fig. 156 "Jubiläumsbeilage" in *Münchener Medizinische Wochenschrift* 80(1933).

Fig. 157 Leven, *100 Jahre klinische Dermatologie*, p. 143.

Fig. 158 E. Hoffmann, "Alois Memmesheimer zum 60. Geburtstag am 14. Juli 1954" in *Dermatologische Wochenschrift* 130(1954):767.

Fig. 159 Nékám, *Deliberationes Congressus Dermatologorum Internationalis IX-I*, vol. 4, p. 59.

Fig. 160 Ibid., p. 412a.

Fig. 161 *Münchener Medizinische Wochenschrift* 80(1933):1458.

Fig 162 Zentner and Bedürftig, *Das große Lexikon des Dritten Reiches*, p. 380.

Fig. 163 A. Thom and G.I. Caregorodcev, *Medizin unterm Hakenkreuz* (Berlin: VEB Verlag Volk und Gesundheit, 1989), p. 72.

Fig. 164 H. Schott (ed.), *Die Chronik der Medizin* (Gütersloh: Chronik Verlag, 1993), p. 327.

Fig. 165 Thom and Caregorodcev, *Medizin unterm Hakenkreuz*, p. 67.

Fig. 166 "Galerie hervorragender Ärzte und Naturforscher," in *Münchener Medizinische Wochenschrift* 87(1940):559.

Fig. 167 H. Jakobi, P. Chroust, and M. Hamann, *Aeskulap und Hakenkreuz: Zur Geschichte der Medizinischen Fakultät in Giessen zwischen 1933 und 1945* (Frankfurt: Mabuse-Verlag, 1989), p. 18.

Fig. 168 M. Berenbaum, *The World Must Know: The History of the Holocaust as Told in the United States Holocaust Memorial Museum* (Boston: Little, Brown, 1993), p. 64.

Fig. 169 Ehring, *Hautkrankheiten*, p. 150.

Fig. 170 Proctor, *Racial Hygiene*, p. 142a.

Fig. 171 Schott, *Die Chronik der Medizin*, p. 382.

Fig. 172 Ibid., p. 50a.

Fig. 173 A. Scholz, F. Ehring, and H. Zaun, *Exlibris berühmter Dermatologen* (Dresden: Institute for the History of Medicine, Carl Gustav Carus Medical Academy, 1995), p.19.

Fig. 174 Schott, *Die Chronik der Medizin*, p. 359.

Fig. 175 Proctor, *Racial Hygiene*, p. 50a.

Fig. 176 Berenbaum, *The World Must Know*, p. 32.

Fig. 177 Jakobi, Chroust, and Hamann, *Aeskulap und Hakenkreuz*, p. 43.

Fig. 178 Pross and Winau, *Nicht misshandeln*, p. 182.

Fig. 179 W. Jaensch (ed.), *Konstitutions- und Erbbiologie in der Praxis der Medizin* (Leipzig: Johann Ambrosius Barth Verlag, 1934).

Fig. 180 Ibid.

Fig. 181 *Dermatologische Wochenschrift* 127(1953).

Fig. 182 Proctor, *Racial Hygiene*, p. 228a.

Fig. 183 Thom and Caregorodcev, *Medizin unterm Hakenkreuz*, p. 256.

Fig. 184 Zentner, *Illustrierte Geschichte des Dritten Reiches*, p. 125.

Fig. 185 Thom and Caregorodcev, *Medizin unterm Hakenkreuz*, p. 257.

Fig. 186 Zentner, *Illustrierte Geschichte des Dritten Reiches*, p. 125.

Fig. 187 Baader and Schultz, *Medizin und Nationalsozialismus*, p. 144.

Fig. 188 Freund and Berg, *Geschichte der Mikroskopie*, vol. 2, p. 16a.

Fig. 189 "Jubiläumsbeilage" in *Münchener Medizinische Wochenschrift* 80(1933).

Fig. 190 Ibid.

Fig. 191 Ibid.

Fig. 192 Zentner, *Illustrierte Geschichte des Dritten Reiches*, p. 57.

Fig. 193 Lorant, *Sieg Heil!*, p. 136.

Fig. 194 Zentner, *Illustrierte Geschichte des Dritten Reiches*, p. 80.

Fig. 195 Pleticha, *Deutsche Geschichte*, vol. 6, p. 224.

Fig. 196 Hanauske-Abel, "Not a slippery slope or sudden subversion," p. 1458.

Fig. 197 Zentner, *Illustrierte Geschichte des Dritten Reiches*, p. 113.

Fig. 198 Lorant, *Sieg Heil!*, p. 283.

Fig. 199 L. Chagoll, *Im Namen Hitlers: Kinder hinter Stacheldraht* (Cologne: Pahl-Rugenstein Verlag, 1979), p. 11.

Fig. 200 Dejas-Eckertz, Ruckhaberle, Tebbe, et al., *Faschismus*, p. 8.

Fig. 201 Ibid., p. 66.

Fig. 202 E. Hiemer, *Der Giftpilz: Ein Stürmerbuch für Jung u. Alt* (Nuremberg: Verlag Der Stürmer, 1938).

Fig. 203 Ibid., p. 8.

Fig. 204 Ibid., p. 34.

Fig. 205 Zentner, *Illustrierte Geschichte des Dritten Reiches*, p. 172.

Fig. 206 *Dermatologische Wochenschrift* 130(1954).

Fig. 207 Weyers, "Dermatology under the Swastika," p. S48.

Fig. 208 N. Klüken, "Rudolf Strempel zum 65. Geburtstag" in *Hautarzt* 7(1956):336.

Fig. 209 O. Gans, "Zum 70. Geburtstag von Prof. Otto Grütz in Bonn" in *Hautarzt* 7(1956):239.

Fig. 210 Schulze, "Die dermatologische Klinik der Universität Rostock," p. 84.

Fig. 211 Lorant, *Sieg Heil!*, p. 224.

Fig. 212 G. Stresemann, *Wie konnte es geschehen? Hitlers Aufstieg in der Erinnerung eines Zeitzeugen* (Berlin: Ullstein, 1987), p. 124a.

Fig. 213 K. Schlenzka and B. Junge, "Schicksale Magdeburger jüdischer Dermatologen im Nazi-Reich. Carl Lennhoff und Otto Schlein" in *Dermatologische Monatsschrift* 175(1989):307.

Fig. 214 Zentner, *Illustrierte Geschichte des Dritten Reiches*, p. 345.

Fig. 215 Pross and Winau, *Nicht misshandeln*, p. 229.

Fig. 216 Ibid., p. 234.

Fig. 217 Jakobi, Chroust, and Hamann, *Aeskulap und Hakenkreuz*, p. 43.

Fig. 218 P. Milde and A.B. Ackerman, "A critical analysis of textbooks of dermatopathology in historical perspective. Part 5" in *American Journal of Dermatopathology* 15(1993):85–95.

Fig. 219 V. Klemperer, *Ich will Zeugnis ablegen bis zum letzten: Tagebücher 1933–1941*, vol. 1 (Berlin: Aufbau Verlag, 1995), p. 2.

Fig. 220 H. Götz, "In memoriam Theodor Grüneberg 1901–1979" in *Hautarzt* 31(1980):465.

Fig. 221 C. Funk, "Heinrich Löhe zum 75. Geburtstag" in *Hautarzt* 3(1952):382.

Fig. 222 A. Proppe, "Hans Theo Schreus zum 60. Geburtstage" in *Hautarzt* 3(1951):431.

Fig. 223 *Dermatologische Wochenschrift* 156(1970).

Fig. 224 W. Doerr, *Semper Apertus. Sechshundert Jahre Ruprecht-Karls-Universität Heidelberg, 1386–1986*, vol. 2: *Das zwanzigste Jahrhundert, 1918–1985* (Berlin: Springer Verlag, 1985).

Fig. 225 L. Arzt, "In memoriam Franz Walter" in *Hautarzt* 2(1951):94.

Fig. 226 Original figure.

Fig. 227 O. Braun-Falco, "Walter F. Lever zum 60. Geburtstag" in *Hautarzt* 20(1969):565.

Fig. 228 Weyers, "Dermatology under the Swastika."

Fig. 229 Courtesy of I. Silberberg-Sinakin.

Fig. 230 Lorant, *Sieg Heil!*, p. 234.

Fig. 231 Pleticha, *Deutsche Geschichte*, vol. 6, p. 215.

Fig. 232 H. Beerman, "Alfred Hollander zum 75. Geburtstag" in *Hautarzt* 25(1974):261.

Fig. 233 Zentner, *Illustrierte Geschichte des Dritten Reiches*, p.325.

Fig. 234 H. Lautsch and H. Dornedden, *Verzeichnis der deutschen Ärzte und Heilanstalten: Reichs-Medizinal-Kalender für Deutschland*, part 2 (Leipzig: Georg Thieme Verlag, 1937), p. 358.

Fig. 235 H. Biberstein, "In memoriam Kurt Wiener" in *Hautarzt* 11(1960):561.

Fig. 236 *Brockhaus Enzyklopädie* in 20 Bänden, 7th ed., vol. 19, p. 122.

Fig. 237 Zentner, *Illustrierte Geschichte des Dritten Reiches*, p. 120.

Fig. 238 Ibid., p. 213.

Fig. 239 Dejas-Eckertz, Ruckhaberle, Tebbe, et al., *Faschismus*, p. 84.

Fig. 240 Pross and Winau, *Nicht misshandeln*, p. 110.

Fig. 241 Proctor, *Racial Hygiene*, p. 148a.

Fig. 242 Ibid., p. 182a.

Fig. 243 Original figure.

Fig. 244 Herzberg and Korting, *Zur Geschichte der deutschen Dermatologie*, p. 54.

Fig. 245 A. Hollander, "The tribulations of Jewish dermatologists under the Nazi regime" in *American Journal of Dermatopathology* 5(1983):19.

Fig. 246 *Dermatologische Zeitschrift* 77(1938).

Fig. 247 *Dermatologische Zeitschrift* 78(1938).

Fig. 248 Hentschel, *So kam Hitler*, p. 87.

Fig. 249 Jäckle, *Schicksale jüdischer und "staatsfeindlicher" Ärztinnen und Ärzte nach 1933 in München*, p. 34.

Fig. 250 Zentner and Bedürftig, *Das große Lexikon des Dritten Reiches*, p. 255.

Fig. 251 Mann, Heuss, and Nitschke, *Weltgeschichte*, vol. 9, p. 746.

Fig. 252 Zentner, *Illustrierte Geschichte des Dritten Reiches*, p. 328.

Fig. 253 Lorant, *Sieg Heil!*, p. 283.

Fig. 254 H. Ollendorff Curth, "Erich Kuznitzky" in *Hautarzt* 11(1960):288.

Fig. 255 Zentner, *Illustrierte Geschichte des Dritten Reiches*, p. 329.

Fig. 256 Mann, Heuss, and Nitschke, *Weltgeschichte*, Bilder und Dokumente, p. 498.

Fig. 257 Zentner, *Illustrierte Geschichte des Dritten Reiches*, p. 328.

Fig. 258 H. Beerman, "In memoriam Emil Meirowsky" in *Hautarzt* 11(1960):335.

Fig. 259 Schlenzka and Junge, "Schicksale Magdeburger jüdischer Dermatologen im Nazi-Reich," p. 307.

Fig. 260 M.B. Sulzberger, "In memoriam George Miller MacKee 1875–1955" in *Hautarzt* 6(1955):431.

Fig. 261 I. Rosen, "Fred Wise" in *Hautarzt* 2(1951):95.

Fig. 262 A. Marchionini, "Marion B. Sulzberger zum 60. Geburtstag" in *Hautarzt* 6(1955):142.

Fig. 263 *Brockhaus Enzyklopädie* in 20 Bänden, 7th ed., vol. 13, p. 316.

Fig. 264 Zentner, *Illustrierte Geschichte des Dritten Reiches*, p. 254.

Fig. 265 Lorant, *Sieg Heil!*, p. 266.

Fig. 266 Nékám, *Deliberationes Congressus Dermatologorum Internationalis IX-I*, p. 245.

Fig. 267 Lorant, *Sieg Heil!*, p. 264

Fig. 268 Berenbaum, *The World Must Know*, p. 45.

Fig. 269 Zentner and Bedürftig, *Das große Lexikon des Dritten Reiches*, p. 140.

Fig. 270 Berenbaum, *The World Must Know*, p. 44.

Fig. 271 "Jubiläumsbeilage" in *Münchener Medizinische Wochenschrift* 81(1934).

Fig. 272 Hubenstorf, "Der Wahrheit ins Auge sehen," p. 18.

Fig. 273 *Wiener Arzt* 5(1995), frontispiece.

Fig. 274 K. Knolle (ed.), *Große Nervenärzte: 21 Lebensbilder*, vol. 1, 2nd ed. (Stuttgart: Georg Thieme, 1970), p. 256a.

Fig. 275 Toellner, *Illustrierte Geschichte der Medizin*, p. 3250.

Fig. 276 "Jubiläumsbeilage" in *Münchener Medizinische Wochenschrift* 81(1934).

Fig. 277 Zentner and Bedürftig, *Das große Lexikon des Dritten Reiches*, p. 193.

Fig. 278 "Jubiläumsbeilage" in *Münchener Medizinische Wochenschrift* 81(1934).

Fig. 279 Courtesy of H.-P. Soyer, Graz.

Fig. 280 Nékám, *Deliberationes Congressus Dermatologorum Internationalis IX-I*, p. 138.

Fig. 281 W.B. Shelley, J.T. Crissey JT, and J.H. Stokes, *Classics in Clinical Dermatology* (Springfield, IL: Charles C. Thomas, 1953), p. 434.

Fig. 282 E. Lesky, *Meilensteine der Wiener Medizin: Große Ärzte Österreichs in drei Jahrhunderten* (Vienna: Verlag Wilhelm Maudrich, 1981).

Fig. 283 A. Wiedmann, "Stephan Robert Brunauer zum 75. Geburtstag!" in *Hautarzt* 13(1962):382.

Fig. 284 L. Arzt, "In memoriam Hans Königstein" in *Hautarzt* 5(1954):336.

Fig. 285 K. Holubar, C. Schmidt, and K. Wolff, *Challenge Dermatology: Vienna 1841–1992* (Vienna: Verlag der Österreichischen Akademie der Wissenschaften, 1993), p. 81.

Fig. 286 Nékám, *Deliberationes Congressus Dermatologorum Internationalis IX-I*, p. 250.

Fig. 287 "Jubiläumsbeilage" in *Münchener Medizinische Wochenschrift* 81(1934).

Fig. 288 Ibid.

Fig. 289 J. Konrad, "Leo Kumer 1886–1951" in *Dermatologische Wochenschrift* 125(1952):97.

Fig. 290 H. Kresbach, "Anton Musger, 1898–1983" in *Hautarzt* 35(1984):272.

Fig. 291 A. Musger, "Albert Wiedmann zum 65. Geburtstag" in *Hautarzt* 17(1966):190.

Fig. 292 J.A. Gammel, "Hugo Hecht" in *Hautarzt* 14(1963):383.

Fig. 293 E.J. Feuerman, "In memoriam Felix Sagher" in *Hautarzt* 34(1983):101.

Fig. 294 C. Calnan, "Henry Haber (1900–1962)" in *American Journal of Dermatopathology* 7(1985):537.

Fig. 295 Stresemann, *Wie konnte es geschehen?*, p. 124a.

Fig. 296 J. Kanopik, "In memoriam Karel Gawalowski (1890–1965)" in *Hautarzt* 17(1966):192.

Fig. 297 F. Kogoj, "In memoriam Anton Trýb (1884–1960)" in *Hautarzt* 12(1961):144.

Fig. 298 *Dermatologische Monatsschrift* 156(1970).

Fig. 299 Zentner and Bedürftig, *Das große Lexikon des Dritten Reiches*, p. 32a.

Fig. 300 Lorant, *Sieg Heil!*, p. 263.

Fig. 301 Ibid.

Fig. 302 Mann, A. Heuss, and A. Nitschke (eds.), *Weltgeschichte*, vol. 9, p. 735.

Fig. 303 Lorant, *Sieg Heil!*, p. 273.

Fig. 304 Ibid., p. 278.

Fig. 305 A. Marchionini, "Lucien Marie Pautrier zum 80. Geburtstag" in *Hautarzt* 7(1956):382.

Fig. 306 Zentner, *Illustrierte Geschichte des Dritten Reiches*, p. 252.

Fig. 307 C. Zentner, *Illustrierte Geschichte des Zweiten Weltkriegs* (Eltville: Bechtermünz Verlag, 1990), p. 8.

Fig. 308 G. Holmsten, *Kriegsalltag 1939–1945 in Deutschland* (Düsseldorf: Droste Verlag, 1982), p. 39.

Fig. 309 A. Vasiljevic, "In memoriam Josip Fleger" in *Hautarzt* 18(1967):95.

Fig. 310 A. Brnobic, "In memoriam Franjo Kogoj, 1894–1983" in *Hautarzt* 35(1984):270.

Fig. 311 U.W. Schnyder, "Tibor Salomon, 1914–1995" in *Hautarzt* 47(1996):69.

Fig. 312 Mann, Heuss, and Nitschke, *Weltgeschichte*, Bilder und Dokumente, p. 498.

Fig. 313 N. Goldenbogen, S. Hahn, C.-P. Heidel, and A. Scholz, *Medizin und Judentum* (Dresden: Verlag des Vereins für regionale Geschichte und Politik Dresden e.V., 1994) p. 21.

Fig. 314 Ibid., p. 23.

Fig. 315 L.S. Dawidowicz, *The War Against the Jews, 1933–1945*, 10th anniversary ed. (New York: CBS Educational & Professional Publishing, CBS, Inc., 1986), p. 113.

Fig. 316 C.E. Orfanos, "Haim A. Cohen zum 75. Geburtstag" in *Hautarzt* 40(1989):466.

Fig. 317 I. Capetanakis, "Christopher Doucas zum 70. Geburtstag" in *Hautarzt* 11(19600:560.

Fig. 318 A. Marchionini, "Viktor Kafka zum 70. Geburtstag" in *Hautarzt* 2(1951):478.

Fig. 319 Lorant, *Sieg Heil!*, p. 331.

Fig. 320 Jakobi, Chroust, and Hamann, *Aeskulap und Hakenkreuz*, p. 153.

Fig. 321 Dejas-Eckertz, Ruckhaberle, Tebbe, et al., *Faschismus*, p. 96.

Fig. 322 Berenbaum, *The World Must Know*, p. 62.

Fig. 323 Dejas-Eckertz, Ruckhaberle, Tebbe, et al., *Faschismus*, p. 167.

Fig. 324 Pleticha, *Deutsche Geschichte*, vol. 6, p. 318.

Fig. 325 Zentner, *Illustrierte Geschichte des Zweiten Weltkriegs*, p. 208.

Fig. 326 Berenbaum, *The World Must Know*, p. 187.

Fig. 327 Lorant, *Sieg Heil!*, p. 312.

Fig. 328 Zentner and Bedürftig, *Das große Lexikon des Dritten Reiches*, p. 32a.

Fig. 329 Holmsten, *Kriegsalltag 1939–1945 in Deutschland*, p. 108.

Fig. 330 Zentner, *Illustrierte Geschichte des Dritten Reiches*, p. 124.

Fig. 331 Chagoll, *Im Namen Hitlers*, p. 73.

Fig. 332 Zentner and Bedürftig, *Das große Lexikon des Dritten Reiches*, p. 635.

Fig. 333 Mann, Heuss, and Nitschke, *Weltgeschichte*, vol. 9, p. 745.

Fig. 334 Jakobi, Chroust, and Hamann, *Aeskulap und Hakenkreuz*, p. 54.

Fig. 335 P.-M. Seiffert, *Die Hamburger Dermatologische Gesellschaft* (Berlin: Grosse, 1985), p. 22.

Fig. 336 Berenbaum, *The World Must Know*, p. 72.

Fig. 337 Ibid., p. 114.

Fig. 338 Chagoll, *Im Namen Hitlers*, p. 140.

Fig. 339 Dejas-Eckertz, Ruckhaberle, Tebbe, et al., *Faschismus*, p. 124.

Fig. 340 Zentner, *Illustrierte Geschichte des Zweiten Weltkriegs*, p. 341.

Fig. 341 Zentner and Bedürftig, *Das große Lexikon des Dritten Reiches*, p. 381.

Fig. 342 Dejas-Eckertz, Ruckhaberle, Tebbe, et al., *Faschismus*, p. 247.

Fig. 343 Ibid., p. 271.

Fig. 344 Berenbaum, *The World Must Know*, p. 198.

Fig. 345 Ibid., p. 203.

Fig. 346 Ibid., p. 147.

Fig. 347 Dejas-Eckertz, Ruckhaberle, Tebbe, et al., *Faschismus*, p. 243.

Fig. 348 Ibid., p. 118.

Fig. 349 Pross and Winau, *Nicht misshandeln*, p. 225.

Fig. 350 E. Brinkschulte (ed.), *Weibliche Ärzte: Die Durchsetzung des Berufsbildes in Deutschland* (Berlin: Edition Hentrich, 1993), p. 133.

Fig. 351 Chagoll, *Im Namen Hitlers*, p. 129.

Fig. 352 Dejas-Eckertz, Ruckhaberle, Tebbe, et al., *Faschismus*, p. 119.

Fig. 353 F. Schmidt-La Baume, "In memoriam Karl Herxheimer" in *Hautarzt* 4(1953):444.

Fig. 354 O. Gans, "Zum 100. Geburtstag von Karl Herxheimer" in *Hautarzt* 12(1961):241.

Fig. 355 Ehring, *Hautkrankheiten*, p. 232.

Fig. 356 Pross and Winau, *Nicht misshandeln*, p. 249.

Fig. 357 Courtesy of P.-J. Unna, Hamburg.

Fig. 358 Ibid.

Fig. 359 Jakstat, *Geschichte der Dermatologie in Hamburg*, p. 114.

Fig. 360 Zentner, *Illustrierte Geschichte des Dritten Reiches*, p. 366.

Fig. 361 Holmsten, *Kriegsalltag 1939–1945 in Deutschland*, p. 82.

Fig. 362 Thom and Caregorodcev, *Medizin unterm Hakenkreuz*, p. 184.

Fig. 363 Zentner, *Illustrierte Geschichte des Dritten Reiches*, p. 125.

Fig. 364 R.L. Baer, "Otto Braun-Falco zum 60. Geburtstag" in *Hautarzt* 33(1982):242.

Fig. 365 Landes and Menzel, *Geschichte der Universitätshautklinik in Frankfurt am Main*, p. 55.

Fig. 366 Lautsch and Dornedden, *Verzeichnis der deutschen Ärzte und Heilanstalten*, p. 285.

Fig. 367 K.W. Kalkoff, "In memoriam Carl Moncorps" in *Hautarzt* 3(1952):143.

Fig. 368 Weyers, "Dermatology under the Swastika," p. S44.

Fig. 369 Holmsten, *Kriegsalltag 1939–1945 in Deutschland*, p. 22.

Fig. 370 Dejas-Eckertz, Ruckhaberle, Tebbe, et al., *Faschismus*, p. 31.

Fig. 371 Zentner, *Illustrierte Geschichte des Dritten Reiches*, p. 373.

Fig. 372 Lorant, *Sieg Heil!*, p. 329.

Fig. 373 Courtesy of P. Milde, Washington, D.C.

Fig. 374 Zentner, *Illustrierte Geschichte des Zweiten Weltkriegs*, p. 229.

Fig. 375 Mann, Heuss, and Nitschke, *Weltgeschichte*, vol. 9, Bilder und Dokumente, p. 506.

Fig. 376 Lorant, *Sieg Heil!*, p. 338.

Fig. 377 Ibid.

Fig. 378 Ibid., p. 337.

Fig. 379 *Dermatologische Wochenschrift* 110(1940).

Fig. 380 B. Bromberger, H. Mausbach, and K.D. Thomann, *Medizin, Faschismus und Widerstand* (Frankfurt: Mabuse-Verlag, 1990), p. 320.

Fig. 381 Weyers, "Dermatology under the Swastika," p. S154.

Fig. 382   B. Beutelspacher, H.U. Brändle, A. Eberhardt, et al., *Volk und Gesundheit: Heilen und Vernichten im Nationalsozialismus* (Frankfurt: Mabuse-Verlag, 1988), p. 32.

Fig. 383   Beutelspacher, *Volk und Gesundheit*, p. 32.

Fig. 384   "Jubiläumsbeilage" in *Münchener Medizinische Wochenschrift* 80(1933).

Fig. 385   A. Proppe, "Horst-Günther Bode zum 60. Geburtstag" in *Hautarzt* 15(1964):463.

Fig. 386   M. Franzblau, "Nazi medical cronies unpunished 50 years later" in *Dermatopathology: Practical and Conceptual* 2(1996):85.

Fig. 387   Proctor, *Racial Hygiene*, p. 256.

Fig. 388   R. Frühwald, "Oskar Kieß" in *Hautarzt* 6(1955):96.

Fig. 389   A. Proppe, "Erich Langer zum 65. Geburtstag" in *Hautarzt* 7(1956):143.

Fig. 390   A. Wiedmann, "J.H. Rille zum 90. Geburtstag" in *Hautarzt* 5(1954):562.

Fig. 391   Original figure.

Fig. 392   Original figure.

NAME INDEX

SUBJECT INDEX

The
first
edition of
Death of Medi-
cine was written by Wolfgang Weyers with a
foreword by A. Bernard Ackerman. The jacket
was designed by Louise Fili. Interior pages
designed by Louise Fili and Mary Jane
Callister / Louise Fili Ltd, New York
City. Published by Ardor Scribendi
and Madison Books. Printed in offset litho-
graphy by Edwards Brothers in Ann Arbor,
Michigan. Printed on Glatfelter Natural and set in
Walbaum, Uniblock,
and Berliner
Grotesk.
1998